Resident Readiness™

Obstetrics and Gynecology

From Dr Hope

Welcome!

to the HVH family

Notice

Medicine is an ever-changing science. As new research and clinical experience broaden our knowledge, changes in treatment and drug therapy are required. The authors and the publisher of this work have checked with sources believed to be reliable in their efforts to provide information that is complete and generally in accord with the standards accepted at the time of publication. However, in view of the possibility of human error or changes in medical sciences, neither the authors nor the publisher nor any other party who has been involved in the preparation or publication of this work warrants that the information contained herein is in every respect accurate or complete, and they disclaim all responsibility for any errors or omissions or for the results obtained from use of the information contained in this work. Readers are encouraged to confirm the information contained herein with other sources. For example and in particular, readers are advised to check the product information sheet included in the package of each drug they plan to administer to be certain that the information contained in this work is accurate and that changes have not been made in the recommended dose or in the contraindications for administration. This recommendation is of particular importance in connection with new or infrequently used drugs.

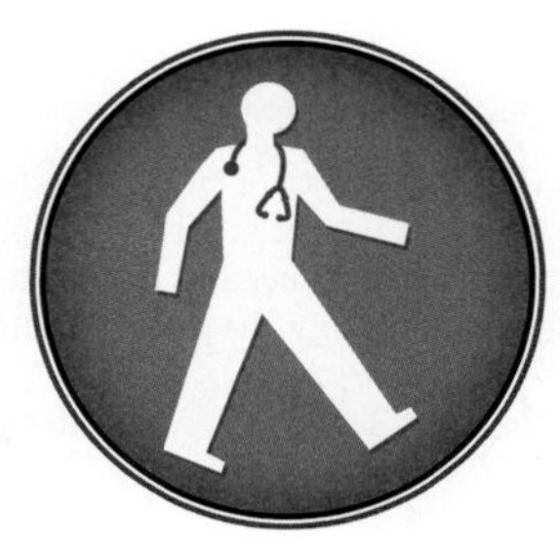

Resident Readiness™
Obstetrics and Gynecology

Debra L. Klamen, MD, MHPE

Associate Dean for Education and Curriculum
Professor and Chair
Department of Medical Education
Southern Illinois University School of Medicine
Springfield, Illinois

Charlie C. Kilpatrick, MD

Associate Professor
Vice Chairman
Department of Obstetrics and Gynecology
Texas Tech University Health Sciences Center
School of Medicine
Lubbock, Texas

Edward R. Yeomans, MD

Professor and Chair
Maternal-Fetal Medicine
Department of Obstetrics and Gynecology
Texas Tech University Health Sciences Center
School of Medicine
Lubbock, Texas

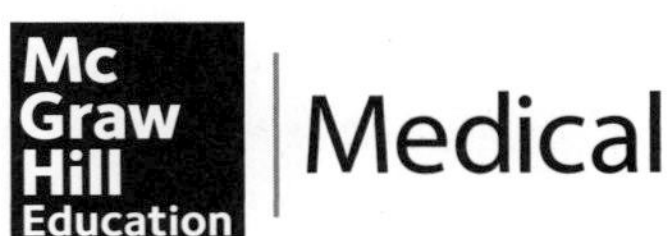

New York Chicago San Francisco Athens London Madrid
Mexico City Milan New Delhi Singapore Sydney Toronto

Resident Readiness™: Obstetrics and Gynecology

1 2 3 4 5 6 7 8 9 0 DOC/DOC 19 18 17 16 15 14

ISBN 978-0-07-178043-8
MHID 0-07-178043-2

This book was set in Minion Pro by Thomson Digital.
The editors were Catherine A. Johnson and Cindy Yoo.
The production supervisor was Richard Ruzycka.
Project management was provided by Shaminder Pal Singh, Thomson Digital.
The designer was Eve Siegel; the cover designer was Anthony Landi.
RR Donnelley was the printer and binder.

This book is printed on acid-free paper.

Library of Congress Cataloging-in-Publication Data

Resident readiness. Obstetrics and gynecology / [edited by] Debra L. Klamen, Edward R. Yeomans, Charlie C. Kilpatrick.
p. ; cm.
Obstetrics and gynecology
Includes bibliographical references and index.
ISBN-13: 978-0-07-178043-8 (pbk. : alk. paper)
ISBN-10: 0-07-178043-2 (pbk. : alk. paper)
I. Klamen, Debra L., editor of compilation. II. Yeomans, Edward R., editor of compilation. III. Kilpatrick, Charlie C., editor of compilation. IV. Title: Obstetrics and gynecology.
[DNLM: 1. Genital Diseases, Female—diagnosis—Case Reports. 2. Genital Diseases, Female—therapy—Case Reports. 3. Perinatal Care—Case Reports. 4. Pregnancy Complications—diagnosis—Case Reports. 5. Pregnancy Complications—therapy—Case Reports. WP 140]
RG103
618.1—dc23

2014001994

To my wonderful husband Phil, who loves me and supports me in all things, especially my crazy passion for horses! To my mother, Bonnie Klamen, and to my late father, Sam Klamen, who were, and are, always there. To my extended family, for their love and understanding. To my students, for keeping me motivated and inspired.—DLK

To all the wonderful medical students I have had the privilege of teaching over the years, your intellectual curiosity inspires me, and most importantly to my amazing wife, Lubna, and my beautiful daughter Maya who together bring joy to my life daily.—CCK

To aspiring obstetrician gynecologists, for whom this book is written, and to my wife, Thuy, for her support.—ERY

CONTENTS

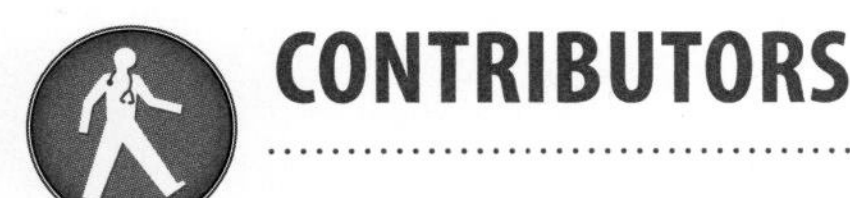

CONTRIBUTORS

Zainab Al-Ibraheemi, MD
Resident
Department of Obstetrics and Gynecology
Texas Tech University Health Sciences Center
Lubbock, Texas
Chapter 4

Candy Arentz, MD, FACS
Assistant Professor
Department of Surgery
Texas Tech University Health Sciences Center
Lubbock, Texas
Chapter 8

Heidi G. Bell, MD
Assistant Professor
Department of Obstetrics and Gynecology
Brody School of Medicine at East Carolina University
Greenville, North Carolina
Chapters 11, 16

Thomas A. Bowman, MD, MBA
Clinical Assistant Professor
Department of Pediatrics
School of Medicine
Texas Tech University Health Sciences Center
Neonatologist, Pediatrix Medical Group
University Medical Center
Lubbock, Texas
Chapter 31

Lubna Chohan, MD
Associate Professor
Department of Obstetrics and Gynecology
Texas Tech University Health Sciences Center
Lubbock, Texas
Chapters 2, 9, 12

James E. de Vente, MD, PhD
Associate Professor
Department of Obstetrics and Gynecology
Brody School of Medicine at East Carolina University
Greenville, North Carolina
Chapter 16

Ammar Dhari, MD
Third Year Resident in Training
Department of Obstetrics and Gynecology
Texas Tech University Health Sciences Center
School of Medicine
Lubbock, Texas
Chapter 14

Laura M. Divine, MD
Resident
Department of Obstetrics and Gynecology
University of Alabama at Birmingham
Birmingham, Alabama
Chapter 15

Jacob M. Estes, MD
Associate Professor, Gynecologic Oncology
Department of Obstetrics and Gynecology
University of Alabama at Birmingham
Birmingham, Alabama
Chapter 15

Naghma Farooqi, MD
Associate Professor
Associate Residency Program Director
Department of Obstetrics and Gynecology
Texas Tech University Health Sciences Center
Lubbock, Texas
Chapters 41, 46

Carol K. Felton, MD, NCMP
Associate Professor
Department of Obstetrics and Gynecology
Texas Tech University Health Sciences Center
Lubbock, Texas
Chapter 10

Tana L. Hall, MD, FACOG
Assistant Professor
Department of Obstetrics and Gynecology
Brody School of Medicine at East Carolina University
Greenville, North Carolina
Chapter 11

Jennifer R. Hamm, MD
Assistant Professor
Department of Obstetrics, Gynecology, and Women's Health
University of Louisville
Louisville, Kentucky
Chapter 36

Roxane Holt, MD
Assistant Professor
Department of Obstetrics and Gynecology
Texas Tech University Health Sciences Center
Lubbock, Texas
Chapters 18, 34

Jaou-Chen Huang, MD
Professor
Department of Obstetrics and Gynecology
Texas Tech University Health Sciences Center
Lubbock, Texas
Chapters 6, 43

Charlie C. Kilpatrick, MD
Associate Professor
Vice Chairman
Department of Obstetrics and Gynecology
Texas Tech University Health Sciences Center
School of Medicine
Lubbock, Texas
Chapters 3, 4, 5, 13, 14, 23, 32, 38, 39, 44, 45

Susan M. Leong-Kee, MD
Assistant Professor
Department of Obstetrics and Gynecology
Baylor College of Medicine
Houston, Texas
Chapter 40

Alita K. Loveless, MD
Assistant Professor
Department of Obstetrics and Gynecology
Texas Tech University Health Sciences Center
School of Medicine
Lubbock, Texas
Chapter 30

Elizabeth Melendez, MD, FACOG
Residency Program Director
Department of Obstetrics and Gynecology
Methodist Health Systems/Methodist Dallas Medical Center
Dallas, Texas
Chapter 24

Jonathan Nathan, MD, MBA
General Surgery Resident
Department of Surgery
Texas Tech University Health Sciences Center
Lubbock, Texas
Chapter 8

Keith H. Nelson, MD
Associate Professor
Department of Obstetrics and Gynecology
Brody School of Medicine at East Carolina University
Greenville, North Carolina
Chapter 16

Lydia D. Nightingale, MD, FACOG
Assistant Professor
Department of Obstetrics and Gynecology
University of Oklahoma Health Sciences Center
Oklahoma City, Oklahoma
Chapter 27

James Marshall Palmer, MD, MS
Assistant Professor
Residency Program Director
Department of Obstetrics and Gynecology
University of South Florida Morsani College of Medicine
Tampa, Florida
Chapter 25

Dana S. Phillips, MD
Associate Professor
Clerkship Director
Department of Obstetrics and Gynecology
Texas Tech University Health Sciences Center
Lubbock, Texas
Chapter 37

Fidelma B. Rigby, MD
Associate Professor
Department of Obstetrics and Gynecology
Virginia Commonwealth University, MCV Campus
Richmond, Virginia
Chapter 22

Jennifer L. Rowland, MD
Staff Physician
Department of Obstetrics and Gynecology
Carl R. Darnall Army Medical Center
Fort Hood, Texas
Chapter 1

Katerina Shvartsman, MD
Assistant Professor
Department of Obstetrics and Gynecology
Uniformed Services University of the Health Sciences
Bethesda, Maryland
Chapter 1

Katie M. Smith, MD
Assistant Professor
Department of Obstetrics and Gynecology
College of Medicine
University of Oklahoma Health Sciences Center
Oklahoma City, Oklahoma
Chapter 42

Kristen R. Uquillas, MD
Resident
Department of Obstetrics and Gynecology
New York University Langone Medical Center
New York, New York
Chapter 33

Sarah Mallard Wakefield, MD
Assistant Professor
Department of Psychiatry
Texas Tech University Health Sciences Center
School of Medicine
Lubbock, Texas
Chapter 35

Abigail Ford Winkel, MD
Assistant Professor
Department of Obstetrics and Gynecology
New York University School of Medicine
New York, New York
Chapter 33

Roger B. Yandell, MD
Associate Clinical Professor
Chief of Gynecology
Department of Obstetrics and Gynecology
Texas Tech University Health Sciences Center
Lubbock, Texas
Chapter 7

Edward R. Yeomans, MD
Professor and Chair
Maternal-Fetal Medicine
Department of Obstetrics and Gynecology
Texas Tech University Health Sciences Center
School of Medicine
Lubbock, Texas
Chapters 17, 19, 20, 21, 26, 28, 29, 46

ACKNOWLEDGMENTS

The Resident Readiness series evolved from ideas that a talented educator and surgeon, David Rogers, had about preparing senior students interested in going into surgery through a resident readiness course. This course was so successful at Southern Illinois University School of Medicine that it spread to other clerkships, and resident readiness senior electives now exist throughout them. The idea for this book series was born by watching the success of these courses and the interest the senior students have in them. It has been a great joy working with Charlie Kilpatrick and Ed Yeomans, completely devoted physicians who retain their humanity for others and passion for education, as well as with the other contributors to this book. I (DLK) am grateful to the Dean, Dr. Kevin Dorsey, whose dedication to education and innovation allowed me to carve out time in my work to be creative. We are greatly indebted to Catherine Johnson from McGraw-Hill, who helped us make the vision of a resident readiness series a reality. Her support and enthusiasm for the project have been unwavering. Likewise, the production manager on the obstetrics and gynecology resident readiness book, Shaminder Pal Singh, has been completely dedicated to the task and is deserving of much thanks. We would also like to thank the many contributors to this book, whose commitment to medical education undoubtedly led to long nights writing and editing in its service. Lastly we appreciate our spouses' forbearance for the hours we spent in front of the computer at home; their patience and understanding are without match.

Debra L. Klamen

INTRODUCTION

Facing the prospect of an internship is an exciting, and undoubtedly anxiety-provoking, prospect. Four years of medical school, after graduation, culminate in a rapid transition to someone calling you "Doctor" and asking you to give orders and perform procedures without, in many cases, a supervisor standing directly over your shoulder.

This book is organized to help senior medical students dip their toes safely in the water of responsibility and action from the safety of reading cases, without real patients, nurses, families, and supervisors expecting decisive action. The chapters are short, easy to read, and "to the point." Short vignettes pose an organizing context to valuable issues vital to the function of the new intern. Emphasis on the discussion of these cases is not on extensive basic science background or a review of the literature; it is on practical knowledge that the intern will need to function well in the hospital and ambulatory setting and "hit the ground running." Many of the cases include questions at the end of them to stimulate further thinking and clinical reasoning in the topic area discussed. References at the end of the cases are resources for further reading as desired.

HOW TO GET THE MOST OUT OF THIS BOOK

Each case is designed to simulate a patient encounter and is followed by a set of open-ended questions. Open-ended questions are used purposely, since the cued nature of multiple-choice questions will certainly not be available in a clinical setting with real patient involvement. Each case is divided into four parts.

Part 1

1. **Answers** to the questions posed. The student should try to answer the questions after the case vignette before going on to read the case review or other answers, in order to improve his or her clinical acumen, which, after all, is what resident readiness is all about.

2. A **Case Review:** A brief discussion of the case in the vignette will be presented, helping the student understand how an expert would think about, and handle, the specific issues at hand with the particular patient presented.

Part 2

Topic Title followed by **Diagnosis** and **Treatment** discussions: In this section, a more generalized, though still focused and brief, discussion of the general issues brought forward in the case presented will be given. For example, in the case of a patient presenting with a vaginal bulge, the case review might discuss the exact treatment of the patient presented, while this part of the book will discuss, in general, the diagnosis and treatment of pelvic organ prolapse. Of note, not all of the cases in the book will fit entirely into this model, so variations do occur as necessary (for example, in the case of women presenting to the clinic for office procedures).

Part 3

Tips to Remember: These are brief, bullet-pointed notes that are reiterated as a summary of the text, allowing for easy and rapid review, such as when preparing a case presentation to the faculty in rounds.

Part 4

Comprehension Questions: Most cases have several multiple-choice questions that follow at the very end. These serve to reinforce the material presented, and provide a self-assessment mechanism for the student.

Section I.
Gynecology

A 46-year-old G3P3 With Heavy Menstrual Bleeding, Interested in Hysterectomy

Katerina Shvartsman, MD and Jennifer L. Rowland, MD

A 46-year-old Caucasian G3P3, with last menstrual period 2 weeks ago, using tubal ligation for contraception, presents to clinic reporting a 6-month history of heavy menstrual bleeding. Her menstrual cycles are every 25 days and last 8 days. She bleeds heavily on days 2 to 4 with passage of clots and requires changing her feminine pad every 2 hours. Her medical history is remarkable for 2 cesarean sections and hypertension. Her blood pressure is 148/94, height 65 in, and weight 180 lb (body mass index [BMI] 30). On pelvic examination, her uterus is enlarged to 12 cm with no adnexal masses or fullness palpated. Her sister recently had a hysterectomy and she is interested in the same management.

1. **What additional information is important in order to be able to counsel this patient about her management options?**
2. **What additional studies may aid in the evaluation of this patient?**

Answers

1. This patient is interested in surgery; however, she needs to be counseled on all possible treatment options. In order to determine potential management options and decide whether the patient is a surgical candidate, a thorough history and physical examination (H&P) needs to be completed.
2. Additional studies to consider in this patient include endometrial biopsy to evaluate for underlying causes of heavy menstrual bleeding (such as endometrial polyps, hyperplasia, endometrial cancer), complete blood count to evaluate for anemia caused by her excessive bleeding, and transvaginal ultrasound or saline-infused sonogram to evaluate for uterine abnormalities (such as leiomyomas or uterine polyps). A pregnancy test should also be performed in any woman of reproductive age with abnormal bleeding.

CASE REVIEW

The diagnosis in this patient is unclear at this time. Currently, all that is known are her symptoms. In order to determine the diagnosis (or differential diagnosis), an appropriate H&P needs to be completed. The H&P needs to be systematically organized and comprehensive.

GYNECOLOGIC HISTORY AND PHYSICAL EXAMINATION

Many institutions have a template already in place, making the process more efficient (see Appendix 1); however, it is important to understand the significance of each component of the H&P. Additionally, when collecting the history, it is helpful to prompt the patient regarding certain diagnoses. For example, specifically ask about common medical disorders such as hypertension, diabetes, and thyroid disease, as patients may omit significant medical issues if their disease is under control.

The components of a gynecologic H&P include:

1. History of present illness (problem-focused history)
2. Comprehensive gynecologic history
3. Health maintenance review
4. Physical examination

The problem-focused history should be specific to the woman's chief complaint. The first sentence serves as an introduction and should contain the patient's age, ethnicity, gravidity, parity, last menstrual period, and reason for her visit. This description should stimulate thought regarding diagnosis and possible treatment. Appendix 2 lists pertinent questions related to several common gynecologic concerns. In this particular patient's case, the history should focus on abnormal vaginal bleeding. Key questions include onset in change of bleeding pattern, frequency, duration, and amount of bleeding.

A comprehensive gynecologic history should include the patient's obstetrical, gynecologic, medical, surgical, social, and family history, as well as allergies and current medications. Every patient may be a potential surgical case; therefore, data that may impact surgical candidacy and postoperative outcome are particularly valuable. Specifically ascertain information regarding:

Hypertensive, diabetic, and asthmatic control

Evidence of obstructive sleep apnea

Evidence of cardiac disease

Personal and family history of venous thromboembolism (VTE) as well as risk factors for VTE

Risk factors for pelvic adhesive disease—prior abdominal surgery, endometriosis, and PID

Confirm that health maintenance is current by reviewing the patient's last Pap smear, mammogram, colonoscopy, bone density study, and immunization history, as applicable, based on her age (see Chapter 36 for guidelines or www.acog.org/wellwoman).

The physical examination should always start with vital signs (BP, HR, RR, Temp) and include the woman's height, weight, and BMI. The gynecologic examination should be tailored to the patient's symptoms, and, at the least, include an abdominal and pelvic examination. The pelvic examination includes 3 elements: (1) inspection of the external genitalia, urethral meatus, vaginal introitus, and perianal region (externally); (2) speculum examination of the vagina and cervix; and (3) bimanual examination of the uterus, cervix, and adnexa. When indicated, a rectovaginal examination should also be performed. Again, keep in mind that each patient is a potential surgical candidate. In this case, the patient is interested in hysterectomy. Key components of her physical examination that may help guide surgical approach (abdominal vs vaginal vs laparoscopic vs robotic) include:

BMI and girth of abdominal pannus

Caliber and laxity of vaginal introitus

Uterine size, shape, position (axis), and consistency

Uterine mobility and descent

Evaluation for adnexal and rectovaginal masses

Treatment

Treatment should be based on the diagnosis, and additional studies may need to be performed. In this case, it would be helpful to:

Verify the patient is not pregnant.

Perform an endometrial biopsy to evaluate the uterine lining for polyps, hyperplasia, or neoplasia.

Order or perform a transvaginal ultrasound to evaluate uterine size or uterine abnormalities such as leiomyomas/adenomyosis or saline-infused sonogram to evaluate the uterus as well as the uterine cavity for submucosal leiomyomas or polyps.

Check a hemoglobin/hematocrit to evaluate for anemia.

Once the data are synthesized, and a diagnosis is made, the patient should be counseled using easy-to-understand terminology about all of her options including risks and benefits and convalescence. (Refer to Chapter 2 for treatment options.) Also, it is important to understand the reason a patient strongly desires or declines certain management options. She may have misconceptions or apprehension regarding particular medications or procedures. It is the physician's role to allay concerns and guide a patient in making a properly informed decision.

If the patient elects to proceed with hysterectomy, a preoperative checklist can be used to anticipate patient needs, improve patient safety, and mitigate medical errors.

At a minimum, the preoperative plan should include:

Planned procedure

Consent form

Review of patient's allergies

Preoperative labs

Antibiotic prophylaxis

DVT prophylaxis

Additionally, the patient should be assessed for 3 major risks: cardiovascular, pulmonary, and thrombotic (DVT). If the patient is found to have a major cardiac or pulmonary condition, she is often referred to an internist specializing in perioperative evaluation and management. Specific guidelines for the management of complicated patients are beyond the scope of this chapter but are readily found in the references provided. Appendix 3 provides a sample checklist to guide preoperative planning.

TIPS TO REMEMBER

- Set the scene with the opening line. Include the patient's age, gravidity, parity, ethnicity if relevant, last menstrual period, current form of contraception, and chief concern. This short introduction stimulates thought regarding differential diagnosis and management.
- Be organized and thorough. Develop a systematic approach to history taking that will translate into a fluid story that is easy to follow.
- Don't be afraid to ask personal or delicate questions relevant to the patient's issues.
- BMI should be part of the vital signs. It plays a significant role in guiding management options.
- If the patient may be a potential surgical case, make sure the history assesses her perioperative risks and the physical examination evaluates for the optimal route of surgery.

COMPREHENSION QUESTIONS

1. During a preoperative physical examination for a patient scheduled for a hysterectomy, a heart murmur is heard. What is the next best step?

    A. Order perioperative antibiotics for bacterial endocarditis prophylaxis.
    B. Proceed to the operating room as planned.
    C. Refer to specialist for further evaluation and recommendation.
    D. Inform the patient that she is too high risk to undergo surgery.

2. What is the appropriate antibiotic prophylaxis for a 45-year-old diabetic with a BMI of 36, undergoing operative hysteroscopy?

    A. Cefazolin 1 g IV within 60 minutes of surgical start
    B. Cefazolin 2 g IV within 60 minutes of surgical start

C. Doxycycline 100 mg po 1 hour before procedure and 200 mg after procedure
D. None

3. When eliciting the patient's allergy history, it is important to ask about which of the following?
A. The patient's reaction to any medications to which she reports being allergic
B. Latex allergy
C. Iodine allergy
D. All of the above

Answers

1. **C.** Recommendations for further management as well as counseling about surgical risks are dependent on the etiology of the patient's murmur. The patient should be evaluated by a specialist who can assist with perioperative guidance. The other answers would be inappropriate without knowing the underlying cause of the murmur.

2. **D.** Antibiotic prophylaxis is recommended in patients undergoing, hysterectomy, but not hysteroscopy. If the patient were scheduled for hysterectomy, then the appropriate answer would be cefazolin 2 g IV, based on her BMI >35.

3. **D.** It is important to know the patient's allergic reactions in order to assess potential cross-reactivity with other medications. For example, patients with an immediate (IgE-mediated) hypersensitivity reaction to penicillin (bronchospasm and wheezing, laryngeal edema and stridor, angioedema, urticarial, hypotension, etc) would be advised not to use a cephalosporin. However, patients with a non–IgE-mediated allergy, such as a mild, nonurticarial rash, may still be candidates to receive a second- or third-generation cephalosporin. Additionally, latex and iodine are commonly encountered in clinical and surgical settings and could cause significant harm in patients who are allergic to these agents.

SUGGESTED READINGS

ACOG Committee on Patient Safety and Quality Improvement. ACOG Committee Opinion No. 526: standardization of practice to improve outcomes. *Obstet Gynecol.* 2012;119:1081–1082.
ACOG Committee on Practice Bulletins—Gynecology. ACOG practice bulletin no. 104: antibiotic prophylaxis for gynecologic procedures. *Obstet Gynecol.* 2009;113:1180–1189.
ACOG Committee Opinion No. 444: choosing the route of hysterectomy for benign disease. *Obstet Gynecol.* 2009;114:1156–1158.

Committee on Gynecologic Practice. Committee opinion no. 534: well-woman visit. *Obstet Gynecol.* 2012;120:421–424.

Gould MK, Garcia DA, Wren SM, et al. Prevention of VTE in nonorthopedic surgical patients: antithrombotic therapy and prevention of thrombosis, 9th ed: American College of Chest Physician evidence-based clinical practice guidelines. *Chest.* 2012;141(2 suppl):e419s–e494s.

Johnson BE, Porter J. Preoperative evaluation of the gynecologic patient: considerations for improved outcomes. *Obstet Gynecol.* 2008;111:1183–1194.

Rahn DD, Mamik MM, Sanses TV, et al. Venous thromboembolism prophylaxis in gynecologic surgery: a systematic review. *Obstet Gynecol.* 2011;118:1111–1125.

Vintzileos AM, Finamore PS, Ananth CV. Inclusion of body mass index in the history of present illness. *Obstet Gynecol.* 2013;121:59–64.

APPENDIX 1

GYNE HISTORY AND PHYSICAL

Name: ____________ Today's Date: ____________ Date of Birth: ____________

Age: ____________ Race/Ethnicity: ____________ Marital Status: ____________

Phone number: ____________ Email: ____________

Address: ____________

Reason for visit: ____________

Obstetrical History

Have you ever been pregnant? ____________

How many times? ____________

Miscarriages: ________ Abortions: ________

Vaginal deliveries ________ C-Section ________

Living children ________

Are you currently pregnant? ☐ Yes ☐ No

Are you currently breastfeeding? ☐ Yes ☐ No

Menstrual History

When was the first day of your last period ___/___/___

Age at first period ________

Length of cycle (#days between periods) ________

How many days does bleeding last? ________

Menstrual flow: ☐ Heavy ☐ Moderate ☐ Light

Do you bleed between periods? ☐ Yes ☐ No

Do you bleed after sex? ☐ Yes ☐ No

Do you have painful periods? ☐ Yes ☐ No

Are you in menopause? ☐ Yes ☐ No

Year menopause occurred: ________

Gynecological History

Are you currently sexually active? ☐ Yes ☐ No

Who do you have sex with? ☐ Men ☐ Women ☐ Both

Are you trying to get pregnant? ☐ Yes ☐ No

What method of birth control do you use:

☐ Tubal ligation ☐ Vasectomy

☐ Intrauterine device ☐ Birth control pills

☐ Depo-Provera ☐ Implant in the arm

☐ Condoms ☐ Other: ________

Do you need birth control? ☐ Yes ☐ No

Do you have a history of:

Gonorrhea or Chlamydia ☐ Yes ☐ No

Herpes ☐ Yes ☐ No

Other sexually transmitted disease ☐ Yes ☐ No

Pelvic Inflammatory disease ☐ Yes ☐ No

Endometriosis ☐ Yes ☐ No

Fibroids ☐ Yes ☐ No

Abnormal pap smear ☐ Yes ☐ No

If yes, when ________ What was the result ________

LEEP or Cone procedure ☐ Yes ☐ No

Medical History: Do you have or have you ever had:

Diabetes ☐ Yes ☐ No

High Blood Pressure ☐ Yes ☐ No

Blood Clots in your legs or lungs ☐ Yes ☐ No

Cancer ☐ Yes ☐ No

Stroke or Heart Attack ☐ Yes ☐ No

Sleep Apnea ☐ Yes ☐ No

High or low thyroid ☐ Yes ☐ No

High Cholesterol ☐ Yes ☐ No

Migraines or Headaches ☐ Yes ☐ No

Asthma or lung disease ☐ Yes ☐ No

Liver or Bowel disease ☐ Yes ☐ No

Depression ☐ Yes ☐ No

Anemia ☐ Yes ☐ No

Other: ____________

Surgical History: (Please list surgeries and year done)

☐ Hysterectomy ________ ☐ Appendectomy ________

☐ Tubal ligation ________ ☐ Gallbladder ________

☐ Breast ________

Other: ____________

Allergies: (include reaction)

None ☐

Medications: ____________

____

Latex ☐ Yes ☐ No

Other (food, herbals, etc) ____________

Medications/Vitamins/Supplements (list dose):

____

____

____

Personal/Social History

Do you smoke ☐ Yes ☐ No

How many packs per day? ___ For how many years? ___

Do you drink >1 alcoholic drink/day ☐ Yes ☐ No

Do you use drugs not prescribed to you ☐ Yes ☐ No

Do you use illegal drugs ☐ Yes ☐ No

GYNE HISTORY AND PHYSICAL *(Continued)*

Personal/Social History

What is your occupation? ______

What is your marital status?

☐ Single ☐ Married ☐ Divorced ☐ Separated ☐ Widowed ☐ Domestic Partner

Have you been physically/emotionally/sexually abused? ☐ Yes ☐ No

Family History

Does anyone in your family have the following. List relationship and age at diagnosis

☐ Breast Cancer? ______ ☐ Heart Disease? ______

☐ Ovarian Cancer ______ ☐ Diabetes ______

☐ Colon Cancer ______ ☐ Bleeding or Blood Clot Problems ______

☐ High Blood Pressure? ______ ☐ Stroke ______

Other: ______

Health Maintenance

Please list most recent date and result of test as applicable

☐ Pap Smear ______ ☐ Colonoscopy ______

☐ Mammogram ______ ☐ Bone Density ______

☐ Flu vaccine ______

Physical Exam (For Medical Use Only)

BP ___/___ **T** ______ **HR** ______ **RR** ______ **HT** ______ **WT** ______ **BMI** ______

Thyroid: ☐ Normal ☐ Abnormal

Heart: ______

Lungs: ______

Breasts:

Right: ☐ Normal ☐ Abnormal ______

Left: ☐ Normal ☐ Abnormal ______

Abdomen: ______

External Genitalia: ______

Vagina: ______

Cervix: ☐ Parous ☐ Nulliparous

Lesion: ☐ Yes ☐ No

IUD string: ☐ Seen ☐ Not seen ☐ N/A

Uterus:

Size: ______

Position: ______

Mobility: ______

Tenderness: ______

Adnexa

Right: ☐ Normal ☐ Abnormal ______

Left: ☐ Normal ☐ Abnormal ______

Diagnosis: ______

☐ **Endometrial Biopsy**

☐ **Ultrasound**

☐ **CBC**

☐ **HCG**

☐ **GC/Chlamydia**

☐ **Pap Smear**

☐ **HPV**

☐ **Type and Screen**

☐ **RX** ______

☐ **RX** ______

Other ______

APPENDIX 2

PROBLEM-FOCUSED QUESTION GUIDE TO SOME COMMON GYNE CONCERNS

Pelvic pain

- When did symptoms first start?
- Location of pain; is it focal (point with 1 finger) or diffuse?
- CODIERS (common mnemonic):

  Character of pain—sharp, dull, gnawing, stabbing, radiating

  Onset—when does it start?

  Duration—how long does an episode last?

  Intensity—how bad does it get?

  Exacerbating factors—what makes it worse (menstruation, sex, exercise, etc)?

  Relieving factors—what makes it better (position, medication, heat, etc)?

  Symptoms associated with pain—nausea, headache, urinary, bowel

Abnormal vaginal bleeding

- When did abnormal bleeding start?
- Amount, duration, frequency of bleeding
- Intermenstrual bleeding or bleeding with intercourse
- Postmenopausal bleeding
- Medication history—hormonal birth control, hormone replacement

Vulvovaginal concern

- Vaginal discharge:

  Onset, consistency, odor, itching, sexual history
- Vaginal dryness:

  Onset, menopausal symptoms, focal or diffuse
- Vulvovaginal pain:

  Onset, lesions, relation to intercourse

Contraception

- Current sexual practice—sexually active? Monogamous? Current partner (male, female, both)?
- What are you currently using?
- What have you used in the past? Any side effects?
- Pregnancy desires?
- Do you use condoms for STD prophylaxis?

APPENDIX 3

SAMPLE PREOPERATIVE CHECKLIST FOR GYNE SURGERY

☐ **Patient has complete medical history and physical examination**

- ☐ Allergies identified
- ☐ Medical factors that may affect anesthesia choices identified (eg, HTN, cardiac disease, sleep apnea, asthma, obesity, malignant hyperthermia)
- ☐ Patient referred for preoperative medical clearance for:

☐ Not applicable	☐ Hypertension	☐ Cardiac disease
☐ Sleep apnea	☐ Hx of DVT	☐ Asthma
☐ Diabetes	☐ Other ________________	

☐ **Patient counseled about risks and benefits of proposed surgery**

- ☐ Consent form signed

☐ **Appropriate preoperative lab work completed or ordered**

- ☐ CBC
- ☐ Type and screen
- ☐ hCG
- ☐ Other: ________________

☐ **Antibiotic prophylaxis ordered to be administered within 60 minutes before incision**

Hysteroscopy/laparoscopy

☐ None

Induced abortion/dilation and evacuation

☐ Doxycycline 100 mg po 1 hour before procedure and 200 mg po after procedure

Hysterectomy/urogynecology procedure

☐ Cefazolin 1 g IV

☐ Cefazolin 2 g IV (if BMI >35 or weight >100 kg or 220 lb)

If immediate hypersensitivity to penicillin:

☐ Clindamycin 600 mg IV plus gentamicin 1.5 mg/kg IV *or*

☐ **Deep vein thrombosis prophylaxis (see Gould et al, 2012 and Rahn et al, 2011 in the section "Suggested Readings" for risk assessment)**

Very low risk

☐ Early ambulation

Low risk

☐ Perioperative intermittent pneumatic compression (IPC)

Moderate risk

☐ IPC *or*

☐ Enoxaparin (40 U) *or* dalteparin (2500 U) sq 2 to 12 hours preoperatively and daily postoperatively until discharge *or*

☐ Unfractionated heparin 5000 U sq 2 hours preoperatively and BID postoperatively until discharge

High risk

☐ IPC *and*

☐ Enoxaparin (40 U) *or* dalteparin (5000 U) sq 2 to 12 hours preoperatively and daily postoperatively until discharge *or*

☐ Unfractionated heparin 5000 U sq 2 hours preoperatively and TID postoperatively until discharge

Highest risk

☐ Same for high risk, consider continuing therapy for 2 to 4 weeks after discharge

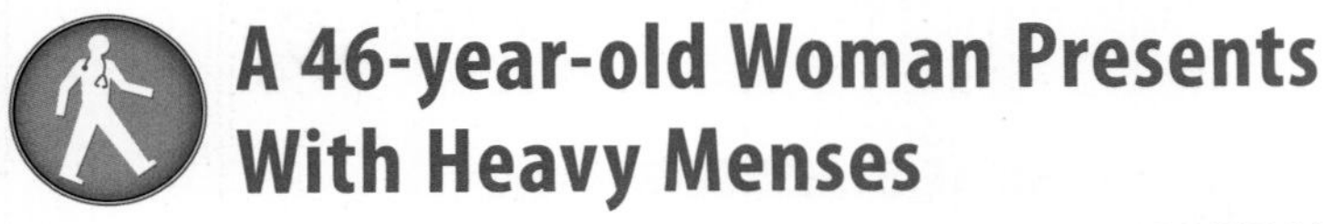

A 46-year-old Woman Presents With Heavy Menses

Lubna Chohan, MD

A 46-year-old gravida 3 para 3 presents as a new patient in your clinic with a chief complaint of "my periods are getting heavier and I am bleeding through my clothes." On taking her history, she has no medical or surgical history, has had 3 vaginal deliveries, denies alcohol or tobacco use, and works full-time in an office. Her gynecologic history shows that her Pap and mammogram are current and her husband had a vasectomy for birth control. In the past, she had regular menses every 30 days lasting 4 days (her heaviest bleeding would require changing a regular tampon every 6 hours).

Over the past year, the patient reports her menses have changed. At times, she will skip a month. More bothersome to her is during her cycles she can bleed for up to 14 days and pass large clots, has to change a super-plus tampon every 1 to 2 hours, and sometimes bleeds through her clothes at work. She notes some occasional hot flushes as well as fatigue.

1. What is the etiology of her bleeding?

2. How would you work up this patient?

3. How would you treat this patient?

Answers

1. Based on the patient's age, recent change in menstrual pattern, and hot flushes, her etiology is likely anovulatory bleeding. Other causes include pregnancy, cervical/endometrial malignancy, intrauterine or cervical polyps, adenomyosis, leiomyomas, thyroid dysfunction, infection, and bleeding disorders.

2. The patient needs a pelvic examination (speculum and bimanual). Recommended laboratory testing includes a pregnancy test, complete blood count (CBC), and thyroid-stimulating hormone (TSH). If she has an abnormal pelvic examination, revealing an enlarged or irregularly shaped uterus, a transvaginal or abdominal ultrasound (depending on the size of the uterus) could be ordered. An endometrial biopsy should be performed to evaluate patients over the age of 45 or in younger patients with an unopposed estrogen history, obesity, or a failed prior treatment for persistent abnormal bleeding.

3. If her pelvic examination and endometrial biopsy are normal and the uterus is of normal size, this patient has a variety of medical and surgical treatment options.

ABNORMAL MENSTRUAL BLEEDING

Most definitions of normal menstruation include a cycle length of 21 to 35 days, duration of 7 days or less, and blood loss of less than 80 mL. Some descriptive terms are listed as follows:

- *Oligomenorrhea*: Intervals between bleeding episodes vary from 35 days to 6 months.
- *Menorrhagia*: Prolonged (more than 7 days) or excessive (greater than 80 mL) uterine bleeding occurring at regular intervals. Also called heavy menstrual bleeding.
- *Metrorrhagia*: Uterine bleeding occurring at irregular but frequent intervals, the amount being variable.
- *Polymenorrhea*: Uterine bleeding occurring at regular intervals of less than 21 days.

Diagnosis

In 2011, a new classification system (PALM-COEIN) was created for causes of abnormal uterine bleeding in nonpregnant reproductive aged women in order to better classify the causes of abnormal bleeding and improve research. The components of PALM are structural and can be measured through either imaging studies or histopathology. The components of COEIN are nonstructural.

PALM:

P: polyp

A: adenomyosis

L: leiomyoma

M: malignancy and hyperplasia

COEIN:

C: coagulopathy (von Willebrand disease, anticoagulation)

O: ovulatory dysfunction (PCOS, thyroid disease, hyperprolactinemia, stress, anorexia, ovulatory disorders occurring during adolescence and menopause transition)

E: endometrial

I: iatrogenic

N: not yet classified

Evaluation

Evaluation is guided by the patient's age, reproductive status, and associated symptoms. These patients require a complete history and physical examination that confirms that the source of bleeding is uterine. Anovulatory bleeding is common in women of this age range. It is also common at the beginning of menarche, in patients with PCOS or who are obese, and during times of great physical stress. Anovulatory bleeding requires exclusion of anatomic abnormalities (ie, leiomyomas), must have a noncyclic bleeding pattern, and must be without other signs of ovulation.

Confirmation of a patient's cervical cytology screening history and sexually transmitted infection history will clue you in to possible involvement of the cervix or to infection (endometritis). Laboratory workup includes a pregnancy test, CBC, TSH, and prolactin. Imaging of the pelvis, specifically sonography, can aid in determining whether there is any evidence of uterine leiomyomas or adenomyosis. Sonography is especially helpful in the obese patient when physical examination is limited by habitus. If intrauterine pathology is suspected (submucosal leiomyomas or intrauterine polyps), a saline-infused sonohysterography provides a more accurate intrauterine image. Endometrial biopsy in patients over the age of 45 with irregular menses (or under the age of 45 with risk factors for endometrial hyperplasia/cancer) will assess for hyperplasia and neoplasia. Simple endometrial hyperplasia has a low risk of progression to endometrial cancer (1%) while complex hyperplasia with the addition of nuclear atypia has the highest risk of progression to endometrial cancer (30%).

Treatment

There are many treatment options for abnormal uterine bleeding. You will have to make a choice depending on the etiology of the bleeding, patient's age and future fertility desire, medical and surgical history, smoking history, and the patient's wishes/work situation (if she is able to take time off of work to recover from surgery). Medical options include nonsteroidal anti-inflammatories (ibuprofen, mefenamic acid), antifibrinolytic therapy (tranexamic acid), progesterone (oral, transdermal, or intrauterine), combined estrogen/progesterone pill, and GnRH agonist (Lupron). Surgical options include hysterectomy (abdominal, vaginal, or laparoscopic), endometrial ablation, and myomectomy in the case of leiomyomas. Another option for leiomyomas is uterine artery embolization, which is performed by radiologists.

TIPS TO REMEMBER

- A complete history and physical examination (including speculum and bimanual) are required.
- Evaluation of abnormal bleeding in women >45 years of age (or younger in those with unopposed estrogen, obesity, and failed medical management or persistent abnormal bleeding) includes an endometrial biopsy to look for evidence of hyperplasia or malignancy.
- Treatment options depend on the underlying cause of the bleeding and include medical management, surgical management, or radiologic management.

COMPREHENSION QUESTIONS

1. Which type of endometrial hyperplasia has the highest progression rate to endometrial cancer?

   A. Simple endometrial hyperplasia
   B. Simple endometrial hyperplasia with atypia
   C. Complex endometrial hyperplasia
   D. Complex endometrial hyperplasia with atypia

2. A 40-year-old G1P1 presents with a 6-month history of irregular menses. Her menses still occur regularly every 29 days and the duration and flow has not changed, but she has new-onset spotting that occurs between her periods and lasts for a few days. Another physician has given her estrogen/progesterone oral contraceptive pills for the past 3 months that has not improved this spotting. Speculum and bimanual examinations do not reveal any abnormalities. You would like to evaluate her for intrauterine pathology, specifically a polyp or submucosal leiomyoma. What is the best imaging study to evaluate this?

   A. Transvaginal ultrasound
   B. Saline-infused sonohysterography
   C. MRI
   D. CT

3. Anovulation is common in all of the following patient ages/characteristics *except* which one?

   A. A 12-year-old with menarche 6 months ago
   B. A 26-year-old with a BMI of 40, new-onset diabetes, and PCOS
   C. A 35-year-old with uterine leiomyomas
   D. A 40-year-old who is training for a marathon
   E. A 47-year-old who is also experiencing hot flushes and vaginal dryness

Answers

1. **D**. The progression rate to endometrial cancer is 1% for simple hyperplasia (mean duration 10 years), 2% to 4% for complex hyperplasia (mean duration 10 years), 23% for atypical hyperplasia (mean duration 4 years), and 29% for complex atypical hyperplasia (mean duration 4 years).

2. **B**. Saline-infused sonohysterography involves passing a small catheter through the cervix and instilling fluid in the uterus during the ultrasound. This allows enhanced endometrial visualization during transvaginal sonogram. Lesions such as an endometrial polyp or submucosal leiomyoma are better visualized in this manner, rather than standard transvaginal ultrasound.

Transvaginal ultrasound is a good screening study to perform if the patient has an abnormal pelvic examination (enlarged or irregularly shaped uterus) or if abnormal uterine bleeding persists despite treatment in someone with a normal pelvic examination. MRI may be useful to guide the treatment of leiomyomas, when considering a myomectomy, or uterine artery embolization.

3. C. Leiomyomas are a structural cause of abnormal uterine bleeding. They should not affect ovulation. A woman at menarche has an immature hypothalamic–pituitary axis causing anovulation. She will have months to years of unpredictable ovulation after menarche. In the first year after menarche, 85% of cycles are anovulatory. Other causes of anovulation are PCOS, thyroid disease, prolactinemia, stress, excessive exercise, eating disorders, and menopausal transition.

SUGGESTED READINGS

Committee on Practice Bulletins—Gynecology. Practice bulletin no. 128: diagnosis of abnormal uterine bleeding in reproductive-aged women. *Obstet Gynecol.* 2012;120(1):197–206.

Deligeoroglou E, Athanasopoulos N, Tsimaris P, et al. Evaluation and management of adolescent amenorrhea. *Ann N Y Acad Sci.* 2010;1205:23–32.

Iram S, Musonda P, Ewies AA. When should the endometrium be investigated? A retrospective non-comparative study of 3006 women. *Eur J Obstet Gynecol Reprod Biol.* 2010;148(1):86–89.

Katz VL, Lentz GM, Lobo RA, et al. *Abnormal Uterine Bleeding. Comprehensive Gynecology.* 5th ed. Philadelphia, PA: Mosby Elsevier; 2007:915.

Munro MG, Critchley HO, Broder MS, Fraser IS; FIGO Menstrual Disorders Working Group. FIGO classification system (PALM-COEIN) for causes of abnormal uterine bleeding in nongravid women of reproductive age. *Int J Gynaecol Obstet.* 2011;113(1):3–13.

Oehler MK, Rees MC. Menorrhagia: an update. *Acta Obstet Gynecol Scand.* 2003;82(5):405–422.

Wallach EE, Vlahos NF. Uterine myomas: an overview of development, clinical features, and management. *Obstet Gynecol.* 2004;104(2):393–406.

Wilkinson JP, Kadir RA. Management of abnormal uterine bleeding in adolescents. *J Pediatr Adolesc Gynecol.* 2010;23(6 suppl):S22–S30.

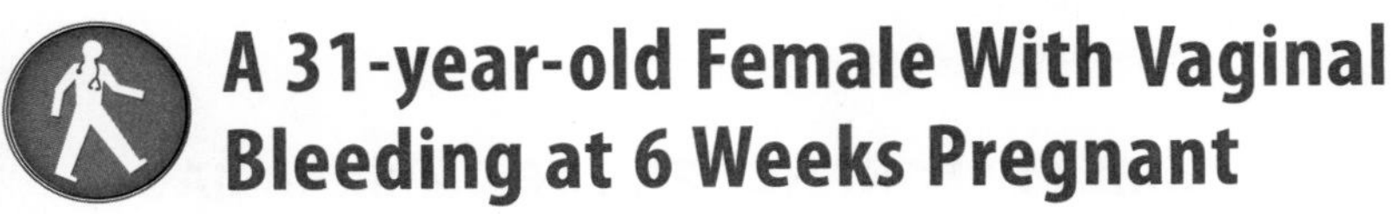

A 31-year-old Female With Vaginal Bleeding at 6 Weeks Pregnant

Charlie C. Kilpatrick, MD

A 31-year-old P1001 at 6 weeks gestation calls the clinic complaining of vaginal bleeding that began last night. She has not sought out prenatal care, as she just had a positive home pregnancy test last week. You ask her to come into the clinic so you can evaluate her. In review of her history she has no medical or surgical history; her first pregnancy went to term without complication and she delivered vaginally. She denies any allergies, and is not taking any medication. She has regular menses, denies abnormal cervical cytology or sexually transmitted infections, and has not had intercourse recently. Her vitals are within normal limits and examination of the pelvis reveals the following: normal external female genitalia, parous introitus, vaginal side wall normal in appearance, parous cervical os, and no active bleeding or discharge; bimanual examination reveals a closed internal cervical os, no cervical motion tenderness, freely mobile uterus, and no adnexal masses appreciated.

1. What is in your differential diagnosis, and what are the next steps you need to take in the management of this patient?

Answer

1. Your top 3 differential diagnoses should include a miscarriage, normal intrauterine pregnancy, and ectopic pregnancy. Your next steps are to obtain a blood type and screen, hemoglobin, quantitative serum beta-human chorionic gonadotropin (hCG), and a transvaginal ultrasound.

CASE REVIEW

The type and screen will allow you to determine this patient's Rh status and whether or not RhoGAM is necessary. A baseline hemoglobin value will alert you to anemia, and gives you a starting point in case her bleeding worsens. A serum quantitative beta-hCG level will confirm that she is pregnant, and the change in this value will help you determine if the pregnancy is normal or abnormal. The transvaginal ultrasound will determine if the pregnancy is intrauterine. The patient is Rh positive, her hemoglobin is 12.4 g/dL, beta-hCG is 1785 IU/mL, and the transvaginal ultrasound reveals a gestational sac measuring 22 mm, embryonic pole of 8 mm, and no cardiac activity. You diagnose her with early pregnancy failure (EPF), and discuss treatment options.

ABORTION/EARLY PREGNANCY FAILURE/MISCARRIAGE

Diagnosis

The definition of abortion is the expulsion or extraction of an embryo or fetus weighing 500 g or less from its mother. An embryonic loss is a loss prior to 10 weeks gestation, while a loss after 10 weeks gestation is a fetal loss. Currently, terminology has more to do with the physiologic process rather than an underlying cause, and as ultrasound improves, the terminology will improve. For example, the term missed abortion assumes the uterus missed recognizing that the intrauterine contents were not viable, while incomplete abortion, incomplete passage of embryonic/fetal tissue, and inevitable abortion, where there is an unstoppable abortive process in place, also have more to do with physical examination findings than the underlying cause.

In a patient with a positive urine pregnancy test, EPF can be diagnosed clinically by noting bleeding, cramping, and an open cervical os with or without tissue present (incomplete or inevitable abortion), or a declining/inappropriate rise in the beta-hCG level in the presence of intrauterine contents (missed abortion). EPF can also be diagnosed with imaging: absence of cardiac activity with a crown rump length ≥7 mm, an empty gestational sac measuring more than ≥25 mm in diameter without an embryonic pole (you will often see this written as fetal pole, but embryonic pole is more accurate), absence of an embryo with a heartbeat ≥2 weeks after a scan that showed a gestational sac without a yolk sac, or absence of an embryo with a hearbeat ≥11 days after a scan that showed a gestational sac with a yolk sac.

The key, when you begin to evaluate first trimester pregnant patients with vaginal bleeding, is to determine if the pregnancy is intrauterine and then whether the pregnancy is normal or abnormal. Each practice location likely has a serum beta level above which they should be able to visualize an intrauterine pregnancy by transvaginal ultrasound. This level is referred to as the discriminatory zone, and often is 1000 to 1500 IU/L. If the beta level is greater than this value and nothing is visualized within the uterus, there should be a strong suspicion of an ectopic pregnancy. Keep in mind the results of the ultrasound depend on the skill of the ultrasonographer and the quality of the equipment as well as other factors (leiomyomas, multiple gestation). If the beta level is below the discriminatory zone and there are no obvious signs of ectopic pregnancy (peritoneal signs on abdominal or pelvic examination, adnexal mass on ultrasound, free peritoneal fluid), then you will need serial beta levels to determine if this is a normal pregnancy. The usual time frame to redraw a beta level is 48 to 72 hours, and you want to employ the same laboratory to perform the beta level.

In a normal pregnancy, the beta level rises in a curvilinear fashion until 41 days of gestation, with 85% of viable pregnancies showing at least a 66% increase in beta level over a 48-hour period, and 99% showing a doubling over a 72-hour period. For a viable pregnancy, the slowest recorded rise of beta-hCG during this early time period is 35% over a 48-hour interval. After this, it rises more slowly until it peaks at around 100,000 IU/L (range of 27,000-230,000 IU/L) at approximately 8 to 11 weeks gestation. After the peak the beta level declines to approximately 12,000 IU/L (range of 2000-50,000 IU/L) at 24 weeks. *Therefore, in the first 6 weeks if the beta declines or does not increase by at least 35% over a 48-hour period, or double in 72 hours, the pregnancy is abnormal.*

Treatment

EPF is the most common complication of early pregnancy with almost 1 in 4 women experiencing it in their lifetimes. This should be communicated to the patient as you begin to answer her questions. Also, this is likely failure of a wanted pregnancy for your patient. Be cognizant of this and treat each patient with respect, kindness, and patience. Patients have a tendency to blame themselves, so try to reassure them that it is not the result of something they did wrong or could have prevented. Most often this is a genetic abnormality, and the strongest risk factors for miscarriage are advancing maternal age and prior miscarriage (alcohol, cigarette smoke, cocaine use, and maternal weight may also be linked).

Medical, surgical, or expectant management can be employed once the diagnosis of miscarriage is certain. If you are certain that the pregnancy is in the uterus but you are not completely sure that the pregnancy is abnormal (ultrasound images are not ideal), a formal transvaginal scan by an experienced sonographer will help. Alternatively, when the imaging is in question, a repeat sonogram in 4 to 7 days is a reasonable course of action. In this situation, when there is confidence of intrauterine products, there is little risk in waiting 4 to 7 days for repeat imaging, and more harm may be done with a hasty medical or surgical treatment plan that may interrupt a viable pregnancy. Miscarriage can be managed with surgery, employing a suction dilatation and curettage under antibiotic cover (doxycycline 100 mg orally BID on the day of surgery). Risks are small but include the risk of anesthesia, hemorrhage, cervical trauma, uterine perforation, infection, and intrauterine adhesions; the latter 2 can affect future fertility. Surgery is the treatment of choice for a patient with a septic abortion. Medical management of miscarriage using prostaglandins has gained widespread use and is very effective. There are many regimens, but 800 μg placed in the vagina, repeated in 48 to 72 hours if expulsion has not occurred, is highly effective. There is very little difference in blood loss, infection rates, or effectiveness between medical and surgical management for missed or incomplete abortion. Expectant management has similar infection rates compared with surgical/medical management with lower overall effectiveness than medical or surgical treatment. RhoGAM should be administered for those patients who are Rh negative to prevent alloimmunization. A 50-μg dose is effective until 12 weeks gestation, but the 300-μg dose is more readily available.

There is debate as to whether an ultrasound is necessary after expectant or medical treatment for miscarriage in order to determine if miscarriage is complete. Some clinicians rely on history and clinical findings (absence of cramping, passage of tissue, decline in bleeding, closed cervical os on examination, declining beta-hCG level) to guide whether the miscarriage has completed. Others employ ultrasound measurements (presence of a gestational sac, or endometrial thickness >15 mm) as evidence of failure. If a clear gestational sac was visualized prior to treatment, then a repeat ultrasound can alert you to the presence or absence of a gestational sac, but the sensitivity of ultrasound in discerning clot from retained products from other intrauterine contents is difficult, and may lead to unnecessary intervention. Currently there is no agreed-upon endometrial thickness layer above which a diagnosis of an incomplete miscarriage is made. A history that elicits passage of tissue followed by cessation of cramping and declining bleeding, combined with a physical examination revealing a closed os, decreased bleeding, and a declining beta level, is sufficient.

Once the miscarriage has completed, pelvic rest for 2 weeks is encouraged, and a delay in pregnancy for 2 to 3 months is common, although the latter is expert opinion more than science. Contraception should be discussed and instructions given to call for any signs/symptoms of an incomplete miscarriage (continued heavy bleeding, cramping, and fever). There is debate on whether beta levels should be followed to a level <2 IU/L for the rare occurrence of gestational trophoblastic disease in patients without tissue available for pathologic confirmation. There are no data to guide one here, but if a declining beta is documented and normal menses resume in 2 to 4 weeks, this is likely unnecessary.

TIPS TO REMEMBER

- Miscarriage is common and this information should be relayed to the patient.
- The goal to managing bleeding in the first 6 weeks of pregnancy is to determine if the pregnancy is intrauterine, and whether it is normal.
- Ultrasound will allow you to determine the location of the pregnancy, especially once the serum beta level has reached your practice location's discriminatory zone.
- If the beta level is below the discriminatory zone, a rise in beta level of at least 35% in 48 hours or a doubling in 72 hours is needed in order for the pregnancy to be considered normal.
- After documenting intrauterine contents, uncertainty as to whether the pregnancy is normal should be verified by an experienced sonographer.
- All treatment options, expectant, medical, and surgical, are acceptable and the decision should be reached after you've had time to discuss with your patient the risks and benefits.
- Clinical signs of a completed miscarriage are a history that elicits passage of tissue followed by the cessation of cramping, a decline in bleeding, a closed cervical os, and a declining beta level. Ultrasound may also be helpful to visualize the presence or absence of a gestational sac after treatment.

COMPREHENSION QUESTIONS

1. Which of the following statements is true?
   - A. Incomplete abortion should always be managed with suction d and c under antibiotic cover.
   - B. Expectant management of miscarriage is associated with higher infection rates than medical/surgical management.
   - C. RhoGAM administration is not necessary in Rh negative patients who experience miscarriage.
   - D. Miscarriage is the most common complication of early pregnancy.

2. A pregnant patient presents at 6 weeks gestation bleeding, Rh positive, Hgb of 12.8, and a beta-hCG of 956 IU/L. Your examination of the abdomen is normal and the cervical os is closed. Ultrasound shows nothing in the uterus. Your next step should be which of the following?
   - A. Misoprostol 800 μg per vagina with follow-up in 48 to 72 hours.
   - B. Surgical management with suction d and c under antibiotic cover.
   - C. Admission to the hospital with repeat beta level in the AM.
   - D. Repeat beta level and ultrasound in 48 to 72 hours in the clinic with bleeding precautions.

3. A pregnant patient presents at 6 weeks gestation with vaginal bleeding, became hypotensive and required an IV fluid bolus before you were called. She is Rh positive, hgb of 11.2, 785 IU/L beta-hCG level, and on examination she has guarding, peritoneal signs, and a closed cervical os with cervical motion tenderness. Radiology is backed up and hasn't had time to get to the ultrasound that was ordered. Your next step should be which of the following?
   - A. Page radiology stat as you suspect this patient has an ectopic pregnancy and needs an ultrasound.
   - B. Admission to the hospital with serial examinations, and repeat beta level in the AM to determine if this is a normal pregnancy.
   - C. Repeat beta level in 48 to 72 hours once you visualize intrauterine contents by ultrasound.
   - D. Take the patient to the OR for suspected ruptured ectopic pregnancy.

4. A pregnant patient presents at 6 weeks gestation with bleeding. She is Rh positive, with a hgb of 11.8, and beta-hCG of 2752 IU/L. Her abdominal examination is within normal limits, pelvic examination reveals a closed os, and no cervical motion tenderness. Transvaginal ultrasound, with experienced sonographer confirmation, shows an empty uterus. Your next step should be which of the following?
   - A. Repeat ultrasound in 4 to 7 days in the clinic.
   - B. Discuss with the patient management options for EPF.
   - C. Repeat beta level in 48 to 72 hours to determine if pregnancy is normal.
   - D. Discuss with the patient management options for ectopic pregnancy.

Answers

1. **D**. Miscarriage is the most common complication in early pregnancy. Incomplete miscarriage can be managed expectantly, medically, or with surgery and infection rates are similar for all 3 methods. RhoGAM is necessary for Rh negative patients in the first trimester for vaginal bleeding or miscarriage to prevent alloimmunization and a 50-µg dose will cover up to 12 weeks gestation.

2. **D**. Repeat beta level in 48 to 72 hours to determine if the pregnancy is normal or not. The uterus is empty on ultrasound, but the beta level is below the discriminatory zone, so you're still trying to figure out if this is a normal pregnancy or not. If imaging revealed a large adnexal mass and free fluid and the patient had peritoneal signs, then you would diagnose an ectopic pregnancy. It's premature to give misoprostol or perform a d and c, and there is no reason to admit the patient to the hospital. If on repeat examination her beta rises appropriately and intrauterine contents are seen, you've got a normal pregnancy.

3. **D**. Take the patient to the OR for suspected ruptured ectopic pregnancy. The beta is below the discriminatory zone, but an examination that reveals hypotension and clinical peritoneal signs in a patient with a positive pregnancy test is an ectopic pregnancy until proven otherwise. This is one of the few times that waiting for any other ancillary test is just increasing morbidity. Admission to the floor, waiting on radiology, and repeating a beta level in 48 to 72 hours will only increase morbidity.

4. **D**. Another ectopic pregnancy! This one is trickier though as the patient is totally asymptomatic. Her beta is above most centers' discriminatory zones (and we listed an experienced sonographer's examination), and the uterus is empty which is an ectopic pregnancy until proven otherwise. Repeating an ultrasound or beta-hCG or discussing management plans for an EPF is not warranted.

SUGGESTED READINGS

Barnhart KT, Sammel MD, Rinaudo PF, Zhou L, Hummel AC, Guo W. Symptomatic patients with an early viable intrauterine pregnancy: HCG curves redefined. *Obstet Gynecol*. 2004;104(1):50–55.

Chen BA, Creinin MD. Contemporary management of early pregnancy failure. *Clin Obstet Gynecol*. 2007;50(1):67–88.

Creinin MD, Harwood B, Guido RS, et al. Endometrial thickness after misoprostol use for early pregnancy failure. *Int J Gynaecol Obstet*. 2004;86:22.

Dighe M, Cuevas C, Moshiri M, et al. Sonography in first trimester bleeding. *J Clin Ultrasound*. 2008;36:352.

Doubilet PM, Benson CB, Bourne T, et al. Diagnostic criteria for nonviable pregnancy early in the first trimester. *N Engl J Med*. 2013;369(15):1443–1451.

Morse CB, Sammel MD, Shaunik A, et al. Performance of human chorionic gonadotropin curves in women at risk for ectopic pregnancy: exceptions to the rules. *Fertil Steril*. 2012;97(1):101–106.

Zhang J, Gilles JM, Barnhart K, et al. A comparison of medical management with misoprostol and surgical management for early pregnancy failure. *N Engl J Med*. 2005;353(8):761–769.

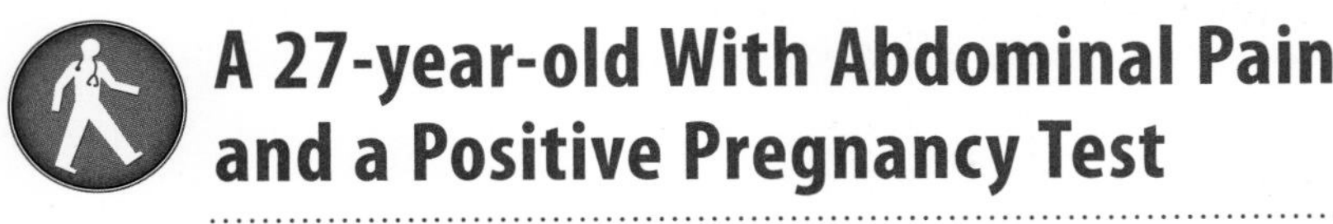

A 27-year-old With Abdominal Pain and a Positive Pregnancy Test

Zainab Al-Ibraheemi, MD
and Charlie C. Kilpatrick, MD

It is just after AM rounds and you are called to see a patient in the emergency room. A 27-year-old G2P0 presents complaining of right lower quadrant pain that began yesterday afternoon. At first the pain was dull, but it has become sharp, a 10/10, and it has spread to her back. She took Motrin, but it didn't help. She is nauseated but has not vomited, has not eaten since yesterday evening, and has no appetite. She also reports some vaginal bleeding, and her LMP was 5 weeks ago. Her past medical history is unremarkable, she has never had surgery, and her prior obstetric history is significant for a miscarriage. Her BP is 108/75, pulse 104, RR 20, and weight 150 lb. She is in mild distress, and prefers to lie in the fetal position when talking to you. Her heart and lung examinations are normal. On abdominal examination there are no scars, decreased bowel sounds on auscultation, tenderness to palpation over the entire abdomen, but more in the right lower quadrant, and when releasing pressure she winces in pain. Pelvic examination reveals normal external genitalia; speculum examination shows blood in the vault, no clots, or discharge, and the cervix appears closed. Bimanual examination reveals positive cervical motion tenderness, right adnexal fullness, and a uterus that is anteverted and small. Her urine pregnancy test is positive, and the quantitative beta hCG level is 3248 IU/L. Abdominal ultrasound performed in the emergency department shows free peritoneal fluid. You perform a transvaginal ultrasound that reveals an empty uterus, free peritoneal fluid, and no adnexal masses.

1. What is in your differential diagnosis?

2. What is your management?

Answers

1. The patient has an ectopic pregnancy that is likely ruptured. A clinical examination that reveals peritoneal signs in the presence of a positive pregnancy test is an ectopic pregnancy until proven otherwise. The differential diagnosis includes appendicitis, urolithiasis, miscarriage, ruptured hemorrhagic cyst, ovarian torsion, pelvic inflammatory disease, and heterotopic pregnancy.

2. The treatment for a ruptured ectopic pregnancy is surgery. The patient went to the OR, and had a laparoscopic right salpingectomy with evacuation of 400 cc of hemoperitoneum. The tube was sent to pathology, and the patient was discharged home after surgery.

CASE REVIEW

Clinical peritoneal signs with the addition of free fluid in the peritoneal cavity on ultrasound suggest tubal rupture and requires surgical treatment over medical treatment for ectopic pregnancy due to the concern for further blood loss and end-organ ischemia. The choice of surgical route (open vs laparoscopic) depends on the skills of the gynecologic surgeon and the patient's hemodynamic stability.

ECTOPIC PREGNANCY

Diagnosis

Ectopic pregnancy is a pregnancy that develops outside the uterine cavity and accounts for 1% to 2% of reported pregnancies in the United States. Even with the ability for earlier detection due to ultrasound, ectopic pregnancy remains a leading cause of maternal mortality in pregnancy. The most common extrauterine sites in order of prevalence are the fallopian tube, ovary, interstitial area, abdomen, and cervix (Figure 4-1). Risk factors for ectopic pregnancy include prior ectopic pregnancy, history of STI, increased number of sexual partners, assisted

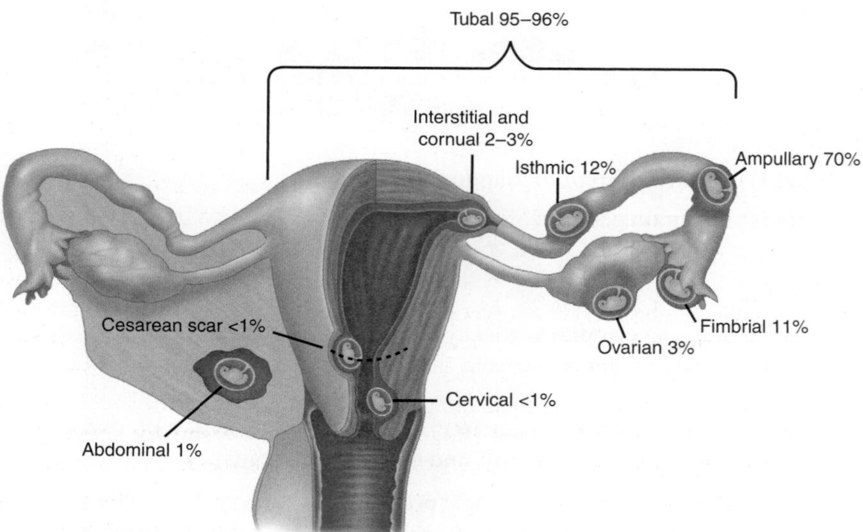

Figure 4-1. Sites of implantation of 1800 ectopic pregnancies from a 10-year population-based study. (Reproduced, with permission, from Cunningham FG, Leveno KJ, Bloom SL, et al. *Williams Obstetrics*. 23rd ed. New York: McGraw-Hill Education; 2010. Fig. 10-1.)

reproductive technology, IUD use, history of tubal surgery including sterilization, pelvic inflammatory disease, smoking, and age >40 years.

The diagnosis of ectopic pregnancy can be made early in gestation with a combination of laboratory and ultrasound findings or later in gestation after tubal rupture by clinical examination and ultrasound findings. History items in women of reproductive age suggestive of ectopic pregnancy are abdominal pain, amenorrhea, and/or vaginal bleeding. In a normal pregnancy, the beta hCG level increase in a viable pregnancy is reviewed in Chapter 3. Briefly, in the first 6 weeks the beta hCG level should double within a 72-hour period (at least demonstrate a 35% increase over a 48-hour period). If this rise in the beta hCG is not demonstrated, then the pregnancy is abnormal. Investigation should then ensue to determine if the pregnancy is intrauterine (see Chapter 3 for more explanation on beta hCG levels in early pregnancy).

Transvaginal ultrasound will allow visualization of the following structures in order of gestation: gestational sac (4.5-5 weeks), yolk sac (5 weeks), and a fetal pole with cardiac activity (5.5 weeks). Tubal rupture is a clinical diagnosis heralded often by signs of hypovolemia (patient complaints of being dizzy, light-headed with signs of hypotension, and tachycardia) and abdominal pain. Often there is not even time to wait for a quantitative beta hCG level, let alone ultrasound finding. Also, remember to evaluate the patient's Rh status and administer RhoGAM when appropriate.

Treatment

Treatment for ectopic pregnancy depends primarily on patient characteristics. Surgery is warranted if the patient is unstable, unable or unwilling to comply with follow-up, or has failed medical management. The choice of surgical route is a clinical one based on the stability of the patient, and the surgical skills of the gynecologic surgeon. Laparoscopy is preferred over laparotomy due to a shorter postoperative recovery time, decreased length of hospital stay, and less postoperative pain. Stability of the patient and obesity play a role in not only the gynecologic surgeon's but also the anesthetist's decision plan. Adding a pneumoperitoneum to an unstable or obese patient increases the degree of difficulty for the anesthesiologist. The pneumoperitoneum adds to the difficulty associated with ventilating an obese patient and limits visualization of the operative field through the laparoscope. In general, in an unstable patient the more expedient route should be undertaken in order to avoid ischemia due to end-organ hypoperfusion. The choice of surgical procedure (salpingostomy where the tube is incised on the antimesenteric border and the ectopic pregnancy removed, vs salpingectomy where the entire tube is removed) depends on patient future fertility desires, the integrity of the tube, and patient compliance with postoperative follow-up. If the patient does not desire future fertility, the tube is ruptured or severely damaged, or the patient cannot follow up postoperatively, salpingectomy is the best option.

The theoretical goal of salpingostomy is to preserve the tube in order to increase chances of future fertility. The difficulty with this approach is that damage to the tube was likely present prior to the ectopic pregnancy (causing the ectopic pregnancy), so in conserving the tube you may be saving a tube that is damaged leading to an increased risk of future ectopic pregnancy. Follow-up after surgery varies by surgical procedure. After salpingectomy, because the entire tube and ectopic pregnancy were removed (which can be verified by reviewing the pathology report), there is little need to follow quantitative beta hCG levels in order to ensure that the ectopic pregnancy has resolved. After salpingostomy, because the entire ectopic pregnancy cannot be guaranteed to have been removed at the time of surgery, you *must* follow beta hCG levels to ensure they decline, and the ectopic pregnancy is resolved.

Medical management, using methotrexate (MTX), is also an option. Patients who are candidates for medical management are those who are compliant, without a ruptured tube, stable, desiring of future fertility, at risk for general anesthesia, and have no contraindications to MTX. Contraindications for MTX use are the following: currently breast-feeding, renal or hepatic dysfunction, blood dyscrasias, and immunodeficiency. MTX is a folic acid antagonist, renally cleared, and is usually given as a single subcutaneous injection based on body weight (50 mg/m^2) after assuring adequate renal (BUN/creatinine), hepatic (liver enzymes, liver function), and bone marrow (CBC with differential) function. Prior to MTX administration counseling to ensure the patient is aware of the follow-up required, side effects of the medication, and likelihood that a second dose is needed (in up to 15% of cases the treatment is not successful) should be undertaken. The last point about failure rate is often overlooked, and is an important point to discuss with your patient. The most predictive clinical factor associated with treatment failure is the beta hCG level. A beta level above 5000 mIU/mL is associated with increased treatment failure. The single-dose regimen begins the day of MTX administration (day 1), with beta levels measured on day 4 and day 7. A 25% decrease from day 1 to day 7 or a 15% decrease from day 4 to day 7 is required to demonstrate clinical effectiveness, after which weekly beta testing can be undertaken. Repeat dosing of MTX is necessary if these decreases are not demonstrated. The patient is followed until the beta hCG level is undetectable (varies by laboratory). Surgery should be considered if 2 doses are given and the desired decrease in beta hCG is not seen.

TIPS TO REMEMBER

- The classic symptoms of ectopic pregnancy are abdominal pain, amenorrhea, and vaginal bleeding.
- In 85% of viable pregnancies the beta hCG level will increase by at least 66% over a 48-hour period, and 99% will double over a 72-hour period.

- Absence of an intrauterine gestational sac and a beta hCG level above your institution's discriminatory zone suggests ectopic pregnancy.
- Women who are diagnosed with ectopic pregnancy and are hemodynamically unstable require surgical treatment.
- MTX is contraindicated in patients who are breast-feeding, unstable, non-compliant, or have active renal, hepatic, or bone marrow disease.
- MTX is less successful when the beta hCG level is >5000 mIU/mL.

COMPREHENSION QUESTIONS

1. A 23-year-old P1 presents with a 24-hour history of heavy vaginal bleeding and lower abdominal pain. Her LMP was 8 weeks ago. Her BP 100/70, P 99, RR 18, and T 37°C. Focused examination reveals peritoneal signs, cervical motion tenderness, and a slightly enlarged uterus. The beta hCG level is 15,092 mIU/mL, hematocrit is 31%, and the patient's pelvic US is as pictured in Figure 4-2.

   What is the most appropriate next step in the management of this patient?

   A. Repeat the beta hCG level in 48 hours.
   B. Administer MTX.
   C. Perform a dilation and curettage.
   D. Perform laparoscopy.

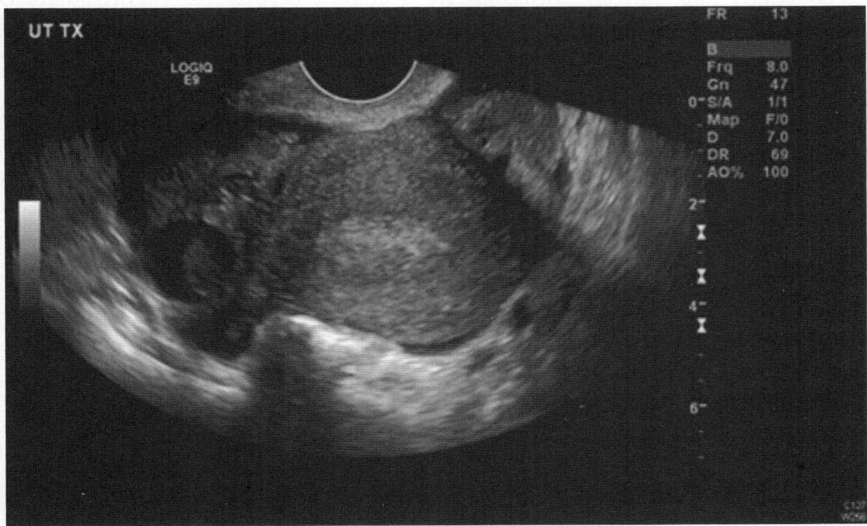

Figure 4-2. Transvaginal ultrasound image

2. A 32-year-old female with a long hx of lupus nephritis and hypertension presents to the emergency department complaining of vaginal bleeding. She has a benign abdominal examination, a beta hCG level of 2234 mIU/mL, and an ultrasound that reveals an empty uterus and a right adnexal mass. You counsel her that she has an ectopic pregnancy and she prefers not to have surgery. The *best* treatment option for her is which of the following?

A. Single-dose MTX at 50 mg/m^2
B. Single-dose MTX at 25 mg/m^2
C. Repeat beta hCG level in 48 to 72 hours
D. Laparoscopic right salpingectomy

3. A 42-year-old woman presents with abdominal pain, vaginal bleeding, and LMP 5 weeks ago. She desired to have her tubes tied after her last pregnancy 7 years ago but did not have it done. On examination she has pain in the left lower quadrant, a beta hCG that is 7265 mIU/mL, and an ultrasound that shows a left adnexal mass and an empty uterus. Her best treatment option is which of the following?

A. Laparoscopic left salpingectomy
B. Single-dose MTX at 50 mg/m^2
C. Laparoscopic left salpingostomy
D. Repeat examination in 48 hours

Answers

1. **D**. The classic clinical manifestations of ectopic pregnancy are amenorrhea, abdominal pain, and vaginal spotting. This patient has a ruptured right tubal pregnancy as evidenced by peritoneal signs on examination, and an ultrasound that reveals an adnexal mass and the presence of free fluid in the pelvis. A dilation and curettage will empty the uterus but not address a pregnancy outside the uterus, a repeat beta hCG would not provide any additional helpful information and delaying would lead to more patient harm, and MTX is contraindicated in cases of tubal rupture.

2. **D**. Even though the patient voiced that she does not desire surgery, keep in mind that MTX is renally cleared. We don't have the results of her renal function, but given her significant renal disease MTX is more dangerous than surgery, and this should be communicated to her. Halving the dose to 25 mg/m^2 is not likely safe and there are no data to support a lower dose for ectopic treatment. A repeat beta hCG level would not address the diagnosis.

3. **A**. This patient has an ectopic pregnancy, and also desires permanent sterilization. There is no need to repeat the beta hCG level, and because the level is >5000 mIU/mL, MTX will be less effective. Surgical management should be

the choice selected and completely removing the tube, a salpingectomy, would accomplish both goals over a salpingostomy, and require less postoperative surveillance. In this case you may even talk to the patient about having the contralateral tube removed at the time of surgery given her desire for no more children.

SUGGESTED READINGS

Barnhart KT, Sammel MD, Rinaudo PF, Zhou L, Hummel AC, Guo W. Symptomatic patients with an early viable intrauterine pregnancy: HCG curves redefined. *Obstet Gynecol.* 2004;104(1):50–55.

Centers for Disease Control and Prevention (CDC). Ectopic pregnancy—United States, 1990–1992. *MMWR Morb Mortal Wkly Rep.* 1995;44:46–48.

Hajenius PJ, Mol F, Mol BW, et al. Interventions for tubal ectopic pregnancy. *Cochrane Database Syst Rev.* 2007;(1):CD000324.

Lipscomb GH, McCord ML, Stovall TG, et al. Predictors of success of methotrexate treatment in women with tubal ectopic pregnancies. *N Engl J Med.* 1999;341:1974.

Morse CB, Sammel MD, Shaunik A, et al. Performance of human chorionic gonadotropin curves in women at risk for ectopic pregnancy: exceptions to the rules. *Fertil Steril.* 2012;97(1):101–106.

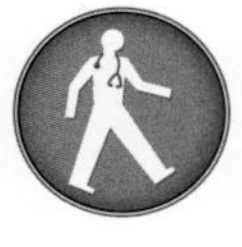

A 21-year-old Female Presents to the Emergency Department With Abdominal/Pelvic Pain

Charlie C. Kilpatrick, MD

A 21-year-old G0 presents to the emergency department complaining of acute-onset abdominal pain, and you are called for a consult to evaluate the patient. The patient reports that the pain began last night before she went to bed, and she thought it was something she ate. She took some antacids and went to sleep but awoke at 0300 with worsening pain and vomited. It is a constant pain that is sometimes sharp, and she is in the fetal position as she tells you this. The pain is "all over" her abdomen but mainly below her belly button with radiation to her right greater than her left. She has never had this pain before. In review of her history she has no medical, obstetrical, or surgical history, and denies any drug allergies. She takes combination oral contraceptive (COC) pills, and occasionally ibuprofen for menstrual cramps. She has irregular menses that last 4 to 5 days, and are crampy in nature. She thinks her last menses was 6 to 7 weeks ago. She denies any history of abnormal cervical cytology, and was diagnosed last year with chlamydia. She was treated for this, and she is no longer with that partner. She has a new male partner of 3 months and they are sexually active, and sometimes use condoms. She is in school, attending the local university in her senior year. She smokes occasionally, drinks socially once or twice a week, and denies illicit drug use.

1. **What is in your differential diagnosis for the abdominal pain, and what are the next steps you need to take in the management of this patient?**

Answer

1. Your differential diagnosis should include miscarriage, ectopic pregnancy, appendicitis, pelvic inflammatory disease (PID), symptomatic ovarian cyst, ovarian torsion, gastroenteritis, and urolithiasis. The list could be much longer, but in a woman of childbearing age, pregnancy and its complications should be investigated first followed by conditions that may require surgical intervention. Your next steps are to review her vital signs and perform a thorough physical examination including a pelvic examination, which includes speculum and bimanual examination to assess for anatomic pathology, urine pregnancy test, screen for sexually transmitted infections (STIs), and consider imaging of the appendix and pelvis.

CASE REVIEW

You complete a sexual history that reveals that she participates in oral and vaginal sex with men (no sex with women, and no anal sex), has had 6 partners in her lifetime, and is not sure about her partners' STD histories or how many partners they have had. She has no urinary frequency or urgency. She is nauseated and vomits again while you are talking to her. Her vital signs are as follows: temperature 101.7°F, pulse 105, BP 122/64, and RR 22. On examination she appears to be in pain. Her lungs are clear to auscultation, cardiac examination reveals an increased rate but no murmurs, gallops, or rubs, and she is reluctant to lie supine for an abdominal examination. She has bowel sounds, and you elicit peritoneal signs with the stethoscope and with palpation. She is tender over the epigastrium and in the right lower quadrant. Extremity examination is normal. You perform a pelvic examination and document the following: normal external female genitalia, shaved mons and labia majora, nulliparous introitus, vaginal sidewalls without lesion, and copious yellow-green discharge. You perform a swab of the endocervical canal to test for gonorrhea and chlamydia, and a saline wet mount of the discharge to look for evidence of trichomoniasis. On bimanual examination she is tender when you move the cervix and begins to cry. You try to evaluate the adnexae, but she has so much voluntary guarding you cannot. You examine the wet mount under the microscope and see trichomonads and numerous white blood cells.

From the history and physical examination you believe she has PID and trichomoniasis, and after discussing with your team and reexamination decide to admit her for IV antibiotics, and to perform tests for other STIs including HIV, syphilis, and hepatitis B. Over the next few days she improves and is sent home with oral antibiotics to complete 14 days of treatment with follow-up in the clinic. Her chlamydia test returns positive, but the rest of the STI testing was negative.

PELVIC INFLAMMATORY DISEASE

Diagnosis

PID is an infection of the upper genital tract: uterus, fallopian tubes, and ovaries. This can lead to endometritis, salpingitis, tubo-ovarian abscess (TOA), peritonitis, and perihepatitis (Fitz-Hugh-Curtis syndrome—see Figure 5-1). The diagnosis of PID is clinical, and is difficult because there is no single diagnostic test. Lower abdominal pain is the most common complaint, and it usually begins around the time of menses. The suspicion of the disease is heightened with increased STI risk factors, prior PID history, or physical examination findings that include the following: peritoneal signs on abdominal examination, pelvic examination that reveals vaginal discharge, and bimanual examination demonstrating tenderness with uterine manipulation or adnexal tenderness or fullness.

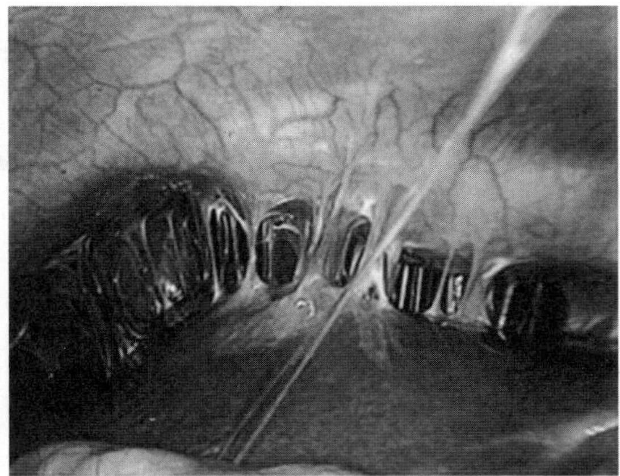

Figure 5-1. Perihepatitis or Fitz-Hugh-Curtis syndrome. Appreciate the adhesions (described as violin string) between the liver and anterior abdominal wall (http://emedicine.medscape.com/article/256448-overview)

The CDC states that the specificity of the diagnosis can be heightened with any 1 of the following: oral temperature >101°F, abnormal vaginal/cervical mucopurulent discharge, abundant WBCs on saline wet mount, elevated erythrocyte sedimentation rate (ESR) or C-reactive protein, and cervical infection with chlamydia or gonorrhea. The most specific criteria to make the diagnosis of PID outlined by the CDC include endometrial biopsy indicating endometritis, laparoscopic evidence of PID, and transvaginal sonogram (or MRI) indicating TOA or thickened fallopian tubes with or without free peritoneal fluid. In general, one should have a high suspicion of disease, especially in areas that have a high prevalence of STIs. A low threshold for diagnosis and treatment of PID is recommended, especially given the little harm associated with PID treatment and the sequelae that can occur with infection.

Treatment

Once you diagnose PID, you must determine whether inpatient or outpatient management is appropriate. Table 5-1 lists indications for inpatient management of PID outlined by the CDC (with the exception of HIV that was added based on clinical experience). Counseling the patient in regard to the potential complications associated with nontreatment of PID, and determining compliance with outpatient treatment is necessary before considering discharge. The treatment regimen should be started as soon as possible to limit the sequelae associated with PID (infertility, ectopic pregnancy, chronic pelvic pain) and should cover the organisms often responsible for the infection (gonorrhea and

Table 5-1. Indications for Inpatient PID Treatment

Tubo-ovarian abscess
Unable to tolerate PO medication
Noncompliant
Pregnancy
Unsure diagnosis (cannot rule out surgical condition)
Not responding to oral treatment
HIV infection

chlamydia). Table 5-2 lists inpatient and outpatient regimens recommended by the CDC. IV treatment can be discontinued 24 hours after clinical improvement, and the patient should then complete an oral antibiotic regimen for a total duration of 14 days. If the clinical picture does not begin to improve within the first 24 hours, imaging of the pelvis is recommended, unless it has already been performed.

Table 5-2. PID Antibiotic Regimens

Inpatient

- Cefotetan 2 g IV Q 12 h *or* cefoxitin 2 g IV Q 6 h *plus* doxycycline 100 mg orally (or IV) Q 12 h
- Clindamycin 900 mg IV Q 8 h *plus* gentamicin loading dose (2 mg/kg), and then maintenance (1.5 mg/kg) Q 8 h

Outpatient

- Ceftriaxone 250 mg IM in a single dose *plus* doxycycline 100 mg orally twice a day for 14 days *with or without* metronidazole 500 mg orally twice a day for 14 days

OR

- Cefoxitin 2 g IM in a single dose and probenecid, 1 g orally administered concurrently in a single dose *plus* doxycycline 100 mg orally twice a day for 14 days *with or without* metronidazole 500 mg orally twice a day for 14 days

OR

- Other parenteral third-generation cephalosporin (eg, ceftizoxime or cefotaxime) *plus* doxycycline 100 mg orally twice a day for 14 days *with or without* metronidazole 500 mg orally twice a day for 14 days

Surgical management (laparotomy or laparoscopy) or interventional radiologic drainage is warranted in those patients not clinically responding to IV antibiotics after 48 hours, or in cases where a large TOA is involved (>8 cm). Prior to the development of more effective parenteral therapy, surgical management for PID was aggressive, and frequently included abdominal hysterectomy with bilateral salpingo-oophorectomy. Recent case series have reported less aggressive surgical procedures (drainage, unilateral salpingo-oophorectomy) or even interventional radiologic drainage with similar short-term outcomes. Deteriorating clinical conditions, such as sepsis or the suspicion of a ruptured TOA, warrant expeditious surgical intervention.

TIPS TO REMEMBER

- PID is a clinical diagnosis, and treatment should begin quickly to limit sequelae.
- A low threshold for the diagnosis and treatment of PID involves relatively little harm with appreciable benefit to the patient.
- The decision to perform inpatient or outpatient treatment is based on clinical factors; ensuring treatment compliance is paramount for outpatient management.
- Inpatient antibiotic treatment should be continued for 24 hours after clinical improvement is demonstrated.
- Surgical management is warranted in light of a worsening clinical picture, sepsis, and/or suspicion of TOA rupture.

COMPREHENSION QUESTIONS

1. Ms D is seen in the clinic complaining of lower abdominal pain that began a few days ago after her menses. She is ultimately diagnosed with PID, and after a discussion in regard to management she opts for outpatient treatment. Two days later she presents to the emergency department with the same chief complaint. The next *best step* is which of the following?

    A. Ultrasound of the pelvis.
    B. Admission to the hospital.
    C. Pain medicine and continued outpatient treatment.
    D. Begin alternative outpatient treatment regimen and ensure partner treatment.

2. Ms B is admitted to the hospital with the diagnosis of PID after a thorough history and physical examination and laboratory evaluation and begun on parenteral treatment Monday afternoon with cefoxitin and doxycycline. Wednesday AM during rounds (over 24 hours later) she is still spiking temperatures to as high

as 102.2°F, and clinically she does not appear to be improving. The next best step in her management is which of the following?

A. To the operating room for surgical management.
B. Add IV metronidazole to improve anaerobic coverage.
C. Continue current parenteral antibiotics and begin more frequent examinations.
D. Imaging of the pelvis.

3. Ms B (from the above scenario) is diagnosed with a 4-cm TOA by transvaginal ultrasound. Thursday AM on morning rounds she has begun to defervesce and her Tmax over the past 24 hours is 100.9. On clinical examination her abdominal tenderness is improving. The next *best step* in her management is which of the following?

A. Continued parenteral antibiotics.
B. Begin oral antibiotics and discharge planning to complete 14 days of total treatment.
C. To the OR for laparoscopic ovarian cyst drainage.
D. To the radiology suite for IR-guided cyst drainage.

Answers

1. **B**. Ms D has demonstrated that she either has not responded to outpatient treatment or has been noncompliant with treatment. Either way, she needs to be admitted and started on parenteral antibiotics. An ultrasound of the pelvis may ultimately be performed but is not the best answer, and pain medicine alone, or an alternative treatment, is not a good clinical choice.

2. **D**. Ms B is not demonstrating improvement after 24 hours of parenteral antibiotics so imaging of the pelvis should be performed to look for evidence of a TOA. Heading to the OR would be a little aggressive at this point, and adding metronidazole or more frequent examinations are not warranted.

3. **A**. After more time and parenteral antibiotics Ms B seems to be improving so surgery or IR management is not necessary, but her symptoms are still present and she is not ready to be discharged home. Continuing the current parenteral antibiotics is warranted.

SUGGESTED READINGS

Chappell CA, Wiesenfeld HC. Pathogenesis, diagnosis, and management of severe pelvic inflammatory disease and tuboovarian abscess. *Clin Obstet Gynecol*. 2012;55(4):893–903. <http://emedicine.medscape.com/article/256448-overview>; Accessed 07.30.13.

Workowski KA, Berman S. Sexually transmitted diseases treatment guidelines, 2010. *MMWR Recomm Rep*. 2010;59:1–110.

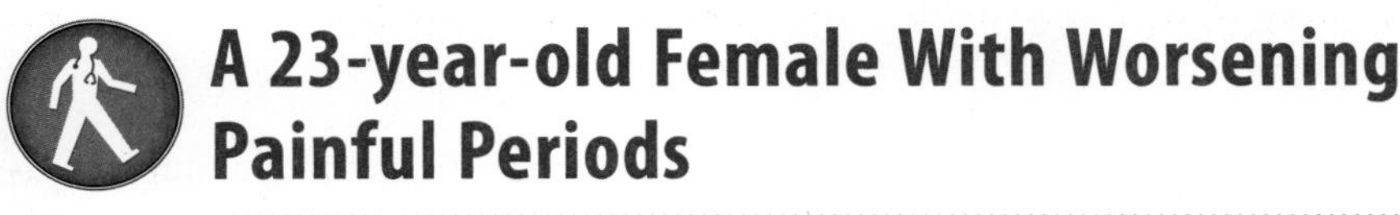

A 23-year-old Female With Worsening Painful Periods

Jaou-Chen Huang, MD

A 23-year-old female presents to the clinic with worsening painful periods. She had menarche at age 12 at which time the periods were not painful, but they have become so over the past 5 years. The pain with menses has intensified over the past 6 months and is no longer relieved by NSAIDs. The pain is cyclic, occurring a few days before the onset of the periods and resolving a few days after menstruation begins. She occasionally experiences diarrhea during menstruation. Her mother had a hysterectomy in her early forties because of pain related to endometriosis. The physical examination is unremarkable. A pelvic ultrasound shows normal ovaries and uterus. The patient is sexually active and uses condoms for birth control.

1. What is the likely diagnosis?

2. What constitutes the initial treatment for this patient?

Answers

1. Based on worsening dysmenorrhea and a positive family history, the likely diagnosis is pelvic endometriosis.
2. Initial treatment consists of continuous birth control pills. If the pain relief is not satisfactory after 2 to 3 months, a diagnostic laparoscopy with possible ablation of endometriotic implants can be planned.

CASE REVIEW

Many gynecological conditions cause painful periods (dysmenorrhea). The progressive nature of this patient's pain and a positive family history support the diagnosis of endometriosis. An empirical treatment with continuous birth control pills can be offered. If there is satisfactory symptom relief, then the treatment continues. If the pain does not improve or worsens despite treatment, then a diagnostic laparoscopy is performed to determine the cause of pain.

ENDOMETRIOSIS

Diagnosis

Endometriosis is the presence of endometrial glands and stroma in locations outside the uterine cavity. The prevalence of endometriosis is ~10% in the general population, but is as high as ~40% in patients complaining of pelvic pain and/

or infertility. The presenting symptoms of endometriosis include painful periods (dysmenorrhea), painful intercourse (dyspareunia), painful bowel movements (dyschezia), irregular uterine bleeding, and/or infertility. The course of endometriosis is progressive. Thus, the intensity of the symptom(s) typically increases over time.

The most common location of endometriotic implants is the pelvis (the pelvic peritoneum). Other locations include the myometrium of the uterus, bladder, and skin (at the episiotomy site or the scar of previous Cesarean section). Rarely, endometriosis is found in distant organs such as the lung. The diagnosis of pelvic endometriosis requires the visualization of classical endometriotic lesions. Histological diagnosis is not usually required.

Two special forms of endometriosis deserve special attention: adenomyosis and endometriomas. Adenomyosis is the presence of endometrial glands and stroma in the myometrium. A diffusely enlarged uterus causing heavy and painful periods in a parous woman in her fourth decade of life is the typical picture. Thus, a patient with adenomyosis may present with symptoms similar to that of a fibroid uterus. An endometrioma is the presence of endometriotic lesions inside the ovary. As a result, cysts form inside the ovary due to trapped "menstrual blood." An endometrioma is also called a "chocolate cyst" because its content has the appearance of melted chocolate. It usually does not cause symptoms until it reaches a critical size, or ruptures. Conditions mimicking an endometrioma include benign and malignant tumors of the ovary. A malignant ovarian tumor may arise from within an endometrioma.

Pathophysiology

The pathogenesis of endometriosis remains elusive, but it can be viewed from two independent but related processes: the *establishment* and the *progression* of the ectopic endometrium. First, the endometrium establishes its presence outside the uterine cavity. Second, it continues to grow reaching a critical mass that causes symptoms.

Dr Sampson's "retrograde menstruation" theory partly explains the first process, that is, the establishment of ectopic endometrium. He ligated the cervices of monkeys and "created" endometriotic lesions in their pelvises. Similar mechanisms likely operate in humans, because endometriosis is a common finding in patients who have Müllerian anomalies and an outflow tract obstruction. However, retrograde menstruation alone is not sufficient to explain the pathogenesis of endometriosis, because menstrual blood is present in the peritoneal cavity in three out of four women during menstruation. Deficient immune surveillance is another factor in the establishment of ectopic endometrium. Less common endometriosis sites (such as those in the bladder, skin, or lung) require different explanations. Once the endometriosis is established, the progression of endometriosis has the following characteristics: (1) dependency on estrogen and resistance to progesterone, and (2) a local microenvironment favoring estrogen production that maintains the feedforward loop.

The ectopic endometrium causes a foreign body reaction, which increases inflammatory mediators (cytokines), prostaglandins, and growth factors in the peritoneal fluid. These soluble factors cause the clinical symptoms. The symptoms of endometriosis include (in decreasing frequency): dysmenorrhea, pelvic pain, dyspareunia, bowel symptoms, bowel pain, infertility, ovarian mass/tumor, dysuria and other urinary symptoms. Mechanical factors such as adhesion may cause some of the above symptoms as well.

Treatment

Treatment options (surgical vs medical) are based on a patient's wishes for future fertility. Medical therapy offers pain relief in 90% of cases, but is not compatible with pregnancy. It has one or more of the following characteristics: low estrogen, high progesterone (typically with progestational agents), and anti-inflammatories. This is because estrogen promotes but progesterone hampers the growth of ectopic endometrium, and symptoms of endometriosis are partly due to elevated inflammatory mediators in the pelvis.

Oral contraceptives contain ethinyl estradiol (a potent synthetic estrogen) and progestin (an agent derived from testosterone, having similar biological activities as the natural progesterone). Oral contraceptive therapy is nicknamed "pseudopregnancy," because birth control pills produce a high estrogen and high progesterone (progestin) environment—similar to that of pregnant women. This "pseudopregnancy" state involves decidualization of both eutopic and ectopic endometrium (endometriotic implants). Gonadotropin-releasing hormone (GnRH) agonists lower the circulating estradiol level to that of postmenopausal women; it produces a reversible menopause (and is thus nicknamed "medical oophorectomy" or "medical menopause"). Under low estrogen conditions both eutopic and ectopic endometrium become atrophic. Similar to birth control pills, progestin-only therapy also decidualizes ectopic endometrium. Danazol is a unique agent which is a derivative of testosterone and contains minute testosterone activity. It produces a state of chronic anovulation. Patients receiving danazol have estradiol levels seen in the early proliferative phase (~60 pg/mL). The low estradiol level and the residual testosterone activity present in danazol keep ectopic endometrium under control. Due to androgenic effects (voice deepening, acne, hirsutism), danazol is not used as often as it used to be, because newer agents with fewer undesirable side effects are available now. None of the medical therapies is compatible with pregnancy, because they cause anovulation. GnRH therapy causes osteoporosis as well (1% bone loss per month). Thus, its use is limited to 6 months—unless it is combined with estrogen add-back to prevent bone loss. Danazol therapy requires regular monitoring of liver function.

Newer agents are being tested for medical treatment of endometriosis. An aromatase inhibitor is one such agent. Combined with birth control pills or progestin, an aromatase inhibitor relieves pain in women who do not respond to conventional medical therapy. Aromatase inhibitors block additional sources of estrogen production such as adipose tissue (the main nonovarian source of estrogen) and endometriotic implants. In reproductive age women, an aromatase inhibitor is used in conjunction with birth control pills to prevent ovarian cysts. Similar to GnRH agonist therapy, osteoporosis is also a concern with aromatase inhibitor therapy.

Surgical treatment of endometriosis is reserved for those who desire pregnancy or those who do not respond to medical therapy. Conservative surgery, removing endometriotic implants and restoring normal anatomy, enhances the cycle fecundity for a finite period of time (usually 6-12 months). Recurrence of symptoms is the rule, unless the surgery is followed by a pregnancy or medical suppressive therapy. Definitive surgical treatment usually is offered to those who have completed their families and/or do not wish to take medical treatment. Preserving the ovary is associated with higher rates of symptom recurrence and repeat surgery.

Surgery for endometriomas and adenomyosis deserves special mention. Surgeries to remove endometrioma may decrease ovarian reserve when the bulk of the ovarian cortex is removed with the cyst wall of the endometrioma. It is still being hotly debated as to the indication of surgery and the type of approach. A surgeon's skill obviously plays an important role in the outcome. Hysterectomy is the usual treatment for symptomatic adenomyosis. Special consideration is made for those who desire fertility by removing the tumor of adenomyosis (adenomyoma).

TIPS TO REMEMBER

- Endometriosis is the presence of endometrial glands and stroma in locations outside the uterine cavity.
- Diagnosis of endometriosis requires visual confirmation of typical lesions; histological proof is not needed.
- Medical therapy can be initiated in patients with symptoms consistent with endometriosis without the need for definitive histological diagnosis.
- Estrogen promotes the growth of endometriotic implants; progesterone and testosterone hamper their growth.
- Medical treatment of endometriosis is effective in most cases. It consists of low estrogen and/or high progesterone (typically using progestational agents). Medical treatment is not suitable for patients desiring pregnancy because it causes anovulation.
- Conservative surgery enhances fecundity, but symptom recurrence is the rule—unless the surgery is followed by pregnancy or medical therapy.

- Definitive therapy is reserved for those who have completed childbearing and/or do not desire future fertility. Preservation of the ovary is associated with higher rates of symptom recurrence and repeat surgery.

COMPREHENSION QUESTIONS

1. Which of the following statements is correct?
   A. Diagnosis of endometriosis requires histological proof.
   B. Medical treatment of endometriosis requires a definitive diagnosis by laparoscopy.
   C. Adenomyosis can easily be differentiated from a fibroid uterus by physical exam.
   D. A malignant ovarian tumor may arise from an endometrioma.

2. Which of the following statements is correct?
   A. The "retrograde menstruation" theory of endometriosis explains the *progression* of endometriotic implants.
   B. GnRH agonist therapy prevents estrogen production inside the endometriotic implants.
   C. Symptoms of endometriosis are partly caused by inflammatory cytokines, prostaglandins, and growth factors.
   D. Preservation of ovaries in definitive surgery for symptomatic endometriosis is *not* associated with higher symptom recurrence.

3. Which medical therapy for endometriosis is associated with the risk of osteoporosis?
   A. Danazol
   B. GnRH agonist therapy
   C. Combination oral contraceptive pills
   D. Nonsteroidal anti-inflammatories

Answers

1. **D.** Diagnosis of endometriosis does not require histological proof. Medical treatment may be initiated in a patient with symptoms consistent with endometriosis without prior diagnosis. Patients with adenomyosis and fibroid uterus may have similar symptoms.

2. **C.** Retrograde menstruation explains the *establishment* of endometriotic lesions in the pelvis, not the *progression* of endometriotic disease. GnRH agonist therapy blocks ovarian estrogen production, not estrogen production by adipose tissue and endometriotic implants (the latter two areas are where aromatase inhibitors function). Preservation of the ovary in definitive surgery for endometriosis is associated with higher risk of symptom recurrence.

3. **B**. GnRH therapy lowers the circulating estradiol level. It may cause osteoporosis. Aromatase inhibitor therapy is also associated with the risk of osteoporosis. Danazol and oral contraceptive pills are not associated with osteoporosis.

SUGGESTED READINGS

Burney RO, Giudice LC. Pathogenesis and pathophysiology of endometriosis. *Fertil Steril.* 2012;98: 511–519.

Falcone T, Lebovic DI. Clinical management of endometriosis. *Obstet Gynecol.* 2011;118:691–705.

Kennedy S, Bergqvist A, Chapron C, et al. ESHRE guideline for the diagnosis and treatment of endometriosis. *Hum Reprod.* 2005;20:2698–2704.

Pavone ME, Bulun SE. Aromatase inhibitors for the treatment of endometriosis. *Fertil Steril.* 2012;98: 1370–1379.

Practice Committee of the American Society for Reproductive Medicine. Endometriosis and infertility: a committee opinion. *Fertil Steril.* 2012;98:591–598.

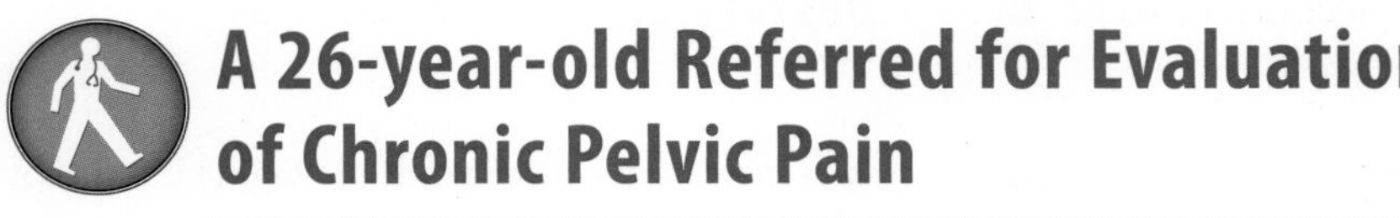

A 26-year-old Referred for Evaluation of Chronic Pelvic Pain

Roger B. Yandell, MD

A 26-year-old G2P0020 with last menstrual period 2 weeks earlier presents to your clinic for evaluation and treatment of pelvic pain of 8 months duration. She was referred from her primary care physician (PCP) after several visits to a gastroenterologist failed to produce any relief of her symptoms. She has a 2-year history of chronic constipation. Her gynecologic history is remarkable for 2 elective first trimester pregnancy terminations. She recently lost her job secondary to frequent absences caused by intractable pelvic pain. Three years earlier she was placed on a selective serotonin reuptake inhibitor by her PCP, but she self-discontinued the medication last year because she felt it was not doing her any good. She describes the pain as 8 to 9/10 in intensity. Laxatives and anticholinergic medicine did not lead to improvement. She appears to be in mild distress from bilateral lower quadrant pain.

1. What do you hope to accomplish at this initial visit?

2. How do you plan to win this woman's trust?

Answers

1. The initial visit for a patient like this seldom leads to a definitive diagnosis. Chronic pelvic pain does not lend itself to a 15- to 20-minute office visit and your front desk staff should not schedule this patient at the beginning of a busy clinic. A detailed history and thorough physical examination should be the goal of the first visit and a follow-up appointment should be given in the next 2 to 3 weeks to review results of any tests that you might order.
2. It is a challenge to win the trust of a patient like this. Typically women with chronic pelvic pain (by definition pain of more than 6 months duration) have already seen several different physicians and they have grown increasingly frustrated. It is not yet clear that the woman's symptoms are gynecologic in origin, so the best you can do is to strive for empathy, thoroughness, and a clear explanation of your plan of evaluation and possible treatments.

CASE REVIEW

Women with chronic pelvic pain may have more than 1 disease process contributing to their symptoms. In the brief presentation you have already learned that she may have irritable bowel syndrome, anxiety over losing her job, depression, and some as-yet-undiagnosed gynecologic disorder. The remainder of this chapter is organized around history, physical examination, and laboratory testing with a goal of making a diagnosis and recommending treatment. It is highly likely that achieving your goal will require several visits.

CHRONIC PELVIC PAIN

Pain, of one type or another, is one of the more common problems that brings women in to see a gynecologist. Fortunately a large number of patients have acute problems that have been present for a short and finite period of time. Because of rapid worsening of symptoms, these patients tend to seek medical care relatively quickly. Women may also present with recurrent or cyclic pain in the form of dysmenorrhea that may be present for a longer period of time. Chronic dysmenorrhea should generally not be considered in the category of chronic pelvic pain because of its relatively straightforward etiology and cyclic nature.

The accepted definition of chronic pelvic pain is pain below the umbilicus that persists for greater than 6 months. One problem is that many physicians will label patients with this diagnosis when they have other problems such as primary/secondary dysmenorrhea or recurrent urinary tract infections.

Regardless of the definition, it is very common for women with pelvic pain to present to the gynecologist for their first visit having already seen a number of other practitioners, including gynecologists, without resolution of the problem. Conversely, others will have been referred after only 1 brief visit to a physician. There are 2 major reasons for these divergent patterns. The first has to do with the perception that pelvic pain in a woman is related to the reproductive tract. This belief is true of patients and physicians alike, leading to prolonged attempts to treat the patient after having made an incorrect diagnosis. Chronic pelvic pain frequently involves the reproductive, gastrointestinal, urologic, musculoskeletal, neurologic, or integumentary systems, and can be significantly affected by psychiatric and psychological issues. The primary source may not be reproductive, but may be significantly affected by normal hormonal fluctuations. This is particularly true of functional bowel disease. All of these organ systems must be considered in order to completely evaluate and manage chronic pelvic pain. The second major problem encountered in evaluating pelvic pain is the sensory innervation of the multiple somatic and visceral structures in this area. In many cases, the patient may have a great deal of difficulty describing or even pointing to the specific site of her pain, thereby complicating the diagnosis.

Sensory Innervation of the Pelvis

As previously stated, there are multiple possible sites in the lower abdomen and pelvis in which noxious stimuli may cause symptoms perceived as chronic pelvic pain. A working knowledge of the sensory innervation of these structures is essential to understanding the sometimes-confusing symptomatology that may be obtained through the history and physical examination. Impulses from afferent somatic nerves follow generally predictable pathways from their respective end-organ sites (skin, muscle, or bone) to the dorsal horn of specific spinal nerve roots. As a result, the patient can more accurately localize painful stimuli in these locations. The visceral afferent impulses travel through sympathetic nerves via preganglionic and postganglionic fibers, where they synapse in one of several plexuses (inferior mesenteric, superior or inferior hypogastric, sacral) or the sympathetic chain before proceeding to 1 or several spinal roots, and finally the dorsal horn of the spinal cord. Because of this more complicated pathway, a single organ may be innervated via several spinal levels. In addition, the somatic and visceral afferents are very poorly myelinated, and pass through the same area of the dorsal horn at any given spinal cord level. This may allow cross-stimulation resulting in referred pain perception in the corresponding somatic structures and vice versa. In addition, the innervation of the pelvic organs overlaps at the spinal level as shown in Table 7-1. There is significant overlap of afferent fibers to multiple organs from T10-L2.

Another extremely important concept in understanding the perception of pain is the *gate theory*, which was originally proposed by Melzack and Wall in 1965. Afferent fibers to multiple organs are constantly sending signals to the brain, yet some of these never reach the level of consciousness. Some are perceived as nociceptive only and others are viewed as painful. This is easily understood by considering bowel activity, which never ceases, yet is seldom felt and rarely painful. Once these nociceptive signals reach the spinal cord, they may be muted or blocked completely from ascending further by feedback loops and

Table 7-1. Afferent Innervation of Pelvic Structures

Abdominal wall and dermatomes:	
• Xiphoid to pubis	T7-T12
• Umbilicus	T10
• Mons pubis	L1
• Perineum	S2-S5
Viscera:	
• Uterus	T10-L1
• Ovary	T10-T11
• Ureters	T10-L2
• Bladder	T11-L2
• Small bowel	T9-T10
• Large bowel	T11-L2

neurotransmitters at this level, effectively "downregulating" their input to the brain, thereby allowing the spinal cord to act as a "gate" or filter. There is also a second mechanism, which involves signals from the brain to the spinal cord, which can enhance this downregulation, again via a mechanism dependent on neurotransmitters. This concept provides a biochemical basis by which psychological states may alter symptomatology and disease processes, and, at least in part, is an explanation of the concept of differing pain tolerance from one person to the next.

Certain circumstances may alter neurotransmitters in the brain, such as depression or other psychiatric disorders, psychological states such as stress, and medications. This may decrease or block the ability of the brain to effect a decrease in afferent impulses allowed to pass through at the spinal cord level, effectively lowering the patient's tolerance to pain. Simply having the pain for extended periods of time may cause chronic stress to the point that this phenomenon can occur. This may be the point at which the patient is considered to fall into the category of chronic pelvic pain syndrome. When this process comes into play, the chronicity of the pain is actually causing the pain to be worse through changes in neurotransmitters, and this issue should be treated separately from the original pain source. The tricyclic antidepressants (usually amitriptyline because of its preferred side effect profile) and the serotonin–norepinephrine reuptake inhibitors have been used with beneficial effects. With coexisting depression it may be acceptable to use SSRIs to achieve the best result. It is also suggested that these medications be referred to as pain modulators as opposed to antidepressants when used for this purpose. It has been our experience that a significant percentage of patients have been told they are "crazy" or that "it is all in your head" and may be very reluctant to take "psychiatric" medications. The use of antidepressants may be interpreted as another physician believing there is really nothing wrong physically. An explanation will usually suffice.

Making a Definitive Diagnosis—History

The previously discussed neurologic factors form the basis of the explanation of the difficulties encountered in trying to determine the specific source of pelvic pain. They may also help in understanding why the amount of pain reported may seem to be excessive in many patients. The gynecologist's main goal is to improve the patient's quality of life and hopefully eliminate her pain completely. This rarely, if ever, occurs in a single visit, and it is important to explain this to the patient. In order to manage the patient's pain successfully, the most important step is to determine any and all problems contributing to the patient's symptoms. Unfortunately it is not uncommon to have 2 or more sources of pain, and in these instances, they tend to have an exponential affect. An in-depth discussion of all the possible disease processes and their management is beyond the scope of this text; however, the reader is referred to several excellent text books dedicated to the topic of chronic pelvic pain (see the section "Suggested Readings"). In addition, management of these patients frequently entails referral to other specialists including urologists, gastroenterologists, psychiatrists, physical therapists, and others for at least some portion of their complete evaluation and care.

The most important aspect in making an accurate diagnosis is a detailed history and physical examination encompassing all of the possible organ systems that may be contributing to the patient's pain. One of the goals is to eliminate possible causes. As previously stated, in a large number of cases the patient will have seen several physicians prior to the first gynecologic visit. Many times, these were busy PCPs who simply could not devote adequate time to obtaining the detail required. In other cases, the physician may have been a specialist who was unable to find any "significant" pathology in his or her field of expertise that fits the presenting complaints. The patient who may have been told by previous physicians that they were not able to find anything wrong with her may be very skeptical that her pain will ever be treated adequately by anyone. She may request the removal of her uterus and/or both ovaries at the outset of the visit. In other cases the patient will have already undergone surgery with little or no long-term improvement. Because of these patients' frustration, one of the first challenges is to begin to develop an atmosphere of trust. An explanation of the multiple possible causes of pelvic pain, maintaining a reassuring attitude, and taking a more detailed history are very helpful in decreasing the patient's level of skepticism regarding her management. An example of the detail required is that many patients, when asked to describe their bowel movements, will state they are normal. This may be the initial response even if they are at times 3 to 4 days apart with intermittent constipation, because that is, in fact, normal for the patient. This certainly may be a symptom of constipation-dominant irritable bowel syndrome or other types of functional bowel disease, and may actually worsen during specific times in the menstrual cycle secondary to hormonal fluctuations. This is a common finding in many women whose chief complaint is severe dysmenorrhea. These women actually have 2 issues that should be addressed individually in order to achieve the best outcome.

The method of asking open-ended questions is generally advantageous in the beginning of the medical history regarding the patient's pain; however, it is rarely adequate. It is very helpful to ask the patient what she believes is causing her pain, if that information has not been offered. Because pelvic pain often tends to wax and wane to some degree with hormonal fluctuations, it is advantageous to relate all aspects of the patient's pain to its timing with her menstrual cycle throughout the history. General questions should be asked regarding the location, duration, character, and intensity. In some instances it is very helpful to have the patient fill out a diary with the above information daily throughout a full menstrual cycle and review this at a subsequent visit. A thorough menstrual and obstetric history, prior surgical history, and medical history must be obtained on all patients. It is very important to ascertain the medications and therapies that the patient has had in the past to treat her pain, in addition to a routine medication list. The following questions are examples of the detail that is required for a full understanding of the patient's pain:

- Is the pain worse during or preceding menstruation or is it totally unrelated? (Although the pain associated with endometriosis and adenomyosis largely occurs during and a few days prior to menstruation, over time adhesions may form that are a separate source of pain from the original cause. The pain may occur daily and/or be associated with physical activity or intercourse once this occurs. Gastrointestinal pain may also be significantly associated with hormonal changes, but most other etiologies are affected to a much smaller degree.)
- Is her pain constant, or does it occur daily at specific times such as late in the day or only after physical activity? (The latter may indicate pelvic adhesions or pelvic organ prolapse.)
- Does bed rest improve the pain?
- Does the pain awaken the patient at night? (This is an unusual finding with gynecologic pathology, but is commonly encountered with gastrointestinal and urologic disorders.)
- Prior to the onset of the patient's pain, was she involved in a car accident or traumatic event, or did she have surgery? (This may indicate neurologic injury with spinal or peripheral nerve compression, pelvic floor muscle or ligamentous damage, muscle spasm marker points, or skeletal injury such as a fractured coccyx or unstable pelvic fracture.)
- Were there any major or stressful life changes that preceded her pain? Are these still ongoing issues?
- Does the pain result in any other problems such as pain in her legs, headaches, or changes in daily activities?

Dyspareunia can be a particularly devastating issue for many women because it may affect so many different aspects of their lives beyond the obvious pain problem. The patient may state that she has been threatened with divorce and is fearful of losing her home and livelihood. This may result in clinical depression or other issues that may need to be addressed separately. The importance of a detailed history in this situation cannot be overemphasized.

- Does the patient continue to have intercourse in spite of the pain, and if so is the frequency of intercourse decreased?
- Is the pain only during intercourse, positional, or does it last for extended periods of time afterward? (Pain lasting for hours and sometimes 1-2 days following intercourse is associated with pelvic venous congestion syndrome, while pain only during intercourse or only in certain positions may

indicate problems with deep pelvic floor muscle spasm, trigger points, or pelvic adhesions.)

- Does the pain largely radiate to the abdominal wall or suprapubic region? (This may indicate scar tissue from the uterus to the abdominal wall and bladder, or interstitial cystitis.)
- Is the pain isolated to the vulva or introitus? (This could indicate a number of different issues including vulvar vestibulitis, vaginismus, urethral syndrome, urethral diverticulum, pudendal neuralgia, or a number of muscular disorders associated with the pelvic floor.)

A history specific to the gastrointestinal tract should always be obtained. The incidence of functional bowel disease has been reported to be as high as 50% in women with chronic pelvic pain as a presenting complaint. In addition to the incidence of diarrhea, constipation, hematochezia, or a past history of any of these issues, it is important to ascertain the frequency and consistency of bowel movements throughout the menstrual cycle because of the significant hormonal effects on the intestine. In many cases the patient reports that any issues she has with diarrhea or constipation are intermittent, and because of this, she may not relate these to her pain. In many instances treatment of even minor abnormalities such as irregular bowel movements may result in improvement in the patient's overall pain score. This can usually be accomplished with minor dietary changes or bulking agents alone. Certainly the possibility of diverticulitis, diverticulosis, and inflammatory bowel disease must be considered when taking the history.

Urinary tract problems are relatively infrequent causes of true chronic pelvic pain. However, a detailed urinary history should be obtained in all patients to exclude this possibility. The history should address urinary frequency, dysuria, hematuria, nocturia, incontinence, urgency, and the incidence of prior infectious processes or urinary tract stones. Two urinary tract problems do cause chronic pain issues and are frequently difficult to definitively diagnose. These are urethral diverticula and interstitial cystitis. In both cases the symptoms include urgency and pain, and can manifest as dyspareunia. The symptoms are intermittent and seemingly unrelated to activities or the menstrual cycle. Patients may have been treated multiple times for urinary tract infections, but on careful review of the laboratory, many of the cultures and urinalysis evaluations were actually negative at the time of treatment. In the case of interstitial cystitis there may be microscopic hematuria, but this is not a dependable finding. Careful physical examination is extremely important if these diagnoses are suspected.

The history to rule out musculoskeletal issues may be somewhat less rewarding than the physical examination. Certainly a detailed history of all prior surgeries, skeletal or orthopedic problems, and trauma is extremely important. As previously discussed, pain that arises from the abdominal wall such as ventral/incisional hernias or neuromas can be more accurately localized and described by the patient in most cases. Neuromas are most frequently associated with prior surgical incisions both temporally and in location. Pain that is more generalized and difficult for the patient to describe is more likely to be referred from pelvic viscera or caused by adhesions to the peritoneum. The possibility of inguinal hernias should also be considered. Pain from muscle spasms in the pelvic floor is a much more common cause of chronic pelvic pain; however, it is very difficult for the patient to describe and localize in many instances. It is usually diagnosed at the time of physical examination.

Neurogenic pain can usually be described and localized fairly well by patients. It tends to follow traumatic events, surgeries, or difficult vaginal deliveries. Neuromas may form adjacent to surgical incisions, episiotomies, or obstetric lacerations. More generalized perineal pain may be secondary to pudendal neuralgia (unilateral), diabetic neuropathy, and chronic infectious processes. The specific symptoms and location of the pain are very important in obtaining the correct diagnosis. The pain may be described as pruritic or burning. Other nerves that affect a smaller and more specific location include the iliohypogastric affecting the anterior suprapubic area, genitofemoral affecting the labia majora, and the posterior femoral cutaneous affecting the lateral perineum to the labia majora. In all cases of perineal pain, dermatoses such as lichen sclerosis must also be considered and the duration and prior treatments (if any) are important.

A thorough psychosocial history is the last topic that should receive special attention in the chronic pelvic pain evaluation. As previously discussed, psychiatric and psychological issues may have a very negative impact on chronic pain. Unfortunately physical, emotional, and sexual abuse of women are underreported and can result in significant emotional issues that many times are not diagnosed or treated. The incidence of chronic depression and posttraumatic stress disorder (PTSD) are significantly elevated in women who have been abused. Women who have PTSD tend to exhibit somatization disorders and both groups are much more likely to exhibit complaints of chronic pelvic pain. This may in part be secondary to the effects on neurotransmitters caused by the psychiatric problems. The treatment of chronic pelvic pain is extremely difficult if these issues are not addressed. Although an attempt should be made to elicit the history initially, many patients will be very reluctant to discuss these topics at the time of initial evaluation. In some cases the patient may have never discussed her abuse with anyone. If this is in any way suspected to be part of the patient's history, this topic should be revisited after several clinic appointments with the hope that the patient may have developed enough trust in her physician to discuss the topic. If the patient has a positive history for psychiatric or psychological problems, a consultation with a psychiatrist may be very beneficial with regards to management of the chronic pain.

The detailed history is an essential part of the evaluation of the patient with chronic pelvic pain; however, this discussion is not intended to be all-inclusive. The history is extensive and can be very time-consuming and difficult to obtain completely in a single encounter. In an effort to be thorough, The International

Pelvic Pain Society has developed a "Pelvic Pain Assessment Form" that is widely used by many practitioners. It is available on the society's Web site with a statement that it may be freely reproduced and distributed.

The Physical Examination

The physical examination performed to evaluate chronic pelvic pain is substantially altered from the standard gynecologic examination of the abdomen and pelvis. The goal is to evaluate each possible source of pain separately without causing painful stimulation that may result in guarding and reflex contraction of pelvic musculature. The evaluation is started by asking the patient to inform the examiner if she experiences pain, and if the pain is in the same location and type as what she has been experiencing. She is then asked to point to the location of her pain with 1 finger if possible. In many cases this will result in a scanning motion over the lower abdomen. In other cases the patient may point to a very specific site on the abdominal wall or vulva. The examination is then begun by gently palpating the abdominal skin and abdominal wall with care taken not to cause displacement of the underlying structures. If pain is elicited at this level, the differential would include neuromas, abdominal wall hernias, and referred pain from underlying visceral structures. If the pain is in or near a prior cesarean section scar, an incisional endometrioma must also be considered. Deep palpation of the abdomen should generally be the last maneuver performed after the pelvic evaluation is completed.

Superficial evaluation of the vulva and introitus is then done to evaluate for inflammatory conditions and hypersensitive areas. If any portion of this evaluation is considered painful, it is advisable to use a Q-tip to palpate the region gently to identify the distribution of the painful sensation. This is also the preferred method to palpate the lesser vestibular glands individually to rule out vestibulitis by moving around the entire introitus in a clockwise manor. A single-digit vaginal examination is then done avoiding the upper vagina and cervix with emphasis on palpation of the levator ani muscles only, to evaluate for muscle spasm and trigger points. This examination is then moved anteriorly to palpate the urethra. If there is any tenderness or fullness noted, an attempt is made to milk the urethra of any content. If purulent material is expressed, this is an indication of a urethral diverticulum and warrants further evaluation by urology. The examining finger is then moved into the upper vagina to palpate the lateral walls to rule out piriformis muscle pain and posteriorly to evaluate for rectal pain. The anterior vagina and bladder are then palpated to evaluate for isolated bladder pain that may be an indication of interstitial cystitis or other sources of purely bladder etiology. Throughout this process the patient is prompted to voice any painful sensations that may be elicited.

A 2-finger digital examination is then performed with attention first to the stretching of the introitus and then to gentle palpation of the cervix. A second somewhat more vigorous palpation of the pelvic floor and bladder may be done at this time prior to gently moving of the cervix to evaluate for motion tenderness.

The examiner's second hand is then placed on the abdominal wall and the bladder palpated separately once again. An attempt is then made to outline the uterus and palpate for pain in the uterine corpus. If this elicits pain, the possibility of endometritis must be considered. The uterus may then be manipulated from side to side and in the anterior posterior plane to evaluate for pelvic adhesions. The ovaries and adnexa are then palpated in a more typical fashion in an attempt to evaluate these separately. Once this is completed, the vaginal speculum is introduced to visually evaluate the vagina and cervix and to obtain cultures if deemed appropriate. This portion of the examination is completed with a rectal examination to assess for isolated rectal pain, and finally a rectovaginal examination to palpate the uterosacral ligaments for nodularity.

Attention is then turned to the abdominal wall again where deep palpation for more cephalad structures is performed. Specific attention is given to palpation of the left lateral abdominal–pelvic wall over the colon, McBurney's point, and the ovarian referred pain point that is one-third of the way from the umbilicus to the iliac crest on each side. The inguinal canals are palpated to evaluate for hernias. The remainder of the physical examination is done in the usual manner with additional attention being given to posture and vertebral alignment to rule out abnormalities associated with posture and other skeletal issues that may produce pelvic pain such as lordosis, scoliosis, and kyphosis.

Laboratory, Imaging, and Management

Following a detailed history and physical examination the physician should have enough information to make a differential diagnosis of the patient's pain. The only laboratory evaluation that should routinely be obtained is a CBC to evaluate the patient's white blood cell count for possible infectious processes, and a urinalysis to evaluate for WBCs, blood, and possible evidence of urinary stones. In many instances these have been evaluated several times prior to the patient's visit. Any other laboratory or imaging studies should be dictated by the findings of the initial evaluation. As an example, in cases of cervical or urethral discharge, cultures should be obtained. If specific uterine or ovarian masses or displacement of these structures is found, pelvic ultrasound may be warranted. In cases of isolated bladder pain or urethral discharge with a differential that includes interstitial cystitis or urethral diverticula, cystourethroscopy is indicated and the patient should be referred to urology for further evaluation. Patients with findings consistent with pelvic floor pain or introital pain may benefit significantly from referral to a physical therapist who is experienced in dealing with pelvic disorders and EMG studies of the pelvic floor musculature.

In situations involving colonic or rectal tenderness, a referral to gastroenterology for colonoscopy may be indicated to rule out diverticulitis, inflammatory bowel disease, or colonic polyps. In the majority of these patients the pain will be functional and the colonoscopy will be negative. Many patients with chronic pelvic pain and a functional bowel component will respond favorably to treatment with psyllium fiber or other bulking agents. It is advisable to start at very low doses (one fourth tsp. daily) and increased by small amounts each week until the patient is having 1 or 2 normal soft bowel movements daily. Starting with larger doses may result in significant diarrhea and worsening of the patient's pain.

Approximately 50% of the patients who present with true chronic pelvic pain will have a purely gynecologic cause. If the pain is elicited with direct palpation of the uterus, the patient should be treated empirically for possible endometritis with doxycycline for 2 weeks. Although the pain is not constant, some patients with uterine pain will show findings consistent with adenomyosis on pelvic ultrasound. This does not confirm the diagnosis. However, if the patient shows no improvement after treatment for endometritis and has completed childbearing, she may benefit from a simple hysterectomy. Unfortunately pain caused by pelvic adhesions or endometriosis can only be diagnosed by laparoscopy; imaging studies prove to be of little value. In this situation the patient may benefit substantially from laparoscopy with appropriate surgical management at that time. It is however very important to delineate the extent to which the surgery will proceed with regards to removal of the uterus, tubes, and/or ovaries in substantial detail prior to moving to this level. Patients need to be counseled extensively on appropriate postoperative expectations. Another option if endometriosis is suspected is a 3-month course of Lupron Depot. It should be remembered that Lupron has also been shown to benefit patients who have functional bowel disease.

A small percentage of patients with chronic pelvic pain will not have an obvious origin, and will continue to have pain that must be managed in spite of a completely negative workup. In some cases, these patients have already had removal of the uterus, tubes, and ovaries. In these situations every effort needs to be made to avoid long-term treatment with narcotic analgesics, even though many will have been on these medications for an extended period of time prior to evaluation. These patients may benefit significantly from a combination of pelvic floor physical therapy, long-term counseling, and biofeedback. Every effort should be made to decrease and ultimately stop narcotics and other addictive substances, because of the high incidence of developing overt dependence in this patient population. The use of pain modulators and nonsteroidal anti-inflammatory medications may be continued indefinitely if used judiciously. Although it has not been used extensively in the absence of a known neurogenic pain component, a 2005 randomized European pilot study did show that gabapentin alone or in combination with amitriptyline was better than amitriptyline alone in the treatment of chronic pelvic pain.

Finally, even though the evaluation and management of chronic pelvic pain is very time-consuming and may last for months or years, it is important to remember that many of these women have pain that may be debilitating and affects almost every aspect of their lives. The vast majority of these patients can be managed successfully and see marked improvement in their symptoms if evaluated and treated appropriately.

TIPS TO REMEMBER

- Don't disparage the efforts of the referring PCP. He or she may not have had the time to devote to an exhaustive workup.
- Take a detailed menstrual history and try to relate the patient's pain and other symptoms to the menstrual cycle.
- Ask the patient what she believes is causing the pain.
- Expand on the patient's psychosocial history.
- Be empathetic—try to win the patient's trust.

COMPREHENSION QUESTIONS

1. Which of the following structures have sensory innervation from the T10 level of the spinal cord?

    A. Ovaries
    B. Small intestine
    C. Ureters
    D. Uterus
    E. All of the above

2. Which of the following statements is *false*?

    A. Emotional states can affect the perception of pain.
    B. Referred pain is caused by abnormalities in the cerebral cortex.
    C. The gate theory suggests that afferent impulses traveling to the brain can be affected by other sensory impulses and by control from the brain itself.
    D. Antidepressant medications can be used to treat chronic pelvic pain.
    E. The availability of neurotransmitters is believed to influence the perception of pain.

3. The physical examination done to evaluate patients with chronic pelvic pain is essentially the same as the normal gynecologic examination except that increased attention should be given to the bladder, the uterosacral ligaments, and the rectal examination. True or false?

Answers

1. **E.** The visceral pelvic organs are all innervated by afferent fibers that come from at least 2 different spinal cord levels. In addition, several different organs may be innervated by afferents from a given level. This phenomenon is one of the reasons women have difficulty discerning the exact origin of painful stimuli in the pelvis.

2. B. The gate theory suggests that there is control of afferent impulses being allowed to proceed to the cerebral cortex at the spinal cord level. However, it goes on to suggest that the brain has direct neural input to the spinal cord to modulate this control. This is felt to be dependent on the availability of neurotransmitters at the level of both the brain and the spinal cord. Emotional states are known to affect the availability of neurotransmitters, thereby increasing the perception of pain. An increase in availability of neurotransmitters is the mechanism through which antidepressants are believed to decrease the perception of pain.

Referred pain is caused by cross-firing between somatic and visceral afferent nerve fibers in the dorsal horn of the spinal cord.

3. False. The physical examination is substantially altered from the standard examination for a number of reasons. Chronic pelvic pain may be caused by any structure in the pelvis and it is common for the patient to have 2 or more sources of pain. The goal is to evaluate all possible sources with this in mind. Because any significant pain caused during the examination may cause reflex guarding and contraction of the abdominal wall and pelvic muscles, the examination needs to be done gently and, to some extent, from the most superficial structures into the deeper organs. The parts of the examination that are likely to produce pain such as deep palpation of the abdominal organs, manipulation of the uterus, and the speculum examination are not done until the end.

SUGGESTED READINGS

Blackwell R, Olive D, eds. *Chronic Pelvic Pain: Evaluation and Management.* New York: Springer-Verlag; 1998.

Howard F, Perry CP, Carter JE, El-Minawi AM, eds. *Pelvic Pain: Diagnosis and Management.* Philadelphia, PA: Lippincott Williams & Wilkins; 2000.

Melzack R, Wall PD. Pain mechanisms: a new theory. *Science.* 1965;150:971.

Sator-Katzenschlager SM, Scharbert G, Kress HG, et al. Chronic pelvic pain treated with gabapentin and amitriptyline: a randomized controlled pilot study. *Wien Klin Wochenschr.* 2005;117:761.

Steege J, Metzger D, Levy B, eds. *Chronic Pelvic Pain: An Integrated Approach.* Philadelphia, PA: WB Saunders Company; 1998.

Vercellini P, ed. *Chronic Pelvic Pain.* Chichester, West Sussex: John Wiley & Sons; 2011.

A 31-year-old With a Breast Lump

Candy Arentz, MD, FACS and
Jonathan Nathan, MD, MBA

A 31-year-old female presents with a breast lump. She reports that she has always had "lumpy" breasts and they have never bothered her. She doesn't do regular breast examinations, but recently noticed 1 lump during her menstrual cycle. She denies any nipple discharge, and has never had any previous imaging or biopsy of her breasts. The patient has no significant medical or surgical history. She has regular menses, menarche at age 12, and is not using birth control, but in the past used combined oral contraceptive (COC) pills. The patient denies any family history of breast or ovarian cancer. On examination, there is a firm, rubbery, mobile mass in the upper outer quadrant of the right breast at 10 o'clock, 4 cm from the nipple. There are no overlying skin changes or evidence of nipple retraction. There are no palpable axillary or supraclavicular nodes.

1. What is your differential diagnosis in this patient?

2. What is the next step in making the diagnosis?

Answers

1. The differential diagnosis in this patient includes benign breast tissue, fibroadenoma, cyst, and breast cancer.
2. The next step in making the diagnosis is imaging of the breast. For young women (less than 40), ultrasound should be the first imaging technique ordered.

CASE REVIEW

The patient will lead you to the diagnosis most of the time. This case in particular addresses one of the most common breast symptoms encountered: a symptomatic breast mass. It is important to work up the mass and ensure that it is not cancer of the breast. Mammography is the standard for breast imaging, and is used as a screening test for breast cancer in women 40 and over. A diagnostic mammogram is appropriate if there is a palpable abnormality. In a diagnostic mammogram additional views are taken as well as views done under compression and magnification. The limitation for mammography is breast density, which is why mammography is not as useful for those under 40. For young women, ultrasound should be the first imaging technique ordered. Ultrasound may also be used in combination to better characterize abnormalities seen on mammography.

The ultrasound reveals a hyperechoic, homogeneous mass with distinct borders. A biopsy is subsequently performed revealing fibrous tissue compressing epithelial cells. You diagnose the patient with a fibroadenoma and discuss monitoring and treatment options.

BENIGN BREAST DISEASE

Diagnosis

Fibroadenomas usually present in women aged 15 to 25 and can grow during periods of increased estrogen levels, such as pregnancy. They can be multiple and change during the menstrual cycle. Usually firm, smooth, and mobile, these are well-circumscribed tumors composed of glandular and stromal tissue. The patient may have known they were there for some time, but they are often found by the practitioner in women with dense breasts. To rule out malignancy they must pass the "triple test": benign examination, characteristic benign appearance on ultrasound, and benign biopsy result. There is some evidence that short-term follow-up of small (less than 2 cm) fibroadenomas is acceptable. A repeat ultrasound 6 months later, for those who are low risk, may confirm the diagnosis of fibroadenoma instead of biopsy if the size remains unchanged.

Benign breast tissue is a diagnosis of exclusion. Often the patient or provider will feel something different in the breast and describe it as a mass. It cannot be overlooked and should be imaged if there seems to be a change or the patient thinks it has changed. Breasts contain fat, fibrous tissue, ducts and lobular tissue; often the difference in density of these will result in some areas being more firm than others. This is usually the case in the upper outer quadrant and along the inframammary crease. Imaging should be ordered, but will likely show dense tissue without a defined mass. Remember approximately 15% of breast cancer can't be seen by mammography, so if suspicion is high, don't stop here.

Cysts are fluid-filled, epithelial-lined masses. They are almost always multiple, bilateral, and varied in size. One may be much more prominent on physical examination, but on ultrasound multiple will be seen. These are normal in premenopausal breasts and represent clogged ducts. Although often painful, simple cysts have no malignant potential. Cysts are usually filled with normal breast secretions that are green to brown in color. Aspiration can be done, but recurrence is high. Biopsy with removal of part of the cyst wall will resolve the cyst in question, but will not prevent others.

A breast abscess can be classified into central and distant from the nipple. Risk factors include breast-feeding, smoking, piercing, and diabetes. Central abscesses are often recurrent and can require surgical excision. Simple abscesses less than 5 cm can be drained percutaneously, but often require multiple aspirations and oral antibiotics. Patients must be reliable and follow-up is needed. For abscesses larger than 5 cm, open incision and drainage is preferred and antibiotics are rarely needed. If the abscess is recurrent, excision of the involved duct may be required.

Breast pain, or mastalgia, is a common complaint without a good treatment. A thorough history should be taken as to the timing of the pain; whether it is cyclical, unilateral, or bilateral; and any history of trauma. Cyclical breast pain resolves with menopause. If the pain is unilateral, it may be musculoskeletal in nature and physical examination of the shoulder, pectoralis muscle, and upper back should be done to rule out referred pain to the breast. A common reason for breast pain is a poorly fitted bra. The breast should be examined for indentations caused by the bra and recommendations made; an underwire bra often causes pain at the inframammary crease or on the lateral aspect near the axilla. Most breast pain can be solved with a well-fitted bra that provides support, and NSAIDs. Removal of caffeine from the diet may have some benefit, but must be removed for up to 6 months before relief is seen. On occasion, medical treatment may be necessary.

Nipple discharge requires a careful history. Is the discharge unilateral or bilateral? Is the discharge from 1 duct or many? What is the color of the discharge? Does it happen spontaneously? If the nipple discharge is bilateral, then a systemic workup should be done including ruling out pregnancy, inspecting the patient's medication list, and checking thyroid and prolactin levels. If the nipple discharge is unilateral, it is more concerning for cancer. A bloody nipple discharge is associated with cancer 20% of the time, but the most common cause of bloody nipple discharge is a benign intraductal papilloma. Workup should be similar to the breast mass workup, but may include a ductogram which is a contrast study through the nipple to look at the architecture of the duct. Excision of the offensive duct may be necessary if imaging is nondiagnostic.

Keep in mind the possibility of breast cancer. The two most common risk factors for breast cancer are female gender and age. If the patient has a new mass, imaging should be performed and the patient should be referred to a breast surgeon if results are inconclusive or the mass is suspicious in appearance. Suspicious lesions contain calcifications, have irregular borders, and are usually new or changed from any previous imaging study.

TIPS TO REMEMBER

- In women under 40, ultrasound of the breast is the preferred imaging technique.
- Fibroadenomas most commonly present between the ages of 15 and 25.
- The "triple test" includes benign breast examination, characteristic benign appearance on ultrasound, and benign biopsy result.
- Unilateral nipple discharge is concerning for cancer.

COMPREHENSION QUESTIONS

1. A 55-year-old woman presents to your office with unilateral bloody nipple discharge. Which of the following statements is *least* accurate?

   A. The patient needs bilateral mammograms to characterize the lesion.
   B. A breast ultrasound may be used in combination with mammogram to characterize the lesion.
   C. The most likely explanation for her symptoms is breast cancer.
   D. The patient may require a ductogram and directed excision of the duct.

2. A 29-year-old diabetic female comes to your clinic with a "bump" on her right breast that has progressively increased in size and pain over the past few weeks. The patient is currently breast-feeding. On examination, there is a 2-cm erythematous mass, 5 cm from the nipple at 9 o'clock. An ultrasound reveals a loculated fluid-filled cavity. What is the next best step in management?

A. Obtain a mammogram.
B. Percutaneous drainage.
C. Open incision and drainage.
D. Excisional biopsy.

3. The above patient undergoes several aspirations and completes several courses of oral antibiotics over the past 6 months. She now presents with a recurrent abscess measuring 8 × 6 cm. What is your next step?

A. Obtain an MRI of the breast.
B. Perform a partial mastectomy.
C. Incise and drain.
D. Reassure.

Answers

1. **C**. The most common cause of bloody nipple discharge is intraductal papilloma. Appropriate workup should include mammogram, and ultrasound may also be used in combination to better characterize abnormalities seen on mammography. A ductogram can also be obtained to locate the papilloma and to help provide directed excision of the duct.

2. **B**. Both diabetes and breast-feeding are risk factors for a breast abscess. Simple abscesses less than 5 cm can be drained percutaneously. For abscess larger than 5 cm, open incision and drainage is preferred. A mammogram would not be helpful, especially in a young female with dense parenchyma.

3. **C**. Breast abscesses larger than 5 cm require open incision and drainage. If the abscess recurs after incision and drainage, excision of the involved duct may be required.

SUGGESTED READINGS

Amin AL, Purdy AC, Mattingly JD, Kong AL, Termuhlen PM. Benign breast disease. *Surg Clin North Am*. 2013;93:299–308.

Bland KI, Copeland RM. *The Breast: Comprehensive Management of Benign and Malignant Diseases*. 4th ed. Philadelphia, PA: Saunders Elsevier; 2009.

Gallapalli V, Liao J, Dudakovic A, Sugg S, Scott-Conner C, Weigelet RJ. Risk factors for development and recurrence of primary breast abscesses. *J Am Coll Surg*. 2010;211:41–48.

Miltenburg DM, Speights VO. Benign breast disease. *Obstet Gynecol Clin North Am*. 2008;35:285–300.

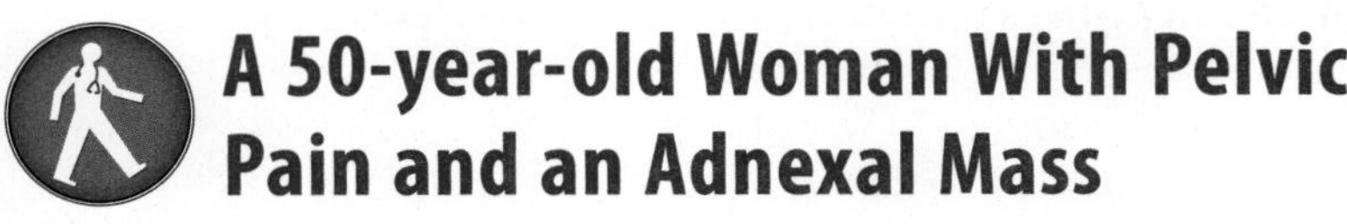

A 50-year-old Woman With Pelvic Pain and an Adnexal Mass

Lubna Chohan, MD

A 50-year-old G2P2 presents to your office with the complaint of right lower quadrant pain for the past 6 months that has been worsening. Her pain occurs daily and is constant. She feels that the pain worsens with movement. Pain medication improves her symptoms. She has regular bowel movements daily and no issues with urinary symptoms. She is still having regular monthly menses but complains that the bleeding is getting heavier.

She had her annual examination done earlier in the year and was found to have a normal mammogram and normal colonoscopy. Her past medical and surgical history are negative.

On examination, there is noted to be a 7-cm mass on the right that is palpable on bimanual and rectal examination. The mass feels mobile. Her uterus is slightly enlarged and irregular contour is noted. She is sent for a transvaginal ultrasound that demonstrates an 8-cm right adnexal mass that is multilocular and cystic. No papillary excrescences or solid components are noted. Her uterus contains some small fibroids. Her CA125 is 25 U/mL.

1. What is your differential diagnosis?

2. What is your management plan for this patient?

Answers

1. Table 9-1 lists the differential diagnosis of adnexal masses, by ovarian and nonovarian origin. The patient listed above likely has an ovarian tumor. The most common type of ovarian tumor is epithelial (either serous or mucinous). Table 9-2 includes the types of ovarian tumors.

2. As this patient is symptomatic from this adnexal mass and also complains of heavier menstrual bleeding, the plan is hysterectomy with bilateral salpingo-oophorectomy (BSO).

CASE REVIEW

The perimenopausal woman in this case presented with pelvic pain and an adnexal mass. An ultrasound was obtained that did not show findings suspicious for malignancy and her CA125, a serum tumor marker, was low. Therefore, she was scheduled for a hysterectomy with BSO. Intraoperatively the mass was sent to pathology for frozen section and the preliminary report was benign ovarian cyst. The uterus, tubes, and remaining ovary were removed laparoscopically (the route of hysterectomy is at the discretion of the operating surgeon). Final pathology result was a benign serous cystadenoma.

Table 9-1. Differential Diagnosis of Adnexal Masses in Women

Ovarian origin: • Physiologic cyst (follicles, hemorrhagic, corpus luteum) • Endometrioma • Theca lutein cyst • Neoplasm (benign, malignant, or borderline) • Metastatic cancer
Nonovarian origin: • Fallopian tube (ectopic pregnancy, hydrosalpinx, tubo-ovarian abscess, cancer) • Pedunculated fibroid • Pelvic kidney • Gastrointestinal origin (diverticular abscess, appendiceal abscess/tumor, inflammatory or malignant bowel disease) • Peritoneal inclusion cyst • Reproductive tract anomaly in adolescents (ie, obstructed uterine horn)

ADNEXAL MASSES

Almost 10% of women will undergo surgical evaluation of an adnexal mass during their lifetime. The lifetime risk of having ovarian cancer is 1 in 70. Only 20% of ovarian cancers are diagnosed as Stage I (5-year survival rate is >90%). The majority of these cancers (65%-70%) are diagnosed in an advanced stage (5-year survival rate is 30%-55%).

Risk factors for malignancy include older age (menopause), BRCA carrier, Lynch II syndrome or hereditary nonpolyposis colorectal cancer, nulliparity, endometriosis, and primary infertility. BRCA1 carriers have a 60-fold increased risk of developing ovarian cancer by 60 years of age and BRCA2 carriers have a 30-fold increased risk. The only treatments shown to decrease the risk of epithelial ovarian cancer include prophylactic oophorectomy and combined oral contraceptives. The longer a woman takes combined oral contraceptives, the greater protection she has from developing cancer.

Diagnosis

Adnexal masses may be diagnosed on a routine pelvic examination (annual examination), imaging study ordered for pelvic symptoms, or an incidental finding on an imaging study (ie, CT scan done to evaluate the appendix shows an adnexal

Table 9-2. Types of Ovarian Tumors (and Their Frequencies)

Epithelial tumor (65%)
• Most common: serous, mucinous, endometrioid
• Less common: clear cell, Brenner
Germ cell tumor (20%-25%)
• Benign cystic teratoma (dermoid)
• Immature teratoma (malignant)
• Dysgerminomas (most common type of malignant germ cell tumor)
• Endodermal sinus tumor (yolk sac tumor)
• Choriocarcinoma
Sex cord stromal tumor (6%)
• Granulosa-theca cell tumor
• Thecomas
• Fibromas (most common benign solid ovarian tumor)
• Sertoli-Leydig cell tumor (androblastomas)
Lipid cell tumor (<0.1%)
Gonadoblastoma (<0.1%)
Soft tissue tumor (not specific to ovary)
Secondary (metastatic) tumors

mass). Once a mass is found, the next step is to evaluate for the likelihood of malignancy, as this will affect your treatment decision.

The first-line imaging study to evaluate an adnexal mass is a transvaginal ultrasound. Results of the ultrasound should include size, unilateral/bilateral, consistency (cystic, solid, mixed), septations, papillary excrescences, mural nodules, and free fluid in the pelvis. Ultrasound findings that are concerning for malignancy are ascites, papillary excrescences, mural nodules, solid consistency, and bilateral masses. Findings that are more consistent with benign pathology include unilocular cyst, thin-walled, and smooth with regular borders.

Other imaging studies that may be used after initially performing a transvaginal ultrasound include CT and MRI. CT scan may be ordered if there is a concern for malignancy. CT may be able to detect findings of metastasis: pelvic/periaortic lymph node enlargement, peritoneal implants, and metastasis to omentum or liver. MRI may be useful in differentiating the origin of a nonadnexal mass, that is, leiomyomas.

The most common tumor marker that is checked when concern is present for ovarian malignancy is CA125. It is expressed in 80% of epithelial carcinomas, but less frequently by mucinous tumors. A level of >35 U/mL is considered elevated. CA125 is not a good screening test for ovarian cancer as it is increased in only 50% of patients with Stage I cancer. Also, there are multiple other conditions that will also cause an elevated CA125: leiomyomas, endometriosis, peritoneal inflammation/PID, hemorrhagic ovarian cysts, pregnancy, inflammatory disease (lupus, inflammatory bowel), and liver disease. Other tumor markers that are specific for certain germ cell tumors include beta hCG, AFP, and LDH.

Adnexal masses may undergo torsion (twisting of an ovary on its ligamentous supports that can result in compromised blood supply). Torsion is diagnosed based on the patient's symptoms as well as ultrasound findings (Doppler may show absence of venous or arterial flow). If torsion is suspected, surgery should be performed.

Treatment

Surgical intervention is appropriate when there is concern for malignancy or the patient is symptomatic from the mass. Ovarian cystectomy is usually attempted in younger women (desiring future fertility) and those in whom the mass is thought to be benign. When there is concern for malignancy, a salpingo-oophorectomy should be performed.

Referral or consultation with a gynecologic oncologist should be considered when there is concern for malignancy: presence of ascites, abdominal or distant metastasis, and postmenopausal women with elevated CA125 or a fixed pelvic mass.

In the asymptomatic woman with ultrasound findings consistent with a benign mass, observation is an appropriate step. Imaging studies are usually repeated in these cases.

TIPS TO REMEMBER

- When an adnexal mass is diagnosed, try to determine whether it is ovarian or nonovarian in origin.
- The most common ovarian tumor is epithelial (serous and mucinous).
- The majority of ovarian cancers are diagnosed in advanced stages.
- Risk factors for ovarian malignancy are older age (menopause), BRCA carrier, Lynch II syndrome or hereditary nonpolyposis colorectal cancer, nulliparity, endometriosis, and primary infertility.
- Interventions that decrease the risk of epithelial ovarian cancer are prophylactic oophorectomy and combined oral contraception.
- The first-line imaging study for adnexal mass evaluation is transvaginal ultrasound.

- Ultrasound findings that are more concerning for malignancy are ascites, papillary excrescences, mural nodules, solid consistency, and bilateral masses.
- CA125 elevation can be caused by ovarian cancer, leiomyomas, endometriosis, peritoneal inflammation/PID, hemorrhagic ovarian cysts, pregnancy, inflammatory disease (lupus, inflammatory bowel), and liver disease.

COMPREHENSION QUESTIONS

1. Adnexal masses that are nonovarian include which of the following?
   A. Appendiceal abscess
   B. Pelvic kidney
   C. Pedunculated fibroid
   D. Ectopic pregnancy
   E. All of the above

2. Risk factors for ovarian malignancy include all of the following *except* which?
   A. BRCA carrier
   B. Multiparity
   C. Older age (menopausal)
   D. Lynch II syndrome

3. Which ultrasound finding is concerning for ovarian malignancy?
   A. Solid consistency
   B. Unilocular
   C. Thin-walled cyst
   D. Smooth borders
   E. Unilateral

4. Which statement is *true* regarding CA125 tumor marker?
   A. Ovarian cancer is the only cause of an elevated CA125.
   B. CA125 is most commonly expressed by mucinous tumors.
   C. CA125 is considered elevated once the level is >100 U/mL.
   D. CA125 is not a good screening test for ovarian cancer.

Answers

1. **E**. Nonovarian origin of adnexal masses includes fallopian tube (ectopic, hydrosalpinx, TOA), gastrointestinal (appendix, diverticular abscess, bowel disease), fibroid, pelvic kidney, peritoneal inclusion cyst, and reproductive tract anomaly.

2. **B**. Risk factors for malignancy include older age, BRCA carrier, Lynch II syndrome or hereditary nonpolyposis colorectal cancer, nulliparity, endometriosis, and primary infertility.

3. **A**. Ultrasound findings that are concerning for malignancy are ascites, papillary excrescences, mural nodules, solid consistency, and bilateral masses.

4. **D**. CA125 is expressed in 80% of epithelial carcinomas, but less frequently by mucinous tumors. A level of >35 U/mL is considered elevated. CA125 is not a good screening test for ovarian cancer as it is increased in only 50% of patients with Stage I cancer. Also, there are multiple other conditions that will cause an elevated CA125: leiomyomas, endometriosis, peritoneal inflammation/PID, hemorrhagic ovarian cysts, pregnancy, inflammatory disease (lupus, inflammatory bowel), and liver disease.

SUGGESTED READINGS

American College of Obstetricians and Gynecologists. ACOG practice bulletin no 83: management of adnexal masses. *Obstet Gynecol.* 2007;110(1):201–214.

Chang HC, Bhatt S, Dogra VS. Pearls and pitfalls in diagnosis of ovarian torsion. *Radiographics.* 2008;28(5):1355–1368.

Liu JH, Zanotti KM. Management of the adnexal mass. *Obstet Gynecol.* 2011;117(6):1413–1428.

Stenchever MA, Droegemueller W, Herbst AL, Mishell DR. *Comprehensive Gynecology.* 4th ed. St. Louis: Mosby Inc; 2001:165–173, 957–990.

A 51-year-old Woman With Hot Flashes, Mood Swings, and Who Is Not Sleeping

Carol K. Felton, MD, NCMP

A 51-year-old G3P3, last menstrual period 2 years ago, presents to the clinic for an annual examination, complaining of mood swings, worsening over the past year, 8 to 10 hot flashes a day, and unable to get a good night's rest. She had all her children vaginally, and her surgical history is noteworthy for a tubal ligation but nothing else. She's had no vaginal bleeding for 2 years, and no other complaints. Her vital signs and physical examination are essentially normal (thyroid, heart, lungs, and abdomen) with the exception of a 1-in loss in height since last year. On pelvic examination she has atrophic-appearing external female genitalia, and the vagina is pale, thin, and bleeds easily with pressure. The vaginal canal is narrowed, the cervix appears normal, and bimanual examination reveals a small mobile uterus with no adnexal masses or fullness appreciated.

1. **What is your diagnosis?**
2. **What could you do for this patient?**

Answers

1. This patient is postmenopausal based on her history (greater than 12 months of amenorrhea without any obvious pathologic/physiologic causes) and her symptom complex. Laboratory tests, specifically a high serum FSH, are not required to make the diagnosis. Since she has come for an annual examination, basic labs may include cervical cytology (based on her history and last cytology performed), urinalysis, and lipid and thyroid profiles (see Chapter 45). Other screening tests may include a mammogram and tests for colon cancer screening.
2. Therapy to alleviate her hot flashes should be considered. The benefits and risks of hormone therapy should be discussed with the patient. Also, since she has lost an inch in height, risk factors for osteoporosis should be sought, diet assessed, and weight-bearing exercise recommended. Follow-up after 3 to 4 months of therapy is important (especially with mood swings and therefore possible depression).

CASE REVIEW

If you were to treat this patient's vasomotor symptoms with estrogen, she would need the addition of progesterone for endometrial protection against hyperplasia. The goal in hormone treatment with estrogen is the lowest dose that will ameliorate symptoms, used for the shortest period of time. Long-term or maintenance use of estrogen for prevention of disease should not be prescribed. A typical estrogen starting dose would be 1 mg estradiol (or its equivalent) and tailored based on the patient's symptoms. Given her loss of height and risk factors, she should have a baseline DEXA scan to assess her bone loss, and must make sure her calcium intake is at least 1200 mg daily (dietary and supplements) and 800 to 1000 IU vitamin D daily. Recommend a healthy well-balanced diet, at least 30 minutes of weight-bearing exercise daily, no smoking, minimization of alcohol intake (≤1 drink per day), and return to clinic in 3 to 6 months to assess the benefits (or complication) of her therapy regimen.

MENOPAUSE

With the "graying of America" medical students and residents will see many women go through the menopausal transition. At least 75% of perimenopausal women have hot flashes, the classic hallmark of menopause. Symptoms vary with climate, diet, body habitus, and lifestyle, racial, and ethnic factors. Sleep disturbances occur in about half of perimenopausal and postmenopausal women. Often, sleep disturbances (inadequate amount of sleep or poor quality) are associated with mood/cognition symptoms. Sleep disturbances can also be associated with physical symptoms and chronic illness, cardiac problems, and mood disorders (depression).

Diagnosis

Menopause is a *clinical* diagnosis determined by the final menstrual period retrospectively determined after 12 months of amenorrhea. The average age for menopause in the United States is 51. It is preceded by a menopausal transition period characterized by hot flashes, mood swings, vaginal dryness, sleep problems, and menstrual irregularity. This can last up to 4 or 5 years before the final menstrual period. There is no specific endocrine marker of menopausal transition. Since the hormonal picture is continually changing, measurements of FSH or estradiol are unreliable in assigning the reproductive stage of an individual woman.

Hot flashes are the most common symptom, commonly occur at night time, and usually abate in 4 to 5 years. Sleep problems are about half as common as hot flashes. Vaginal dryness is first noticed during sexual intercourse as decreased lubrication, and then symptoms extend to everyday function. Menstrual irregularity can be very disturbing and is usually due to anovulation, but exploration for the cause should be undertaken (see Chapter 1). The risk of depression also increases in the perimenopausal transition compared with the premenopausal period.

Treatment

To start with, you should evaluate for risk factors (obstetric and gynecological history, surgical history, current and past medical conditions and medications, family and social histories) and counsel to modify risk factors (such as diet, exercise, substance use—tobacco, alcohol, drugs).

Hormone therapy use is determined by considering the patient's current and past health and prior surgeries. There appears to be a window of opportunity for optimal benefits and minimal risks for starting hormone therapy, and this time is best during the later menopause transition or early post menopause. The only FDA-approved indication for *systemic* hormone therapy is vasomotor symptoms; *local* estrogen therapy is indicated for symptomatic vaginal atrophy. For those women with a uterus, a progestin should accompany estrogen in order to prevent hyperplasia or cancer of the endometrium.

Hormones may be given continuously, cyclically, orally, transdermally, or locally. Many women are asking for "bioidentical hormones"—hormones that are chemically identical to those produced by women. These do come in pharmaceutical grade FDA-approved preparations, containing 17β-estradiol and/or progesterone.

TIPS TO REMEMBER

- The menopausal transition, or perimenopause, is a period characterized by many changes typically beginning 4 years prior to the onset of menopause.
- Menopause is defined retrospectively after 12 months of amenorrhea.
- The average age of menopause in the United States is 51, and it is characterized by vasomotor symptoms, sleep disturbances, depression, and vaginal dryness.
- Systemic hormone therapy is FDA approved to treat hot flashes, and topical estrogen is indicated in the treatment of vaginal atrophy (dryness).
- A discussion with your patient on the risks and benefits associated with hormone therapy based on her underlying medical problems prior to initiation, and duration of treatment, is recommended.
- Progesterone should be added to estrogen in patients with a uterus.

COMPREHENSION QUESTIONS

1. The average age of menopause in the United States is which of the following?

   A. 42 years
   B. 46 years
   C. 51 years
   D. 55 years
   E. 59 years

2. Which of the following symptoms is the most common in the menopause transition?

A. Sleep disorders
B. Vaginal dryness
C. Hot flashes
D. Mood swings
E. Skin thickening

3. What is the biggest risk of unopposed estrogen therapy?

A. Uterine fibroids
B. Endometrial hyperplasia/adenocarcinoma
C. Endocervical adenocarcinoma
D. Cervical squamous cell carcinoma

Answers

1. C. The average age to enter the menopause in US women is 51 years, with a range of 45 to 55 years.

2. C. Hot flashes are the most common sign of menopausal transition, occurring in 75% of US women. The frequency of hot flashes, as well as the other signs/symptoms, varies with race/ethnic/cultural backgrounds, body size (BMI), climate, and diet.

3. B. Unopposed estrogen continues to stimulate proliferation of the endometrium and can lead to hyperplasia and even adenocarcinoma if continued. Fibroid growth is limited in menopause and cancers of the cervix (both squamous cell and adenocarcinoma) at this time are thought to be of viral (human papillomavirus) origin rather than hormonal.

SUGGESTED READINGS

Compounded menopausal hormone therapy questions and answers. US Food and Drug Administration Web site. <http://www.fda.gov/Drugs/GuidanceComplianceRegulatoryInformation/PharmacyCompounding/ucm183088.htm>. Accessed 1/15/2013.

Hormone therapy: is it right for you? <MayoClinic.com/www.mayoclinic.com>. Accessed 1/10/13.

North American Menopause Society. The 2012 hormone therapy position statement of the North American Menopause Society. *Menopause*. 2012;19(3):257–271.

Pinkerton JV. Menopause matters: the truth about bioidentical hormone therapy. *Female Patient*. 2012;37:16–20.

Schierbeck LL, Rejnmark L, Tofteng CL, et al. Effect of hormone replacement therapy on cardiovascular events in recently postmenopausal women: randomised trial. *BMJ*. 2012;345:e6409.

The North American Menopause Society (NAMS). *Menopause Practice: A Clinician's Guide*. 4th ed. Ohio: NAMS; 2010. ISBN 978-0-9701251-9-4.

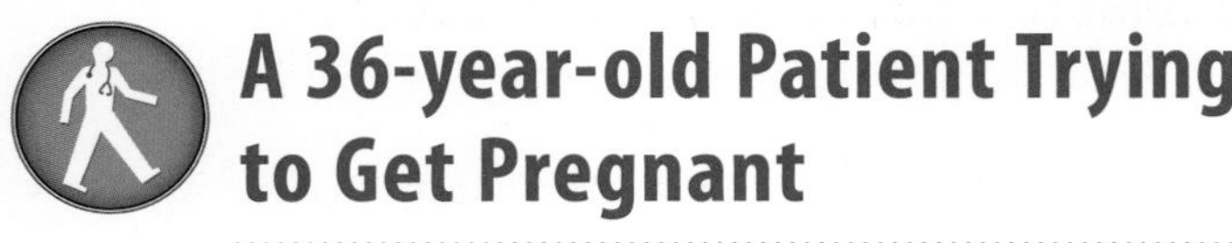

A 36-year-old Patient Trying to Get Pregnant

Heidi G. Bell, MD and
Tana L. Hall, MD, FACOG

A 36-year-old G0 presents to your office for her regular annual examination. Last year, she shared that she was excited about her upcoming marriage and that she and her husband were planning to conceive as soon as possible. She has now been married and having regular unprotected intercourse for 8 months without conception and is concerned about her chances of having children. She is taking a prenatal vitamin, tracking her periods, is healthy without underlying medical problems, and taking no other medications.

1. How would you counsel this patient?

2. What constitutes reasonable workup and management in this patient?

Answers

1. Approximately 84% of couples will conceive within the first 12 months of unprotected intercourse, and 92% within the first 2 years. Usually, after a year of attempting pregnancy without success an evaluation of the etiology should be undertaken. At this patient's age, greater than 35, you recommend an infertility evaluation as it's been over 6 months of trying to conceive without success.
2. There are 3 main components of an infertility evaluation that should be explored by history, physical examination, and laboratory or radiologic studies. You can explain to the patient that there are 3 basic requirements for pregnancy to occur:
   a. Ovulation
   b. Healthy sperm
   c. Normal pelvic anatomy

INFERTILITY

When seeing your first infertility patients in gynecology clinic, try not to get overwhelmed with the plethora of tests and evaluations available. Causes of infertility are generally ovulatory dysfunction (40%), male factor (27%-30%), tubal/uterine pathology (22%), and other or unexplained infertility (5%-16%). By keeping the evaluation and information organized under the 3 major requirements needed to produce a pregnancy, the history and evaluation becomes more manageable and logical.

Diagnosis

Commonly defined as the inability to conceive after 12 months of unprotected intercourse, an infertility evaluation can be offered sooner for the following reasons: maternal age >35, known or suspected ovulatory or sperm dysfunction, and suspicion of tubal or uterine pathology. Approximately 1 in 7 couples is infertile if your patient is 30 to 34, 1 in 5 if she is 35 to 40, and 1 in 4 is infertile if she is 40 to 44 years of age. The initial history and physical examination should focus on evaluating the 3 main fertility requirements.

Ovulation

Begin with simple queries concerning ovulation. Is the patient ovulating, and ovulating regularly? If not, why not? Much of this can be answered in the history of present illness, or addressed with some of the following questions: When was her last menstrual cycle? How long did her cycle last? Are her cycles regular? Some patients may document when they have their menstrual cycles. If their menstrual cycles are normal on history, the patient is likely ovulating. However, confirmatory testing of ovulation may still be necessary.

If menstrual history is grossly abnormal, no additional evaluation is required to establish a diagnosis of anovulation (or oligoovulation at best). The patient should be evaluated for causes of anovulation. This includes looking for signs and symptoms of polycystic ovarian syndrome (PCOS), obesity, thyroid dysfunction, premature ovarian failure, or a prolactinoma. Initial lab studies may include free and total testosterone, DHEA-S, TSH, FSH, and prolactin levels.

Tests to confirm ovulation include basal body temperature (BBT) testing (although this is often time consuming and does not reliably predict the time of ovulation), mid-luteal phase progesterone ("day 21" only if there is a 28-day cycle), and urine luteinizing hormone (LH) predictor kits for home use. In the meantime rather than timed intercourse when ovulation is suspected, which can often be stressful, regular intercourse twice weekly or every 2 to 3 days should ensure coitus during the interval of highest fertility.

Healthy Sperm

Simple questions and semen analysis can help the gynecologist determine appropriate urology referral. Male factor has been quoted to be responsible for as many as 50% of infertility cases, although it is classically thought to account for about 30%. The history should focus on eliciting reasons to refer, including sexual dysfunction, varicocele, history of undescended testes, history of testicular trauma, infection history (mumps especially), medical conditions such as diabetes or cystic fibrosis, gonadotoxin exposure, and previous surgeries. Having previously fathered a child does not guarantee current fertility, but should also be discussed in an initial history. Performing a semen analysis is a fairly simple and cost-effective method for initial screening for male factor infertility, although abnormal results do not confirm the diagnosis and should be repeated.

Normal Pelvic Anatomy

Begin with questions that may uncover abnormal pelvic anatomy. A history of lower (gonorrhea or chlamydia) or upper (pelvic inflammatory disease or tubo-ovarian abscess) genital tract infections, uterine leiomyomas that could impinge on the uterine cavity (submucosal leiomyomas), surgery on the tubes (ectopic pregnancy, tubal reanastamosis), or surgery in the pelvis (endometriosis, pelvic adhesive disease) may clue you in to an abnormal pelvic anatomy. Physical examination of the pelvis should include a careful speculum examination with STI testing based on risk factors, bimanual examination to assess for any uterine, adnexal, or uterosacral ligament tenderness (the latter is suggestive of endometriosis), and rectovaginal examination. Any abnormalities on history or physical examination can be followed up with appropriate imaging. Imaging of the pelvis is best performed with transvaginal ultrasound (if the uterus has not enlarged to a point that it is an abdominal organ). In cases of infertility you may want or need more specific imaging. The location of leiomyomas is best assessed with MRI of the pelvis, the intrauterine cavity with sonohysterogram or hysterosalpingogram (HSG), and the fallopian tubes with HSG. The HSG utilizes dye inserted into the uterus followed by x-ray to determine the uterine cavity morphology as well as whether the dye makes its way through and out the tubes.

Treatment

Treatment of infertility should be guided by the specific diagnosis obtained on thorough history, physical examination, and indicated laboratory or radiologic workup. Cigarette smoking, douching, excessive caffeine, alcohol (more than 4 drinks per week), lubricant use during intercourse, and obesity are associated with higher rates of infertility and should be avoided if possible. About 40% of infertility is due to ovulatory dysfunction, which is commonly treated by general gynecologists. Suspected male factor infertility can be referred to urology, while anatomic abnormalities are best handled by a reproductive endocrinology and infertility (REI) subspecialist, or those with a specific interest and experience in hysteroscopic or laparoscopic tubal/endometrial surgery.

Any underlying causes of ovulatory dysfunction should be treated medically (thyroid dysfunction, prolactinoma, PCOS). Patients should also be counseled to abstain from alcohol, tobacco use, and high levels of caffeine use that have all been associated with subfertility.

Ovulation induction with clomiphene citrate for 3 to 6 cycles can be attempted by the general obstetrician/gynecologist before REI referral (considering the patient's age). Clomiphene (one of several available selective estrogen receptor antagonists) works by blocking the negative feedback of estrogen on FSH at the pituitary level, causing increased signaling for ovulation induction. Twinning may be as high as 7%, but higher-level multiples are fairly rare.

TIPS TO REMEMBER

- Eighty-five percent of couples will conceive in the first year.
- Approximately 1 in 7 couples is infertile if the patient is 30 to 34, 1 in 5 if she is 35 to 40, and 1 in 4 is infertile if she is 40 to 44 years of age.
- Causes of infertility are generally ovulatory dysfunction (40%), male factor (27%-30%), tubal/uterine pathology (22%), and other or unexplained infertility (5%-16%).

COMPREHENSION QUESTIONS

1. What should be evaluated in *every* patient concerned about fertility?
   A. HSG
   B. Ovulatory status
   C. Folic acid levels
   D. BBT patterns

2. After careful history and physical examination you determine that your patient has had tubal ligation reversal surgery about a year ago, and still has not been able to achieve pregnancy. Which of the following imaging studies would be appropriate to evaluate tubal patency (whether or not the tubes are open)?
   A. Sonohysterography
   B. Dynamic MRI
   C. Transvaginal ultrasound
   D. HSG

3. When should ovulation induction with clomiphene citrate be considered?
   A. Semen analysis reveals low sperm count.
   B. Ovulatory dysfunction.
   C. Endometriosis is suspected.
   D. Oligoovulation due to hypothyroidism.

Answers

1. **B**. Ovulatory status should be part of the basic initial workup. History and physical examination should point to the diagnosis and help to evaluate underlying causes. HSG should be reserved for the suspicion of anatomic pathology, folic acid blood levels are unnecessary, and BBT patterns have limited utility.

2. **D**. HSG utilizes dye injected into the uterine cavity followed by x-ray imaging to determine whether there is spillage of dye through the tubes. If the dye isn't seen to exit out the tubes into the peritoneal cavity, the tubes can be considered blocked. Sonohysterography best images the uterine cavity and can be utilized to uncover uterine pathology (submucosal leiomyoma or intrauterine polyp), while pelvic MRI is most sensitive to determine leiomyoma location. Transvaginal ultrasound cannot always locate the fallopian tubes, nor tell you whether they are blocked.

3. **B**. Anovulation can be addressed with clomiphene citrate in many cases. If there is a treatable underlying medical cause for anovulation, such as hypothyroidism, it should be evaluated for and treated appropriately. Endometriosis and abnormal sperm counts will not generally be affected by ovulation induction.

SUGGESTED READINGS

American Urological Association, Jarow J, Sharlip I. Optimal evaluation of the infertile male: AUA best practice statement. Revised 2010. <http://www.auanet.org/content/media/optimalevaluation2010.pdf>. Accessed January 2013.

Fritz MA. The modern infertility evaluation. *Clin Obstet Gynecol.* 2012;55(3):692–705.

Fritz MA, Speroff L. Female infertility. In: Fritz MA, Speroff L, eds. *Clinical Gynecologic Endocrinology and Infertility.* 8th ed. Philadelphia, PA: Wolters Kluwer Health/Lippincott Williams & Wilkins; 2012:1137–1191

Lobo RA. Infertility: etiology, diagnostic evaluation, management, prognosis. In: Lentz GM, Lobo RA, Gershenson DM, Katz VL, eds. *Comprehensive Gynecology.* 6th ed. Philadelphia, PA: Elsevier Mosby Inc; 2013:869–895.e4.

National Collaborating Centre for Women's and Children's Health (UK). *Fertility: Assessment and Treatment for People With Fertility Problems.* London: RCOG Press; 2004. NICE Clinical Guidelines, No. 11. <http://www.ncbi.nlm.nih.gov.jproxy.lib.ecu.edu/books/NBK45935>. Accessed January 2013.

Practice Committee of the American Society for Reproductive Medicine. Diagnostic evaluation of the infertile female: a committee opinion. *Fertil Steril.* 2012;98(2):302–307.

A 32-year-old Multiparous Patient Desires Laparoscopic Tubal Ligation

Lubna Chohan, MD

After counseling a 32-year-old G4P4 on birth control options, she desires a laparoscopic bilateral tubal ligation. You feel that she is a good candidate for this surgery as she has a normal BMI (22) and no prior surgeries or medical problems. Her baseline blood pressure is 110/65 and pulse is 70.

On the day of her procedure, you are the primary surgeon. Once she undergoes general anesthesia, she is positioned in dorsal lithotomy position. The operating table is level (flat). You make a small 5-mm incision at the umbilicus and use a Veress needle to obtain entrance into the peritoneal cavity. Once you place the Veress needle, the opening CO_2 pressure is 14 mm Hg. You suspect that you are not in the peritoneal cavity due to the high opening pressure. You remove the Veress needle and reinsert it. On the second attempt, your opening CO_2 pressure is 4 mm Hg. You feel comfortable that you are in the abdominal cavity. You insufflate the peritoneal cavity and remove the Veress needle. You then introduce a 5-mm optical trocar with an attached camera and confirm peritoneal entry.

You begin to survey the pelvis when anesthesia notifies you that the patient is acutely tachycardic with a pulse in the 120s and hypotensive at 80/40. After a few minutes, anesthesia tells you that the patient is becoming more unstable with a worsening pulse and blood pressure.

1. What is your diagnosis?

2. How would you manage this patient?

Answers

1. Secondary to the acute change in the patient's vital signs, a vascular injury may be present. Of the injuries associated with laparoscopic surgery, vascular injuries can be the most life-threatening. If you damage a major vessel, such as the aorta, vena cava, or iliac vessels, you will not likely see blood filling the abdomen/pelvis due to the vessels' location in the retroperitoneal space. Often, after the Veress needle is placed, you may observe blood coming out the top of the needle. This is a sign that you have a vascular injury.

2. Suspecting a vascular injury in an *unstable* patient, the most appropriate course of action is to perform an emergent laparotomy. Notify the operating room (OR) team that there is a vascular injury and that you are converting the surgery to a laparotomy. Stay calm. Anesthesia should be starting additional IV access. Call for blood products in the room or activate your massive transfusion protocol and an emergency intraoperative consult to the surgery team (vascular surgery,

trauma surgery, or general surgery, whoever is readily available). While this is going on, you need to continue with the laparotomy and hold pressure on the source of bleeding until help arrives. Start transfusion once the blood products arrive. You have a patient with unstable vital signs due to acute blood loss. You should transfuse based on her vital signs and how much blood you estimate is lost. Do *not* wait for a stat H/H to return to decide upon transfusion.

LAPAROSCOPY

There are many advantages to the laparoscopic approach, compared with a more traditional open approach. These advantages include decreased postoperative pain and narcotic use, faster recovery and return to daily activities, earlier return of bowel function, a shorter hospital stay and inpatient hospital costs, decreased wound infection rates, and earlier ambulation with a decreased risk of thromboembolic events.

Entrance Techniques

Veress needle

The Veress needle is a spring-loaded needle that is placed blindly into the peritoneal cavity, relying on a surgeon's feel. While inserting the needle at the umbilicus, you will feel 2 "pops" or hear 2 "clicks." This corresponds with perforating 2 layers of tissue: the fascia and then peritoneum. When placing the Veress needle, the patient should be in a flat/level position. If she is in Trendelenburg position, the relationship of the umbilicus (more cephalad) to the great vessels changes and may increase your risk of vascular injury.

The angle of the Veress needle should vary based on the patient's BMI. The position of the umbilicus is on average 0.4 cm caudal to the aortic bifurcation in normal weight women (BMI <25), 2.4 cm caudal in overweight women (BMI 25-30), and 2.9 cm caudal in obese women (BMI >30). For this reason, the angle of the Veress needle insertion should vary from 45° in relation to the anterior abdominal wall in nonobese women to 90° in obese women.

After the Veress needle is placed and prior to CO_2 insufflation, it is helpful to attach a water-filled syringe to the Veress and first withdraw. If fecal matter returns, the tip of the Veress is likely in the bowel indicating bowel injury. If blood returns, you are likely in a vessel indicating vascular injury. If nothing is returned, saline is injected and should flow freely. You can then disconnect the syringe and place a few drops of saline in the Veress port, and then elevate the anterior abdominal wall creating a suction that will draw the saline into the peritoneal cavity. This is referred to as the "hanging drop test." These confirmatory tests are less reliable than the opening CO_2 pressure. Once the CO_2 gas is attached and flowing, the initial (opening) CO_2 pressure should be low (less than 10 mm Hg, and ideally less than 5 mm Hg). If the initial opening pressure is higher than 10 mm Hg, this is likely a result of preperitoneal Veress placement (the needle perforated the fascia but not the peritoneum). When successful abdominal entrance is noted with the Veress, generally continue insufflating until a pressure of 15 mm Hg is reached. At this time, the Veress needle is removed and the trocar can then be placed blindly, noting again 2 "pops" indicating peritoneal placement, or in a manner described below with an optical trocar.

Open technique (Hasson trocar)

This technique does not employ a Veress needle. It involves making a small abdominal incision (usually infraumbilical or subumbilical), and then passing a blunt-tipped cannula into the abdomen. The skin is first incised, followed by the fat and fascia. The fascia is fixed with suture, and then dissection continues until the peritoneum has been entered. The Hasson trocar is placed into the peritoneal cavity and secured by fascial sutures.

Optical trocar

An alternative technique to the 2 options previously mentioned includes the optical trocar (your laparoscope is placed in the trocar) with insertion under direct visualization. Your entry angle is the same as for the Veress needle. With optical trocar insertion, you will be able to visualize each layer of tissue as you traverse it. Once the peritoneum is entered, remove the obturator (inside of the trocar), and attach gas to create a pneumoperitoneum. This technique can be performed after or in lieu of Veress needle insufflation.

There is not 1 entry technique/device that is superior. They all can have complications. Factors to consider when choosing an entry include prior surgical history (potential for intra-abdominal adhesions), obesity, presence of an umbilical hernia (possible bowel presence, difficulty maintaining pneumoperitoneum due to fascial defect), pregnancy, or abdominal mass. The choice of entry technique is left to the discretion of the surgeon.

Entry Location

Although the abdominal cavity is commonly entered near the umbilicus, there will be instances that you will choose to enter at a different location. This may occur due to concern of periumbilical adhesions or a pelvic mass that may be ruptured if you place your initial trocar at the umbilicus. Another entry site includes Palmer's point (left upper quadrant entry). Prior to entry at Palmer's point, the stomach should be emptied by nasogastric suction. Entry point is 3 cm below the left subcostal border in the midclavicular line. Patients who may not be good candidates for entry at Palmer's point include those who may have adhesions in the left upper quadrant (prior gastric surgery) or those with significant hepatosplenomegaly.

Complications

Vascular: As described in the case above, these injuries are the most acutely life-threatening, especially with involvement of the aorta, vena cava, or iliac vessels. The aortic bifurcation is found at the level of the umbilicus in a patient of normal weight (and more cephalad to the umbilicus in obese women). When placing a trocar or Veress needle at the umbilicus, the angle of insertion should vary based on the patient's BMI. Keep in mind that the left common iliac vein is located below the aortic bifurcation and can be injured as well. In thin patients, the distance between the anterior abdominal wall and underlying retroperitoneal vessels may be as little as 2 cm. While you have a thin patient under general anesthesia, gently place your fingers in her umbilicus and you can often feel the underlying major vessels pulsating and appreciate their close proximity.

During placement of lateral trocars, injury to the inferior epigastric vessels can occur, especially in the obese. The inferior epigastric artery can usually be seen laparoscopically as it runs along the abdominal wall peritoneum, reliably located 6 cm from the midline. The lateral trocars should be placed greater than 6 cm from the midline to avoid vascular injury to the inferior epigastric artery.

Bowel: A gastrointestinal injury can have a mortality rate as high as 3.6%. Injury can occur at the time of entry, tissue dissection, or lysis of adhesions. There is also the possibility of thermal injury, or devascularization. If there are omental or intestinal adhesions around the umbilicus noted after initial entrance into the abdomen, you can move the camera to another port in order to fully evaluate the umbilical trocar and ensure no bowel damage. If you note a thermal injury to the bowel, but no enterotomy, it is important to carefully evaluate the entire bowel or consult general surgery. Some bowel injuries are not recognized at the time of the initial surgery and this delay in diagnosis contributes to the morbidity and mortality of this injury.

Urinary tract: Risk factors for bladder injury include a distended bladder during insertion of a suprapubic trocar, prior surgery causing bladder adhesions leading to a more cephalad position, or endometriosis. If you are unsure of the bladder margins, you can delineate the bladder by distension with saline. Other than a visible cystotomy, a bladder injury should be suspected if you note clear fluid in the pelvis or gas distending the Foley catheter drainage bag. To evaluate for a cystotomy, backfill the bladder noting for leakage of fluid. The ureter is most susceptible to injury when ligating the uterine and ovarian artery. It is important to visualize the ureter prior to performing these 2 surgical procedures. Postoperatively, direct visualization of the interior of the bladder and ureteral efflux with diagnostic cystoscopy should be considered when the integrity of either is in question.

TIPS TO REMEMBER

- A good laparoscopic surgeon should be aware of her/his limitations and know when to call for assistance.
- Your patient's BMI and distribution of abdominal fat should guide your entry into the peritoneal cavity; a more acute angle is used in thinner patients.
- An initial CO_2 pressure that is <10 mm Hg usually indicates correct placement of the Veress needle in the peritoneal cavity.
- There is not 1 peritoneal entrance technique that is without risk.
- The most life-threatening vascular injuries involve the aorta, vena cava, and iliac vessels.
- In thin patients, the distance between the umbilicus and underlying great vessels may only be 2 cm.

COMPREHENSION QUESTIONS

1. Of the following statements, which is most accurate regarding Veress needle placement?

   A. When inserting the Veress needle into the peritoneal cavity at the level of the umbilicus, you will feel 3 "pops."

   B. An opening CO_2 pressure <10 mm Hg is reassuring that you have correct placement of the Veress needle in the peritoneal cavity.

   C. In an obese patient, you should angle the Veress needle at 45° to the anterior abdominal wall.

   D. In a thin patient, you should angle the Veress needle at 90° to the anterior abdominal wall.

   E. If you notice bleeding from the Veress needle after insertion, your next step should be to insufflate the patient with CO_2 gas.

2. Factors to consider in choosing an entry technique (Veress, open, or Optiview) for laparoscopy include which of the following?

   A. The patient's BMI or distribution of abdominal fat

   B. Prior surgical history

   C. Presence of an umbilical hernia

   D. Presence of an abdominal mass

   E. All of the above

3. In regard to laparoscopic complications, all of the following are true *except* which one?

   A. An unrecognized bowel injury at the time of laparoscopic surgery will increase morbidity and mortality.
   B. Gas (carbon dioxide) in the Foley catheter drainage bag during laparoscopy is an indication of bladder injury.
   C. Thermal injury to the bowel, if identified, should be addressed at the time of surgery.
   D. Vascular injury to the inferior epigastric artery is common at the time of umbilical Veress needle placement.
   E. Backfilling the bladder with saline may help to recognize a bladder injury.

Answers

1. **B**. An opening CO_2 pressure <10 mm Hg is consistent with correct placement in the abdominal cavity. With Veress needle insertion near the umbilicus, there should be 2 "pops" that correspond to the fascia and peritoneum. Veress needle insertion should be angled at 45° for a thin patient and 90° for an obese patient. If blood is seen coming out the top of the Veress needle, you have a vascular injury. Do *not* insufflate the patient—if you do, this can cause a life-threatening air embolism.

2. **E**. All of these factors should be considered when choosing your entrance device as well as the entry location. In a patient with multiple prior laparotomies or with a vertical midline incision extending to the umbilicus, you may choose not to enter the abdomen at the umbilicus for fear of abdominal adhesions near the umbilicus. You may choose instead to enter in the upper abdomen. With an umbilical hernia, there could be bowel contents in the hernia sac that could be injured with placement and the fascial defect (depending on the size) may make maintenance of a pneumoperitoneum difficult. You may choose instead to use another entry technique. For patients with an abdominal/pelvic mass or who are pregnant, the size of the mass/uterus needs to be considered. If the mass extends 2 cm superior to the umbilicus, you would likely choose not to enter the abdomen at the umbilicus for fear of rupturing the mass that is directly below you (or perforating a pregnant uterus). You may choose instead to enter in the upper abdomen.

3. **D**. Damage to the inferior epigastric vessels, although more common, is less morbid, and usually occurs when the lateral lower quadrant trocars are placed. The inferior epigastric arteries are reliably located 6 cm from the midline.

SUGGESTED READINGS

Ahmad G, O'Flynn H, Duffy JM, et al. Laparoscopic entry techniques. *Cochrane Database Syst Rev.* 2012;2:CD006583.

Baggish MS, Karram MM. *Atlas of Pelvic Anatomy and Gynecologic Surgery.* 2nd ed. Philadelphia: Elsevier Inc; 2006:1029–1033.

Krishnakumar S, Tambe P. Entry complications in laparoscopic surgery. *J Gynecol Endosc Surg.* 2009;1(1):4–11.

Rock JA, Jones HW. *TeLinde's Operative Gynecology.* 10th ed. Philadelphia: Lippincott Williams & Wilkins; 2011:332–334.

Tinelli A. *Laparoscopic Entry.* London: Springer; 2012.

Vilos GA, Ternamian A, Dempster J, et al. Laparoscopic entry: a review of techniques, technologies, and complications. *J Obstet Gynaecol Can.* 2007;29(5):433–465.

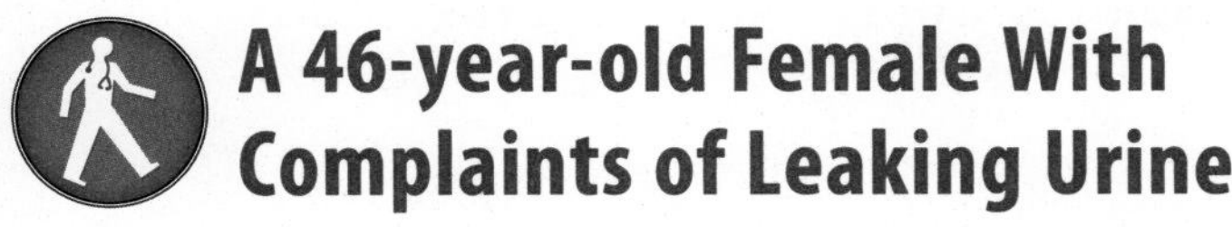

A 46-year-old Female With Complaints of Leaking Urine

Charlie C. Kilpatrick, MD

A 46-year-old P3013 presents to the clinic complaining of leaking urine. She has noticed this for a number of years, but recently it has become more frequent and bothersome. She has no significant past medical or surgical history, and delivered all 3 of her children vaginally. She denies any allergies, is not taking any medication, does not smoke, and drinks alcohol occasionally. She has regular menses that last 3 to 5 days. Her menses are not painful or heavy, and she denies intermenstrual bleeding. She has no history of abnormal cervical cytology or sexually transmitted infections, and has a healthy sexual relationship with her spouse of 20 years. She complains of leaking urine with coughing, sneezing, and heavy lifting. She urinates about 5 times a day, and once at night, and feels as though she empties her bladder completely when she does urinate. She denies urinary urgency as well as incontinence of flatus or feces. Her vital signs are within normal limits and examination of the pelvis reveals the following: normal external female genitalia, parous vaginal introitus and cervix, cervical os without lesion or discharge, and no tenderness to palpation of the anterior vaginal wall. Bimanual examination reveals a normal sized uterus that is freely mobile, no suprapubic tenderness, and no adnexal fullness. With Valsalva, there is some bulge in the anterior vaginal wall but it is not close to the hymen, and posteriorly you notice no bulge. With coughing she demonstrates leakage of urine, and you note that the urethra is mobile. Rectovaginal examination is within normal limits, without evidence of enterocele or rectocele, and the tone of the external anal sphincter is normal.

1. What is in your differential diagnosis?

2. What are the next steps you need to take in the management of this patient?

Answers

1. Your differential diagnosis should include stress urinary incontinence, urgency incontinence, mixed incontinence, overactive bladder, urethral diverticulum, urinary tract infection, vaginal discharge, and vesicovaginal fistula.

2. Few ancillary tests are needed in the assessment of urinary incontinence, and in this case a urinalysis and postvoid residual volume (PVR) will suffice. Some may also use a bladder diary, recording intake and urine output for 48 hours, when the history is not clear.

CASE REVIEW

Urinary incontinence affects greater than 25% of the general population, and prevalence increases with age. Other risk factors for incontinence besides age include medication use, obesity, mental or physical impairment, and increasing parity. More than 250,000 women underwent surgery for stress urinary incontinence in the United States in 2010, and the cost of incontinence is estimated to be in billions of dollars annually. Common terminology for female incontinence is listed in Table 13-1. The rest of this chapter will review diagnostic steps and treatment recommendations for female urinary incontinence.

URINARY INCONTINENCE

Diagnosis

The diagnosis of urinary incontinence necessitates a detailed history to include the following: daytime frequency, episodes of incontinence, urgency symptoms,

Table 13-1. Terminology for Common Female Incontinence Symptoms

Term	Description
Urinary incontinence	Complaint of involuntary loss of urine
Stress incontinence	Complaint of involuntary loss of urine on effort or physical activity, or on sneezing or coughing
Urgency incontinence	Complaint of involuntary loss of urine associated with urgency
Mixed incontinence	Complaint of involuntary loss of urine associated with urgency and also with effort or physical exertion or on sneezing or coughing
Nocturia	Complaint of interruption of sleep 1 or more times because of the need to urinate. Each episode is preceded and followed by sleep
Urgency	Complaint of a sudden compelling desire to pass urine that is difficult to defer
Overactive bladder syndrome	Urinary urgency, usually accompanied by frequency and nocturia, with or without urgency urinary incontinence, in the absence of other pathology
Anal incontinence	Complaint of involuntary loss of feces or flatus
Fecal incontinence	Complaint of involuntary loss of feces
Flatal incontinence	Complaint of involuntary loss of flatus

nocturia, and other voiding symptoms. The key is to determine which symptoms bother the patient most, because many patients suffer from a number of incontinence types. If you cannot elicit a good history or the patient's history is unclear, a voiding diary may help. A voiding diary is performed over 2 days, requires a "hat" (which can be placed over the toilet and is marked to record volume), and should also include amount and type of intake (especially caffeinated beverages), episodes/volume of continence/incontinence, hours of sleep, and nocturia episodes. There are even mobile phone apps available to record this information. Quality of life symptoms should be elicited; there are numerous validated questionnaires available for use. The diagnosis of urgency urinary incontinence is an affirmation to whether leakage of urine occurs with urgency. Stress urinary incontinence is likely if the patient states that she leaks urine with coughing and sneezing (or other physical activity), and a bladder stress test may help to confirm this. Many patients have mixed urinary incontinence (stress and urgency).

Physical examination should include a pelvic examination noting the presence or absence of pelvic organ prolapse (see Chapter 44), and urethral hypermobility. A neurologic examination is warranted in cases where incontinence develops acutely or when there is an underlying neurologic abnormality (recent cerebrovascular accident, multiple sclerosis). The only laboratory testing usually necessary is a urinalysis for hematuria and infection (presence of leukocyte esterase or nitrites). Leakage of urine with coughing should be assessed. Prior to testing for stress incontinence, the patient's bladder should be full, and if not the bladder can be backfilled with 300 mL. You should ask the patient to cough, noting urethral hypermobility and leakage of urine. A positive test is one in which urine leaks immediately with coughing. A delay in leakage may indicate a cough-induced bladder muscle contraction. Determining the PVR (the amount of urine present in the bladder after voiding) can be performed with a bladder scanner or in and out urethral catheterization. This is helpful in complicated cases of urinary incontinence, when planning surgery for urinary incontinence, or in women who report that it is difficult to empty their bladder fully. Routine urodynamic testing for the evaluation of incontinence in women is not recommended and the instances when urologic referral is necessary are beyond the scope of this chapter.

Treatment

Treatment is directed at the type of incontinence that is most bothersome. Lifestyle factors including weight loss and avoiding inciting factors may help limit incontinence episodes. Behavioral methods such as pelvic muscle exercises, bladder training, and biofeedback are also first-line, noninvasive strategies that may improve quality of life. If these are not successful, surgical treatment for stress urinary incontinence has high success rates. The most frequent procedure is placement of a suburethral sling in a retropubic or transobturator fashion. The former is associated with more postoperative obstructive voiding or urgency symptoms while the success rates of both are similar. These procedures are associated with complications including infection at the time of surgery, damage to adjacent organs, urinary retention, and erosion of the mesh into the vagina.

First-line treatment options for urgency incontinence begin with noninvasive steps as outlined above, and if not helpful, second-line options include antimuscarinic medication (by increasing bladder capacity and decreasing urgency). There are side effects associated with these medications: dry mouth, constipation, decreased cognition, blurry vision, drowsiness, and tachycardia, and they are contraindicated in patients with acute angle closure glaucoma and gastric retention. Third-line treatment options in patients who have not responded to behavioral and anticholinergic therapy include neurologic stimulation therapy and botulinum toxin injection into the bladder.

TIPS TO REMEMBER

- Urinary incontinence is common, and questions concerning bladder function should be part of a woman's yearly examination.
- Assessment for stress urinary incontinence relies mainly on a history and physical examination, demonstrating leakage of urine with Valsalva.
- Many patients will have mixed incontinence (stress and urgency), so it is important to determine which is more bothersome in order to guide treatment.
- First-line treatment options for stress and urgency incontinence include lifestyle and behavioral therapy.
- Second-line treatment options for urgency incontinence include antimuscarinic medications and, for stress incontinence, surgical therapy.

COMPREHENSION QUESTIONS

1. Which of the following is *not* a proven risk factor for urinary incontinence?
   A. Parity
   B. Age
   C. Obesity
   D. African American race

2. The patient in the clinical scenario above has what type of urinary incontinence?
   A. Mixed incontinence
   B. Stress incontinence
   C. Urgency incontinence
   D. Valsalva incontinence

3. You begin with lifestyle changes and behavioral therapy that help some with her incontinence, but she is back in the office requesting other treatment options. What would be the next treatment option in this patient?

   A. Anticholinergic medication
   B. Suburethral sling
   C. Botulinum toxin bladder injection
   D. Vaginal estrogen cream

Answers

1. **D**. African American race is not a risk factor for urinary incontinence, and in fact non-Hispanic white women have the highest rates of incontinence. Age, increasing parity, obesity, physical/mental impairment, and certain medication usage are established risk factors for incontinence.

2. **B**. The patient in the scenario reports leaking urine with coughing and sneezing, but denies the urgency to empty her bladder or leaking urine with an urge to urinate. Therefore, she has stress incontinence. Since she does not have urgency incontinence, she does not have mixed incontinence, and Valsalva incontinence is not a term used to describe incontinence.

3. **B**. The next option in a patient with stress urinary incontinence would be a suburethral sling. Antimuscarinic medications are a second-line treatment option in a patient with urgency incontinence, and botulinum toxin injection in the bladder is for patients who don't respond to or cannot tolerate antimuscarinics. Vaginal estrogen cream has not been shown to reliably improve stress incontinence symptoms and would not be a good choice.

SUGGESTED READINGS

Griffiths AN, Makam A, Edwards G. Should we actively screen for urinary and anal incontinence in the general gynaecology outpatients setting?—A prospective observational study. *J Obstet Gynaecol.* 2006;26(5):442.

Haylen BT, de Ridder D, Freeman RM, et al; International Urogynecological Association; International Continence Society. An International Urogynecological Association (IUGA)/International Continence Society (ICS) joint report on the terminology for female pelvic floor dysfunction. *Neurourol Urodyn.* 2010;29(1):4–20. doi:10.1002/nau.20798 [review].

Holroyd-Leduc JM, Tannenbaum C, Thorpe KE, Straus SE. What type of urinary incontinence does this woman have? *JAMA.* 2008;299(12):1446.

Madhuvrata P, Cody JD, Ellis G, et al. Which anticholinergic drug for overactive bladder symptoms in adults. *Cochrane Database Syst Rev.* 2012;1:CD005429.

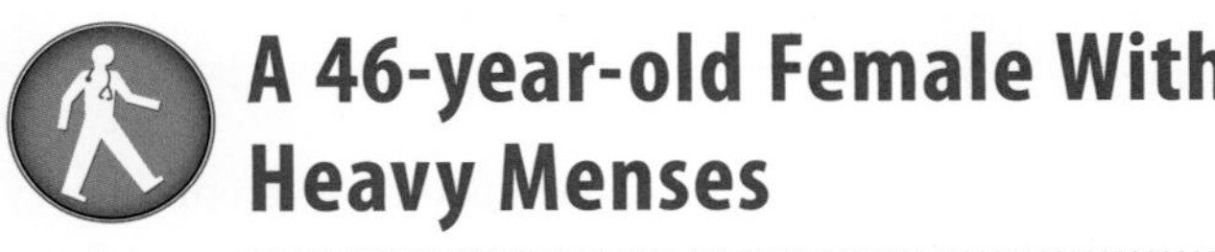

A 46-year-old Female With Heavy Menses

Ammar Dhari, MD and
Charlie C. Kilpatrick, MD

Ms R, a 46-year-old woman, is your next patient in the clinic. She is being seen today after having presented to the emergency center 2 months ago with a complaint of heavy irregular bleeding. At that time she was found to have a hemoglobin of 6.7 g/dL and was given 2 U of packed red blood cells. She underwent an endometrial biopsy and transvaginal ultrasound, and was sent home on oral iron and continuous oral contraceptive pills (COCs). Her medical and surgical histories are unremarkable; she has no drug allergies, does not smoke, and drinks alcohol occasionally. Her obstetric history is significant for 3 normal vaginal deliveries; her largest infant weighed 7 lb and 2 oz. Her gynecologic history is negative for abnormal cervical cancer screening, and she denies any sexually transmitted infections. She urinates 3 to 4 times per day and denies urinary urgency, but does leak when she coughs and sneezes. She finds this annoying since this happens 1 to 2 times per week, depending on physical activity. She denies any bulge or pressure in the vagina.

She has looked over the treatment options that you discussed with her before she was discharged from the emergency center: medical management with COCs and iron, endometrial ablation, or hysterectomy. After careful consideration she has decided that she desires a hysterectomy.

1. **What other information do you need in order to begin to plan for her hysterectomy?**
2. **How do you determine which route of surgery for hysterectomy would be best in this patient?**

Answers

1. In general, it's not a good idea to meet a patient for the first time and suggest surgery. Unless the surgery needs to be performed expeditiously, you want to make sure that the patient is a good candidate for surgery and has considered the risks, benefits, and alternatives to surgery. In this case, given the irregular bleeding she was experiencing, the results of the endometrial biopsy should be reviewed to ensure there is no evidence of endometrial hyperplasia or cancer. A thorough history and physical examination with emphasis on the pelvic examination, review of the ultrasound findings, and repeat hemoglobin to determine whether her anemia has resolved are all prudent next steps when considering hysterectomy. Demonstrating urine leakage with Valsalva and ensuring a normal postvoid residual volume would also be helpful as the 2 of you may decide on surgical correction of what appears to be stress urinary incontinence.

2. The route of surgery for hysterectomy can be determined by a careful history and physical examination. History items that will influence your decision are the following: surgical history (number and type of surgeries, or surgeries associated with postoperative complications), gynecologic history (prior pelvic inflammatory disease, endometriosis, suspicion of gynecologic pathology), and items that would make surgery or postoperative healing more difficult (obesity, smoking, diabetes). Physical examination findings that will guide you are the size and mobility of the uterus, descent of the uterus on examination, and the presence of any adnexal masses or enlargement. Your goal is to provide the patient with the least invasive method to address her complaint. In this case, her complaints are heavy irregular menses leading to symptomatic anemia, and stress urinary incontinence.

CASE REVIEW

You should expand on this patient's history and perform a pelvic examination with your attending in the clinic. She has no history of pelvic inflammatory disease or endometriosis, and no prior abdominal surgery. Her repeat hemoglobin is 10.8 g/dL, and her ultrasound reveals the following: 9.4 × 7.8 × 5.2 cm uterus, 2.3 × 1.8 × 3.2 cm subserosal uterine leiomyoma at the level of the uterine fundus, right ovary measures 3.2 × 2.9 × 3.0 cm, and left ovary 2.8 × 3.1 × 3.2 cm. No pelvic masses are noted and no free fluid is visualized. With the bladder full the patient leaks urine with coughing, the urethra is mobile, and after emptying her bladder she has 20 mL left in the bladder by bladder scan. On pelvic examination she has normal external female genitalia, a parous introitus, and the vaginal side walls and cervix are without lesion or discharge. The cervix is of normal size, and there is some old blood in the vaginal vault. There is no obvious prolapse of the anterior or posterior vaginal wall with Valsalva and she does not complain of a bulge in the vagina. Bimanual examination reveals a freely mobile uterus, approximately 10 cm in its greatest vertical dimension, with no appreciable lateral spread (about 4 cm in either direction of the midline), slightly anteverted, and without any evidence of uterosacral nodularity or tenderness. The posterior cul-de-sac does not feel obliterated, and rectovaginal examination confirms the absence of posterior fullness or pain. The tone of the external anal sphincter is normal.

In 3 weeks, you perform a vaginal hysterectomy, suburethral sling, and cystoscopy. She does well and is discharged home the next day.

ROUTE OF HYSTERECTOMY

Hysterectomy remains the most commonly performed gynecologic procedure. Over 600,000 hysterectomies were done in the United States in 2012 with the abdominal approach being the most common route. Indications for hysterectomy usually fall into a number of broad diagnostic categories: uterine leiomyoma, abnormal uterine bleeding, pelvic organ prolapse, pelvic pain or infections (eg, endometriosis, pelvic inflammatory disease), and malignant or premalignant conditions.

Selecting a Surgical Route

Surgical removal of the uterus can be achieved via 1 or a combination of the following routes: abdominal, vaginal, laparoscopic, and robot-assisted laparoscopic. Deciding on which route is influenced by many factors: anatomy of the vagina, pelvis, and uterus (size and shape), presence of accompanying pathology (leiomyomas, ovarian cysts, endometriosis, prior abdominal surgery), suspicion of malignancy, surgeon's experience and training, availability of resources, nature of the procedure (emergent vs elective), and preference of the thoroughly informed patient.

In general, a surgeon should choose the procedure that maximizes patient safety and minimizes morbidity and recovery time for the patient. Recent developments in gynecologic surgery have expanded the minimally invasive options for hysterectomy. Less invasive procedures are typically preferable to more invasive procedures. The American College of Obstetricians and Gynecologists (ACOG) advises surgeons to use the vaginal approach whenever possible.

Several factors have been proposed as relative contraindications for vaginal hysterectomy: large uterus, nulliparity, prior cesarean section, narrow pubic arch (<90°), and narrow vagina. However, many studies have disputed those contraindications. Nulliparous women often have a vaginal caliber sufficient for a vaginal approach; decreased mobility can be overcome and improved once division of the uterosacral and cardinal ligaments is achieved. Large uteri can be dealt with by uterine size reduction techniques such as wedge morcellation, uterine bisection, and intramyometrial coring. Recognized contraindications for the vaginal route include suspicion of intraperitoneal malignancy, need for access to the peritoneal cavity, suspected peritoneal adhesions, inability to position the patient for vaginal hysterectomy, and suspected inability to access the uterine artery blood supply. Figure 14-1 is a picture of the uterus firmly attached to the anterior abdominal wall, due to dense peritoneal adhesions. Studies have shown that vaginal hysterectomy is associated with decreased overall complications (decreased postoperative infection, decreased surgical site infection, decreased ureteral and bladder injury rate), decreased need for blood transfusion, decreased postoperative recovery time, shorter postoperative hospital stay (less cost), and less postoperative narcotic use when compared with the abdominal route.

There is some debate among surgeons as to what is meant by the term "laparoscopic hysterectomy." A total laparoscopic hysterectomy refers to the entire surgical case being performed through the laparoscope to include ligation of the uterine vessels, separation of the uterus from the vagina, and reapproximation of the vaginal cuff through the laparoscope. If the laparoscope is used only for visualizing the pelvis, adhesiolysis, and ligating the utero-ovarian or

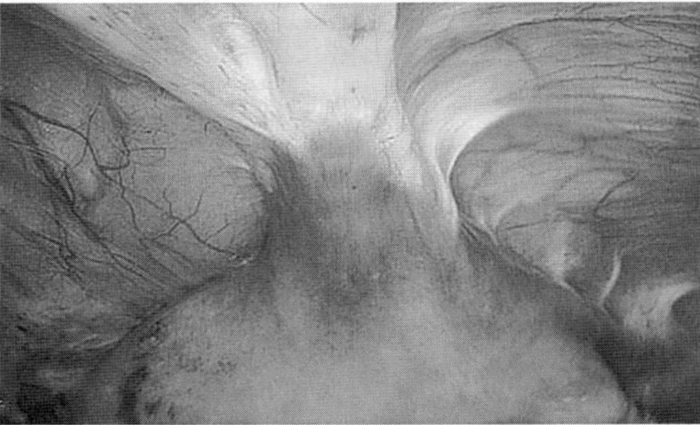

Figure 14-1. Laparoscopic view of the uterus adherent to the anterior abdominal wall, after cesarean delivery.

infundibulopelvic ligaments, then the procedure is termed a laparoscopic-assisted vaginal hysterectomy (LAVH).

The ACOG has listed the following conditions as potential indications for laparoscopic assistance to facilitate vaginal hysterectomy: adhesiolysis, treatment of endometriosis, management of large leiomyoma(s), and ligation of infundibulopelvic ligaments in preparation for oophorectomy.

An abdominal hysterectomy involves the same technique as a total laparoscopic hysterectomy, but the abdominal incision is larger in order to allow adequate visualization of the pelvic cavity. The larger incision and exposure of the peritoneal cavity to the "outside world" is what is generally thought to delay postoperative recovery and increase length of hospital stay. There are many instances when an abdominal approach is preferred, most of which have to do with the technical difficulty of the hysterectomy itself.

The use of a robot is a relatively new technique for performing hysterectomy. It has gained popularity among gynecologic oncologists due to its perceived ease of use compared with the laparoscope, although there is little evidence to support this. The concern for a prolonged learning curve (about 70 cases) and cost (roughly $2000 more per case compared with laparoscopic approach) has prevented the endorsement of the robot by ACOG for use at the time of hysterectomy for benign disease.

Preoperative Counseling

Since many intraoperative and postoperative issues can be anticipated preoperatively, the surgeon should use this time to review the patient's history and physical examination, identify physical limitations, gather required information to plan surgery, optimize medical status, and counsel the patient about what to expect from the procedure and during recovery. In doing so, preoperative evaluation may result in a shorter hospital stay with fewer complications and greater patient satisfaction.

As with any other operative procedure, informed consent should be obtained and the patient's expectations should be discussed in detail. This includes alternative treatments, risks and benefits of the procedure, the expected duration of the procedure, and recovery period. Table 14-1 lists possible complications for hysterectomy that can be used as a guide to review preoperatively with the patient.

Table 14-1. Complications Associated With Hysterectomy

Type	Incidence	Treatment
Intraoperative		
Hemorrhage requiring transfusion	2%	Obtain hemostasis, transfusion
Bladder injury	1%-2%	Closure in 2 layers, cystoscopy, bladder drainage, consider urology consult
Ureteral injury	1%-2%	Repair, ureteral stent, urology consult, retrograde pyelogram
Bowel injury	<1%	Repair, run the entire bowel, consider general surgery consult
Vascular injury[a]	<1%	Repair, general/vascular surgery consult
Postoperative		
Urinary retention[b]	5%-15%	Bladder drainage and rest
Surgical site infection[c]	3%	Open the wound, antibiotics, wound care
Urinary tract infection	2%	Oral antibiotics
Small bowel obstruction	1%	NPO, nasogastric drainage, imaging, replete electrolytes, possible reexploration
Deep tissue infection	<1%	Imaging, drainage, consider interventional radiology consult
Venous thromboembolic event	<1%	Anticoagulation, consider internal medicine consult
Fistula (vesicovaginal, rectovaginal)	<1%	Repair, may need urology/colorectal surgery consult

[a]At the time of Veress needle or trocar insertion during laparoscopic hysterectomy.
[b]Depends on the route of surgery and concomitant procedures performed. In general, the more bladder dissection/manipulation, the more retention postoperatively.
[c]After abdominal or laparoscopic hysterectomy.

Postoperative Care

The important elements of postoperative care are to ensure that the patient has adequate pain control, is able to void and completely empty her bladder, is ambulating without difficulty, and is tolerating liquids or a diet without nausea/vomiting. Once she meets these milestones, you can usually safely discharge her to home. Some advocate outpatient vaginal hysterectomy, but you will not likely encounter this at most centers.

Initial pain control will likely be intravenous and consist of NSAIDs, acetaminophen, narcotics, or some combination of the 3. Once liquids are tolerated, you can switch to oral medications for pain, and continue to work on patient ambulation. The first time out of bed the patient will likely require assistance, and until she is ambulating without difficulty venous thromboembolic prophylaxis should be continued. The nausea often associated with general anesthesia can sometimes make advancement of oral liquids and food difficult. Hysterectomy, unless there was extensive bowel manipulation due to adhesions or bowel injury, has minimal effect on postoperative bowel function, so there is little reason to wait for bowel sounds or passage of flatus prior to advancement of diet. Postoperative follow-up should be scheduled in 1 or 2 weeks, and precautions regarding common postoperative complications should be communicated to the patient.

TIPS TO REMEMBER

- Selection of the route for hysterectomy should take into account history and physical examination findings, with vaginal hysterectomy the preferred route when possible.
- Preoperative counseling should include the risks, benefits, and alternatives to hysterectomy.
- Benefits of the vaginal approach compared with an abdominal approach include the following: decreased length of postoperative hospital stay, decreased cost, decreased postoperative pain and healing time, and decreased injury to the bladder and ureter.
- Postoperative care after hysterectomy ensures the patient can adequately empty her bladder, ambulate, tolerate a liquid or regular diet, and has adequate pain control.

COMPREHENSION QUESTIONS

1. A 43-year-old healthy female P3 with 3 prior cesarean deliveries presents with a long history of regular heavy menses. This began about 4 years ago, and she was begun on COCs and NSAIDs during her cycle that did not improve her

symptoms. Two years ago you performed an endometrial ablation, and her cycles improved for about 6 months, but are heavy again. She is tired of the heavy menses and is requesting a hysterectomy. Pelvic examination is as follows: normal external genitalia, nulliparous introitus, vagina and cervix without lesions, old blood in the vault, and the cervix is hard to visualize as it is very high in the vagina. Bimanual examination reveals a small nonmobile uterus, and normal adnexa without masses or fullness. The *best* choice for route of hysterectomy in this case is which of the following?

A. Abdominal hysterectomy
B. LAVH
C. Vaginal hysterectomy
D. Total laparoscopic hysterectomy

2. A 44-year-old healthy female presents complaining of irregular, heavy menses after having tried COCs for 6 months without improvement. At a prior visit you performed an endometrial biopsy, which was normal. She has been reading about her options and would prefer a hysterectomy over endometrial ablation. You would like to perform a vaginal hysterectomy. Which of the following factors would be a contraindication for the vaginal route?

A. Leiomyomatous uterus
B. Inability to abduct the hips
C. Obesity
D. Previous cesarean delivery

3. Which of the following is *not* considered an advantage of the vaginal route versus the abdominal route for hysterectomy?

A. Decreased length of postoperative hospital stay
B. Decreased length of postoperative recovery time
C. Decreased ureteral injury rate
D. Decreased surgical technical difficulty

Answers

1. **D.** From the examination of the pelvis (limited mobility of the uterus, cervix high in the vaginal vault that may preclude access to the uterine arteries) and her history (3 previous cesarean deliveries with suspicion of intraperitoneal adhesions, no vaginal deliveries), attempting this case through the vagina would be technically challenging. Laparoscopic assistance is used when there is suspected ovarian pathology or a need to survey the pelvic cavity (pelvic pain, endometriosis, adhesions, etc) and still requires access to the cervix through the vagina. The advantage of a total laparoscopic route versus an abdominal route is a decreased length of postoperative stay and recovery time for the patient and in this case is the best route for surgery.

2. **B**. Previous cesarean delivery, leiomyomas, and obesity are not contraindications for vaginal surgery. The most important factors in choosing the vaginal route are the mobility of the uterus and whether you can access the posterior cul-de-sac. Also, the patient should be able to abduct the hips in order to be placed in lithotomy position.

3. **D**. Vaginal hysterectomy has been associated with all of the choices except D. For experienced vaginal surgeons the vaginal route may be deemed technically easier, but as with any surgical case the skills and experience of the surgeon determine which is technically easier.

SUGGESTED READINGS

ACOG Committee Opinion No. 444: choosing the route of hysterectomy for benign disease. *Obstet Gynecol.* 2009;114(5):1156–1158. <http://www.cdc.gov/reproductivehealth/WomensRH/00-04-FS_Hysterectomy.htm>. Accessed July 8, 2013.

Kovac SR. Clinical opinion: guidelines for hysterectomy. *Am J Obstet Gynecol.* 2004;191(2):635–640.

Wright JD, Ananth CV, Lewin SN, et al. Robotically assisted vs laparoscopic hysterectomy among women with benign gynecologic disease. *JAMA.* 2013;309(7):689–698.

Zakaria MA, Levy BS. Outpatient vaginal hysterectomy: optimizing perioperative management for same-day discharge. *Obstet Gynecol.* 2012;120(6):1355–1361.

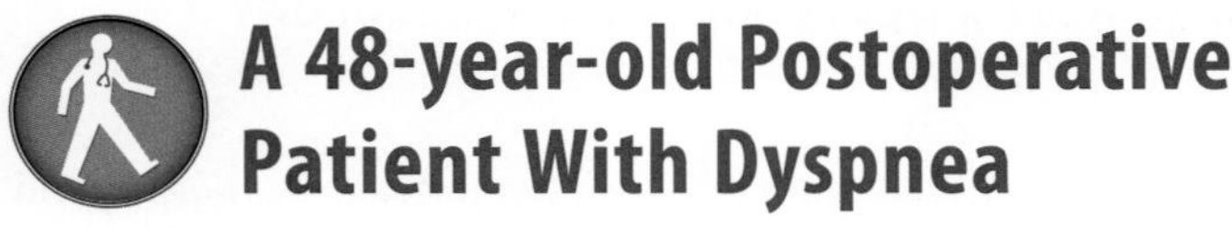

A 48-year-old Postoperative Patient With Dyspnea

Laura M. Divine, MD and
Jacob M. Estes, MD

You are called to evaluate a 48-year-old female with difficulty breathing. Three days ago she underwent exploratory laparotomy and right salpingo-oophorectomy for suspected ovarian torsion. She is obese (BMI 40) and has a history of hypertension and coronary artery disease. On examination, she is afebrile, with a pulse of 115, respiratory rate of 32, and blood pressure 151/83. Her oxygen saturation by pulse oximetry is 87% on room air. You appreciate wheezing on lung examination. Her abdominal examination is benign and the wound is healing well. The rest of the examination is within normal limits.

1. What is in your differential diagnosis?

2. What are the next steps in the management of this patient?

Answers

1. Your differential diagnosis should include pulmonary embolus (PE), myocardial infarction, pulmonary edema of either cardiogenic or noncardiogenic origin, pneumonia, and atelectasis.

2. Supplemental oxygen should be started immediately given her oxygen saturation of 87%, and her tachypnea and dyspnea. Further workup is needed to diagnose pulmonary embolism. Suggested studies include arterial blood gas, electrocardiogram, chest radiograph, and diagnostic imaging such as computed tomographic pulmonary angiogram (CT-PA) or ventilation/perfusion (V/Q) scan. Other labs such as cardiac enzymes, D-dimer, and serum creatinine may also be helpful.

CASE REVIEW

In a teaching hospital, the first physician to evaluate a patient on the floor will be a first- or second-year resident. You may inherit this role if you are on a fourth year, "Sub-I" rotation. It is important for the initial responder to recognize "sick" from "not sick," and, if the patient is sick, to convey this to your upper level resident/attending quickly. In this case, 4 L of oxygen by nasal cannula improves her oxygenation status, and you begin workup for PE given that she has a number of risk factors. You order a D-dimer level that returns at 678 ng/mL and then a CT-PA that reveals a right lower lobe embolus in the pulmonary artery. You begin anticoagulation and ultimately your patient improves. She meets postoperative milestones allowing discharge to home, and will follow up soon after to gauge her healing and to monitor for adequacy of anticoagulation.

POSTOPERATIVE COMPLICATIONS

Diagnosis and Treatment

You will diagnose and manage numerous postoperative complications throughout your career. They can be frustrating for patient and physician alike. The only way to truly avoid complications is not to operate. The major categories of postoperative complications include the following: genitourinary, respiratory, surgical site infections, thromboembolic, and procedure-specific complications.

Common genitourinary complications include postoperative urinary retention and infection of the lower/upper urinary tract. Many of the surgeries you will perform will be in close proximity to the genitourinary system. The bladder will need to be identified in almost every surgical procedure you perform in obstetrics and gynecology, and manipulation of the bladder often leads to bladder dysfunction and urinary retention. The upper urinary tract is important to identify during hysterectomy and other procedures. The key to managing postoperative urinary retention is recognition and then bladder drainage and rest or patient self-catheterization. Symptoms of urinary retention are suprapubic pain with decreased urinary output, and the diagnosis is made by physical examination, and a large urinary volume obtained with catheterization of the bladder. Infectious complications of the urinary tract are often a result of catheterization of the urinary tract or prolonged bladder drainage and may not be apparent until after discharge from the hospital. If the upper urinary tract is involved, symptoms can include fever, shaking chills, and costovertebral angle tenderness. Physical examination and urine dip or microscopic urinalysis will help to confirm the diagnosis.

Respiratory complications include atelectasis, pneumonia, hypoxemia, pulmonary edema, and acute respiratory failure. Atelectasis is common after surgery under general anesthesia and presents with low-grade fever, decreased pulse oximetry, and decreased breath sounds on lung examination. Treatment is supportive with early use of incentive spirometry and ambulation. Pneumonia will present with fever, sputum production, leukocytosis, and a chest film demonstrating pulmonary infiltrates. Treatment is targeted at common hospital-acquired organisms and should be started promptly. Pulmonary edema may be cardiogenic or noncardiogenic, and presents in a manner similar to our patient with difficulty breathing, tachypnea, tachycardia, and decreased oxygen saturation. Auscultation of the lungs will reveal crackles, and a chest film will reveal alveolar edema. An arterial blood gas can help to quantify the level of hypoxemia, and diuretics are often administered while conducting a thorough search for the underlying etiology. This may include an electrocardiogram, cardiac enzymes, meticulous review of the patient's fluid balance, and echocardiogram. Invasive monitoring is rarely needed.

Surgical site infections include deep tissue infections and superficial wound infections. Deep tissue infections are less common than superficial infections, and would include an intraperitoneal abscess or cellulitis/abscess of the vaginal cuff after hysterectomy. Diagnosis is made by eliciting peritoneal signs on physical examination and by imaging of the abdominopelvic cavity. CT scan with contrast is useful. Treatment will depend on the size of the abscess and the response of the patient to IV antibiotics. Sometimes reexploration or assistance from interventional radiology is necessary. Cellulitis or abscess of the cuff after hysterectomy will present postoperatively with pain in the vagina or abdomen, sometimes with nausea and vomiting, and a malodorous vaginal discharge. Speculum examination will reveal foul-smelling purulent discharge from the cuff of the vagina, and bimanual examination will reveal a tender vaginal cuff and/or abscess. Treatment involves removing sutures in the cuff to allow abscess drainage, IV antibiotics if cellulitis is present, and consideration of imaging to delineate the size/nature of the infection. Deep tissue infections are best managed in the hospital. Superficial infections present with pain at the incision site and subjective fevers. On physical examination the wound will appear erythematous, tender to touch, and will sometimes have purulent material draining from the incision. Treatment consists of opening the wound with debridement of nonviable tissue and, in many cases, administration of antibiotics. Antibiotic selection should include coverage for methicillin-resistant *Staphylococcus aureus* (MRSA).

Thromboembolic complications include both PE and lower extremity deep venous thrombosis, but we will focus on the former. The clinical presentation of PE is highly variable and nonspecific. Clinical suspicion is necessary to facilitate prompt diagnosis and therapy; laboratory tests can then confirm the diagnosis. An elevated plasma concentration of D-dimer indicates recent or ongoing intravascular coagulation, and a level above 500 ng/mL, especially in a patient with high clinical suspicion, warrants imaging. The major imaging tests employed in the evaluation of a patient with suspected PE include V/Q scanning, CT-PA, ultrasonography, and conventional PA. Chest radiography or x-ray can be useful in excluding other diagnoses such as pneumonia, and in the setting of PE will be nonspecific and may include atelectasis or pleural effusion. In addition, the clinical picture of productive cough and fever may help to confirm the diagnosis of pneumonia. Current recommendations for acute PE suggest initial therapy with subcutaneous low-molecular-weight heparin (LMWH) or fondaparinux. Patients with few risk factors for bleeding have a 1% to 2% rate of bleeding complication, while those at high risk have a 13% rate. The majority of bleeding complications are related to the surgical incision with resultant local hematoma formation. In cases of more severe bleeding, conservative management with transfusion and reversal of anticoagulation is employed first. Severe hemorrhage could necessitate reoperation, putting the patient at further risk of blood loss, infection, and related complications. Thus, the decision to begin anticoagulation on a patient in the immediate postoperative period must be made on an individual basis. This patient diagnosed with a PE related to surgery should receive at least 3 months of anticoagulation. The stress of surgery and a hospital stay can also cause and/or exacerbate underlying psychiatric conditions such as anxiety in many patients. Tachycardia, tachypnea, and shortness of breath are all manifestations of anxiety. While anxiety may be treated with reassurance and possibly anxiolytics, the consequences of missing a serious medical condition make anxiety a diagnosis of exclusion.

Prevention

Postoperative complications are inevitable, but there are preventive strategies that will help to decrease their incidence. Your teaching hospital will likely employ numerous preventive measures. Both hospitals and physicians are evaluated in regard to their incidence of postoperative complications.

The biggest risk factor for postoperative genitourinary infection is bladder instrumentation. In order to prevent genitourinary infectious morbidity, hospitals limit postoperative bladder catheterization to 24 to 48 hours after surgery unless there are specific written reasons as to why prolonged drainage is necessary (bladder injury, immobilization, etc).

Measures to decrease postoperative pulmonary complications include preoperative smoking cessation, chest physical therapy, optimization of underlying pulmonary disease, selection of surgical procedures that avoid the upper abdomen, aggressive postoperative lung expansion, and decreased use of postoperative narcotic pain medicine. Cessation of smoking >7 weeks prior to surgery and preoperative chest physical therapy have shown statistically significant decreases in postoperative pulmonary morbidity. Postoperatively the use of incentive spirometry and continuous positive airway pressure (CPAP) has been shown to decrease pulmonary morbidity that may begin as atelectasis, and progress to pneumonia. Your goal is to encourage early ambulation and ensure that the entire lung volume is expanded, to limit the use of postoperative narcotics (because they decrease respiratory drive), and to consider a minimally invasive surgical approach, which, in turn, will decrease postoperative pain.

Prophylactic antibiotics have contributed to decreasing surgical site infections in obstetric and gynecologic surgical procedures. Prior to performing surgery, a "time-out" is conducted in which all the members of the surgical team stop what they are doing and review important surgical details. At many hospitals the administration of preoperative antibiotics is one of the items on the checklist.

Table 15-1. Sample Perioperative Checklist

Sign In (Before Induction of Anesthesia)	Time-Out (Before Skin Incision)	Sign Out (Before the Patient Leaves the Operating Room)
Anesthesia/RN confirm:	OR team member confirms (all other activities to be suspended):	RN confirms:
Identity, procedure, procedure site, and consent	Confirmation of procedure, incision site, and consents	Name of surgical procedure performed
Site marked	Images available	Instrument count correct
Difficult airway or aspiration risk	Site is marked and visible	Equipment problems
Patient allergies	Surgeon states: critical steps, case duration, anticipated blood loss	Specimens properly labeled
Possible EBL >500 cc? If so, blood available	Anesthesia states: antibiotic administration before incision	Postoperative care concerns, recovery issues
Briefing performed	Scrub nurse: sterilization is confirmed	
	Introduction of team members	

Table 15-1 is a sample perioperative checklist that includes a list of suggested items to use for "time-out."

Prevention of thromboembolic complications may include early ambulation, pneumatic compression devices, and prophylactic anticoagulation beginning in the preoperative period and continuing into the postoperative period.

TIPS TO REMEMBER

- Postoperative complications are going to occur, and preoperative steps can be taken to decrease their incidence.
- Following gynecologic surgery the most common categories of complication include genitourinary, respiratory, infectious, and thromboembolic.
- Clinical suspicion is necessary to facilitate prompt diagnosis and therapy of postoperative PE.
- Initial treatment for acute PE is subcutaneous LMWH or fondaparinux.

COMPREHENSION QUESTIONS

1. All of the following can reduce postoperative pulmonary complications, except which one?

   A. Postoperative pain control that relies solely on narcotic medications
   B. Inspirex use in the postoperative state
   C. Preoperative chest physical therapy
   D. Preoperative smoking cessation >7 weeks prior to surgery

2. You have finished in the operating room after a long day. You are called to see the first patient you operated on this morning (total laparoscopic hysterectomy) due to abdominal pain. She is in the recovery room, has normal vital signs, has ambulated, has urinated 150 cm^3, and is tolerating clear liquids, but her pain is not well controlled.

   On examination she is very tender just above the pubic bone. She also thinks that she did not empty her bladder completely, but the nurse said she used the bed pan to urinate. What is your next step?

   A. Take her back to the operating room as she must have a bowel or bladder injury.
   B. CT scan of the abdomen/pelvis to look for evidence of surgical injury.
   C. Complete blood count to look for evidence of anemia and/or infection.
   D. In and out catheterization of the bladder.

3. What is the initial treatment of a pulmonary embolism in a patient without significant contraindications?

   A. LMWH
   B. Warfarin
   C. Filter in the inferior vena cava
   D. Thrombolytics
   E. Embolectomy

Answers

1. **A.** Preoperative smoking cessation (>7 weeks) and chest physical therapy have been shown to reduce postoperative respiratory complications. Postoperatively, the use of the inspirex to ensure complete lung expansion helps to decrease post-operative atelectasis and hypoxemia. Narcotic medications have a tendency to decrease respiratory drive, and therefore decrease lung expansion, so the goal should be a multimodal pain control regimen minimizing narcotic use.

2. **D.** The scenario is not an uncommon one. The patient has pain due to an overdistended urinary bladder. The urine output recorded by the nurse is likely "overflow," meaning the bladder is so distended that it has reached its capacity and is leaking. Imaging, a trip back to the OR, or blood work is not needed. Catheterization of the bladder will alleviate the situation, and then you must determine whether bladder rest is needed.

3. **A.** LMWH is the initial treatment of choice in patients without risk factors. It is easy to administer, has a manageable half-life, and has predictable pharmacokinetics.

SUGGESTED READINGS

Fedullo PF, Tapson VF. Clinical practice. The evaluation of suspected pulmonary embolism. *N Engl J Med.* 2003;349(13):1247–1256.

Guyatt GH, Akl EA, Crowther M, et al. Executive summary: Antithrombotic Therapy and Prevention of Thrombosis, 9th ed: American College of Chest Physicians Evidence-based Clinical Practice Guidelines. *Chest.* 2012;141(2 suppl):7S–47S.

Haynes AB, Weiser TG, Berry WR, et al. Changes in safety attitude and relationship to decreased postoperative morbidity and mortality following implementation of a checklist-based surgical safety intervention. *BMJ Qual Saf.* 2011;20(1):102.

Møller AM, Villebro N, Pedersen T, Tønnesen H. Effect of preoperative smoking intervention on postoperative complications: a randomised clinical trial. *Lancet.* 2002;359:114.

Section II.
Obstetrics

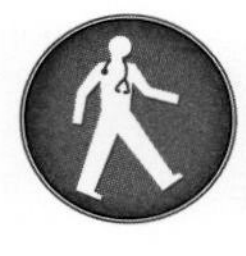

A 27-year-old Postpartum Patient Admitted to the Surgical Intensive Care Unit

Heidi G. Bell, MD, Keith H. Nelson, MD, and James E. de Vente, MD, PhD

A 27-year-old G3P2002 is brought to your Surgical Intensive Care Unit (SICU) where you are rotating as an intern. She is at 30 weeks of gestation and was involved in a rollover motor vehicle collision today. She sustained a femur fracture that has been surgically corrected. Her blood pressure is 110/70, pulse 120, and respiratory rate 16. She complains of leg and abdominal pain. Fetal heart rate by auscultation is in the 150s. There is no vaginal bleeding.

1. What is your assessment of the patient's vital signs?

2. What are some of the most important principles of management for this patient?

Answers

1. The patient is tachycardic. These changes may be due to pain and anxiety, but a pregnant patient typically does not become tachycardic until she has lost more blood than would be required in a nonpregnant patient, and this possibility should be examined carefully. The fetal heart rate is in the normal range.

2. The changes in physiology during pregnancy are profound and important to understand when taking care of critically ill obstetric patients (see Table 16-1). They begin to occur in the first trimester—do not be fooled just because a patient doesn't yet have a large gravid uterus. These changes can be categorized into 4 main responses to the pregnancy:

   - Support of the fetus (volume, nutrient and oxygen supply, and clearance of fetal waste)
   - Protection of the fetus (from starvation, toxins, and the maternal immune system)
   - Preparation of the uterus for labor
   - Protection of the mother from blood loss at delivery

   These 4 responses can often be predicted by the learner reasoning through 3 fundamental physiologic alterations:

   - Hypercoagulability
   - Immunosuppression
   - Smooth muscle relaxation

Table 16-1. Quick Facts for Review on the Elevator Up to Evaluate the Pregnant Patient in the ICU

- Compensated respiratory alkalosis, with normal ABG values: pH 7.4-7.53, pco_2 25-33 mm Hg, HCO_3 18 mEq/L
- Respiratory rate does *not* change
- Cardiac output increases by 50%
- GFR increases by 50%
- Heart rate may increase slightly, but rarely above 100
- White blood cell count may be increased to as high as 14,000 in the normal pregnant patient

CASE REVIEW

Unless there is a fellowship in maternal trauma/critical care at your program, maternal trauma/critical care cases will be rare. There are a few facts about maternal physiology that you will need at your fingertips to care for critically ill pregnant patients:

- Arterial blood gas (ABG): pregnancy is a state of compensated respiratory alkalosis:
  - pH 7.4 to 7.53 (nonpregnant 7.38-7.42).
  - pco_2 25 to 33 mm Hg (nonpregnant 38-42)—if above 35 in the pregnant patient, consider intubation!
  - Bicarbonate 16 to 22 mEq/L (nonpregnant 22-26)—a decreased capacity to buffer acidosis.
- Cardiac output: increased to about 6 L/min (nonpregnant 4 L/min)
- Heart rate: increased by up to 20% near term (but rarely above 100 bpm)

Rarely do educators advocate rote memorization, but in emergency situations there is critical information that you will need—the items above are only the minimum that you need to care for a critically ill patient.

In our sample case, the elevated heart rate is concerning because a tachycardic response to hypovolemia requires greater blood loss in a pregnant patient than in a nonpregnant patient. Blood volume increases by about 50% in pregnancy, which can mask the physiologic signs of hypovolemia caused by hemorrhage until life-threatening blood loss has occurred. The patient presented in this case should be examined carefully, observed closely, and have laboratory testing performed promptly to evaluate for the possibility of obstetric hemorrhage complicating her orthopedic injury. While she is being monitored, she should be correctly positioned with left lateral uterine displacement.

MATERNAL PHYSIOLOGY IN PREGNANCY

Basic Principles

Maternal physiology is altered to protect and nourish the fetus and guard the mother from cardiac injury during delivery. A reasonable rule of thumb if you are asked about a physiologic change in pregnancy is "it increases by about 50%." This guideline applies to cardiac output, glomerular filtration rate (GFR), blood volume, and many other parameters. It may be simpler to learn the exceptions as we examine organ systems affected by pregnancy. The basic principles of immunosuppression, hypercoagulability, and smooth muscle relaxation are also a good way to remember physiologic modifications of pregnancy. The learner should be aware that during the labor and delivery process specifically, there is a whole different set of changes that occur in maternal physiology, especially with regards to the cardiovascular system, which are beyond the scope of this chapter.

Cardiovascular system

The maternal cardiovascular system tries to protect itself from blood loss at delivery. Blood volume increases by about 50%. Red cell volume only rises by 33% compared with a greater increase in plasma volume, so the apparent effect is referred to as the physiologic anemia of pregnancy. Cardiac output increases by about 50%. Systemic vascular resistance (and therefore blood pressure) decreases in early pregnancy, nadirs around 14 to 24 weeks, and then increases progressively to approach prepregnancy levels at term. Lateral displacement of the gravid, third-trimester uterus by positioning a mother on her left side rather than supine can increase cardiac output by as much as 14%.

Hematologic system

The principle of hypercoagulability will help you remember that most clotting factor levels increase during pregnancy. White blood cell counts increase and may still be normal at 14,000/mL. Most sources use 5000 to 12,000/mL as normal levels in pregnancy. Platelet counts may drop slightly but should not be interpreted differently during pregnancy than in the nonpregnant patient.

Respiratory system

As discussed at the beginning of the section "Case Review," pregnancy is a state of compensated respiratory alkalosis. This change supports fetal oxygenation and waste removal since the maternal pco_2 falls below that of the fetus to facilitate CO_2 exchange from fetus to mother. Mucosal edema and hypervascularity of the airways may make pregnant patients more difficult to intubate.

Many pregnant women perceive an increased work of breathing due to loss of abdominal muscle tone necessitating greater use of accessory muscles. Total lung capacity and functional residual capacity decrease because of decreased reserve volumes and diaphragmatic elevation, but minute ventilation, alveolar ventilation, and tidal volume all increase by 30% to 50%. Respiratory rate does *not* change despite the overall effect of hyperventilation. Tachypnea in the pregnant patient should be evaluated just as in the nonpregnant patient.

Genitourinary system

The GFR increases by about 50%. Smooth muscle relaxation in the ureter leads to physiologic hydronephrosis and an increased risk for pyelonephritis. Glucosuria will occur in about 1 in 6 normal women during pregnancy, but diabetes should still be considered when it is seen. Serum creatinine levels may fall to 0.5 mg/dL or lower, so values above 0.9 mg/dL should prompt evaluation for underlying renal disease.

Gastrointestinal system

Smooth muscle relaxation is the primary driver of the following physiologic changes in pregnancy:

- Increased gastroesophageal reflux due to relaxation of the lower esophageal sphincter
- Delayed gastric emptying time (which may increase risk of aspiration pneumonitis with anesthesia)
- Decreased gallbladder contractility causing cholestasis and/or an increased prevalence of gallstones
- Increased constipation due to relaxation and slowing of the colon

There is also increased blood flow to the liver, which combined with an increased GFR causes increased clearance and decreased half-lives of medications during pregnancy. Liver enzyme levels remain essentially unchanged with the exception of alkaline phosphatase, which is produced in large amounts by the placenta.

Endocrine system

During normal pregnancy, the pituitary gland may enlarge by as much as 135% of the nonpregnant size (a notable exception to the "increases by 50%" rule). This has clinical implications in patients with pituitary adenomas and also predisposes patients to pituitary necrosis in severe postpartum hemorrhage since the blood supply is a portal system. The thyroid gland enlarges and increases production of thyroid hormones by 40% to 100%. Thyroid-stimulating hormone (TSH) levels may decrease (another exception to the 50% rule) during pregnancy due to high levels of human chorionic gonadotropin (hCG), which shares the same alpha subunit as TSH and may therefore stimulate thyroid receptors. Overall, however, pregnancy should be a clinically euthyroid state, since thyroid-binding globulin also increases and therefore free T3 and T4 levels should remain the same.

Pregnancy is also a state of relative glucose intolerance, leading to gestational diabetes in some women. Largely due to the effects of human placental lactogen

(HPL) from the placenta, maternal insulin resistance increases in order to increase glucose availability to the fetus.

Musculoskeletal system

A woman's center of gravity in pregnancy changes before the uterus is visually apparent. Relaxation of tendons and ligaments and lordosis induced by the pregnancy will modify a patient's posture and balance. The bones and ligaments of the pelvis undergo relaxation, which can lead to pain in the symphysis pubis or hips and cause the characteristic gait seen in gravid patients.

Immune system

The physiologic effects of immunocompromise are seen as the fetus, which is functionally an allograft, is protected from the maternal immune system. The major change is an alteration of the balance away from cell-mediated immunity toward humoral immunity. This shift leads to increased susceptibility to intracellular pathogens and may lead to improvement in cell-mediated immunopathologic diseases such as rheumatoid arthritis. The apparently counterintuitive increase in white blood cells is due to recirculation of previously marginalized leukocytes. These marginalized leukocytes may also explain the shift in white cell differential toward more immature forms.

TIPS TO REMEMBER

- Physiologic changes in pregnancy are governed by hypercoagulability, immunocompromise, and smooth muscle relaxation.
- Increased maternal tolerance to acute blood loss requires increased vigilance in patients following trauma.
- Most physiologic alterations in pregnancy relate to support and protection of the fetus, preparation of the mother for delivery, and protection of the mother from delivery-related blood loss.

COMPREHENSION QUESTIONS

1. A hospitalized patient reports shortness of breath in labor and is found to be tachypneic with a respiratory rate of 30. Oxygen is administered by non-rebreather face mask at 10 L/min and an ABG is drawn. The lab calls with the following result:

pH 7.30
po_2 60 mm Hg
pco_2 40 mm Hg
HCO_3 12 mEq/L

The most appropriate management of this result is which of the following?

A. Administration of furosemide
B. Intubation
C. Reassurance and observation
D. Repositioning in decubitus position

2. Smooth muscle relaxation causes which of the following symptoms in normal pregnancy?

A. Constipation
B. Decreased gastric emptying time
C. Decreased incidence of gastroesophageal reflux
D. Glucose intolerance
E. Hypothyroidism

3. Which of the following laboratory or physiologic parameters is *abnormal* for a pregnant patient?

A. Alkaline phosphatase 200 U/L
B. Heart rate 96 bpm
C. Respiratory rate 24 breaths/min
D. Serum creatinine 0.5 mg/dL
E. Glucosuria

Answers

1. **B**. This is one of the few facts that *must* be understood and remembered by anyone who will be in a position to take care of pregnant women who are critically ill. A pregnant woman may be truly in danger of respiratory failure with ABG values that the lab will report as "normal." Furosemide may be a reasonable intervention, but this patient is really in respiratory distress/pending failure and should be intubated at this time. Reassurance and observation is not a reasonable option with this ABG in pregnancy. Repositioning will help to oxygenate the fetus, but not the mother.

2. **A**. Constipation is caused by smooth muscle relaxation in the colon, leading to increased transit times through the colon and increased water absorption from stool. Gastric emptying time is increased, reflux is increased due to relaxation of the lower esophageal sphincter, glucose intolerance is not mediated by smooth muscle relaxation, and hypothyroidism is not normal in pregnancy.

3. **C**. Respiratory rate does not change appreciably during pregnancy, so a pregnant patient with tachypnea should be evaluated just as a nonpregnant patient. Increased alkaline phosphatase, decreased serum creatinine, and decreased pco_2 will be reported by most commercial labs as "abnormal," although they are

normal in the pregnant patient. Blood pressure may drop in the midtrimester of pregnancy below baseline values, but should primarily be evaluated with the individual patient's baseline values in mind. Glucosuria may be present in up to 1/6 pregnant women due to increased GFR.

SUGGESTED READINGS

Clark SL, Cotton DB, Lee W, et al. Central hemodynamic assessment of normal term pregnancy. *Am J Obstet Gynecol.* 1989;161:1439–1442.

Maternal physiology. In: Cunningham GF, Leveno KJ, Bloom SL, Hauth JC, Rouse DJ, Spong CY, eds. *Williams Obstetrics.* 23rd ed. New York, NY: The McGraw-Hill Companies Inc; 2010:107–135.

Norwitz ER, Robinson JN. Pregnancy-induced physiologic alterations. In: Belfort M, Saade G, Foley M, Phelan J, Dildy G, eds. *Critical Care Obstetrics.* 5th ed. Chichester, UK: John Wiley and Sons Ltd; 2010:30–51.

Sibai BM, Frangeih A. Maternal adaptation to pregnancy. *Curr Opin Obstet Gynecol.* 1995;7:420–426.

Yeomans ER, Gilstrap LC. Physiologic changes in pregnancy and their impact on critical care. *Crit Care Med.* 2005;33(10S):S256–S258.

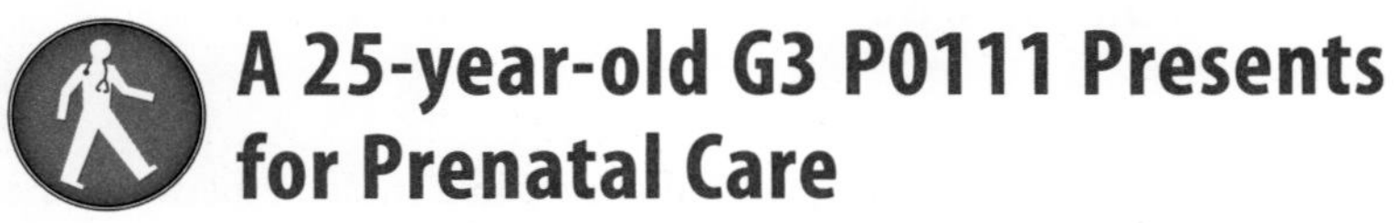

A 25-year-old G3 P0111 Presents for Prenatal Care

Edward R. Yeomans, MD

A 25-year-old African-American woman G3 P0111 presents for her first prenatal visit at 16-weeks gestational age by uncertain last menstrual period (LMP). She smokes 1 pack of cigarettes per day, but denies other types of substance abuse. Review of labs drawn at a nurse screening visit 2 weeks earlier is remarkable for O-negative blood type with a positive antibody screen. You are an intern meeting this patient for the first time.

1. What issues require immediate action based on this brief history?

2. What percent of women initiate prenatal care after the first trimester?

Answers

1. At the time of this first visit, you are responsible for performing a detailed history and physical examination (H&P) and reviewing laboratory data. Assuming that no additional issues are discovered, your encounter with this patient must address at least 4 points:
   a. Establish gestational age.
   b. Obtain information regarding her past obstetric history.
   c. Counsel the patient to stop smoking.
   d. Identify the antibody and request a titer.
2. Twice as many African-American women present for prenatal care after the first trimester as Caucasians (24% compared with 12%). Such late presentation means missing an opportunity to accurately determine gestational age in a woman with an unsure LMP. The opportunity to offer first trimester screening for aneuploidy has also been lost.

CASE REVIEW

With a few noteworthy exceptions, the new OB H&P requires the same structured approach as any other H&Ps. Those exceptions are illuminated by the present case. The most important piece of information that affects later pregnancy management is an accurate estimate of gestational age. Many pregnancies are dated by the LMP. The estimated date of delivery (EDD) is calculated from the LMP by subtracting 3 months from the LMP and adding 7 days (Naegele's Rule). However, this woman did not know her LMP. Physical examination can add some useful information, for example, a fundus palpable midway between the symphysis pubis and the umbilicus would be consistent with 16 weeks. It would be reasonable to order an ultrasound (US) examination to establish dates in this case. The US estimate of gestational age can be used to order a quad screen for open neural tube defects and aneuploidy between 15 and 21 weeks if the patient desires screening. If the patient is close to 16 weeks, the accuracy of the sonogram is ±10 days. In contrast, a first trimester US is accurate to within ±4 days. (For further details, please refer to Chapter 18.)

The past obstetric history of this patient is also important and provides a clue to her positive antibody screen. Her first pregnancy was a ruptured ectopic at 8 weeks, but she did not receive RhoGAM after the surgery. In her second pregnancy, she was weakly positive for anti-D antibody and she had a spontaneous preterm vaginal delivery at 34 weeks. Her antibody screen this time is highly likely to be anti-D again, but the titer will be important for management. If it is ≥16 (titers were formerly expressed as ratios such as 1:2, 1:4, 1:8, but are now expressed as a whole number using only the denominator; the higher the number, the greater the amount of circulating antibody), then serial Doppler assessment of peak systolic velocity in the fetal middle cerebral artery may be indicated.

Finally, cigarette smoking increases the risk of a number of adverse outcomes including preterm birth, preterm premature rupture of membranes, placenta previa, and abruption of the placenta. At this first visit, the patient should be advised to stop smoking. This issue should then be assessed at subsequent visits. She should be told that smoking may have contributed to her previous preterm birth and that it will again be a factor if her behavior continues during the current pregnancy. Based on her prior spontaneous preterm birth, she should be counseled regarding 17-hydroxyprogesterone injections.

PRENATAL CARE

The provision of comprehensive prenatal care is important to residents at all levels of training. Fourth-year students planning to pursue a career in obstetrics and gynecology should familiarize themselves with a standard prenatal record such as the one prepared by the American College of Obstetricians and Gynecologists. This record is quite detailed and relevant information may be missed by a cursory or careless H&P. Once the form has been completed (these days often electronically), it should be reviewed at each subsequent visit to avoid overlooking important checkpoints. A wise precaution given to me many years ago is "bad prenatal care may be worse than none."

The case used to introduce the topic of prenatal care illustrated some important elements, but residents should address all of the items listed in Table 17-1 at the first visit. Subsequent visits are much quicker; an organizational scheme for a return OB visit is shown in Table 17-2. Finally, relevant OB labs are provided in Table 17-3.

Table 17-1. Outline of First Visit

Menstrual history
Past obstetric history
Past medical/surgical history
Genetic screening
Infections/immunization
Physical examination
Problem list[a]
Dating criteria

[a]This should be updated as pregnancy progresses.

Table 17-2. Return OB Visit

Ask patient for new complaints/questions
Check weight, blood pressure, dipstick urine
Measure fundal height
Listen to fetal heart tones
Ascertain presentation by abdominal examination (at ≥26 weeks)
Document fetal movement (at ≥20 weeks)
Review lab/ultrasound data
Schedule return appointment

Table 17-3. OB Labs

Blood type and Rh status
Antibody screen
Hemoglobin/hematocrit
Test for syphilis, rubella, hepatitis B, HIV
Gonorrhea, chlamydia, Pap
Urinalysis/culture
Special tests: quad screen, glucose challenge test, cystic fibrosis test
Screen for group B *Streptococcus* (35-37 weeks)

From the labs listed in Table 17-3, it is apparent that screening for various types of infection is an important component of prenatal care. An exhaustive discussion of the various infectious diseases for which screening is recommended is beyond the scope of this chapter. Instead, the change in approach to screening for 2 specific infections will be considered. First, syphilis screening with serologic testing has long been a standard element of prenatal care. High-risk women should be screened again in the third trimester. However, the time-honored approach of screening with a nonspecific test (either RPR or VDRL), followed by a specific test (MHA-TP or FTA-ABS) for only those women with a positive nonspecific test, has changed. Since 2009, the initial test is a *Treponema*-specific IgG test. Since this test is applied to a large group of predominantly low-risk women, residents and fully trained physicians will occasionally be confronted with a false-positive IgG. Complex algorithms have been published to assist with this task.

Second, group B beta-hemolytic *Streptococcus* (GBS) is arguably the most important bacterial perinatal pathogen. Intrapartum administration of antibiotics was shown in a classic article to reduce vertical transmission from mother to infant. The question that arose following the publication of that article was how best to identify women who need treatment. It was shown in large studies that routine screening of all pregnant women (as shown at the bottom of Table 17-3) is more effective than a risk factor–based approach, and that is the current recommendation. Intravenous penicillin G has emerged as the treatment of choice and algorithms have been published to guide treatment of culture-positive women with allergy to penicillin. Screening for infection has added to the complexity of modern prenatal care. Even so, there are more than 20 perinatal infections for which screening is *not* recommended.

A strong case can be made for constructing and regularly updating a problem list for all prenatal care with at least 2 columns: problem on the left and intervention on the right. For example, a problem might be "Rh negative" and the intervention would be to "administer RhoGAM at 28 weeks."

The overall effectiveness of prenatal care is striking: it has contributed to a reduction in maternal mortality, stillbirth, neonatal death, and preterm birth. It allows for education of young (and old) mothers and helps to foster development of a strong and trusting doctor–patient relationship. Mastering the provision of comprehensive and compassionate prenatal care is an important goal of students entering the field of obstetrics and gynecology and one of the key chapters in this book on resident readiness.

TIPS TO REMEMBER

- Familiarize yourself with a standard Prenatal Care form such as the one promoted by the ACOG.
- When screening discloses the presence of or risk for a perinatal infection, read about the particular infection and adhere to published guidelines.

- Use the short, but frequent visits for prenatal care to educate your patients and build a strong doctor–patient relationship.
- Make, use, and update a problem list. This feature is incorporated into many current electronic health records.

COMPREHENSION QUESTIONS

1. What is the accuracy of an US-estimated gestational age of 16 weeks?
    A. ±4 days
    B. ±10 days
    C. ±14 days
    D. ±21 days

2. In the case presented, why should an US be ordered before requesting a quad screen?
    A. To look for evidence of hemorrhage
    B. To look for choroid plexus cysts
    C. To establish gestational age since the interpretation of the quad screen is gestational age dependent
    D. To perform a fetal anatomic survey

3. Which of the following infections should *not* be screened for at the initial OB visit?
    A. Gonorrhea
    B. Chlamydia
    C. Syphilis
    D. Group B *Streptococcus*

Answers

1. **B.** This answer is taken straight from the chapter. The other choices apply to different gestational ages:

    A: Crown–rump length measurement at 6 to 13 weeks

    C: Second trimester US at 20 to 26 weeks

    D: Third trimester US at ≥26 weeks

2. **C.** The interpretation of a quad screen is critically dependent on gestational age. The woman in the case presentation did not know the date of her LMP, so US is a necessary step in establishing gestational age. A quad screen, appropriately named, consists of assaying 4 substances in maternal blood: beta hCG,

alpha-fetoprotein, unconjugated estriol, and inhibin A. Results are valid only if drawn between 15 and 21 weeks.

Choice A—this patient gave no history of bleeding.

Choice B—choroid plexus cysts can be seen at 16 weeks, but have no bearing on the quad screen.

Choice D—the anatomic survey should be performed at 20 to 22 weeks.

3. **D**. Group B *Streptococcus* should be screened for at 35 to 37 weeks (Table 17-3). All the others should be screened at entry to care.

SUGGESTED READINGS

American Academy of Pediatricians, American College of Obstetricians and Gynecologists. American College of Obstetricians and Gynecologists' Antepartum Record and Postpartum Form. In: *AAP/ACOG Guidelines for Perinatal Care*. 6th ed. Elk Grove Village, IL: American Academy of Pediatricians, American College of Obstetricians and Gynecologists; 2007:463–476 [Appendix A].

American College of Obstetricians and Gynecologists: Committee Opinion No. 279. Prevention of early-onset group B streptococcal disease in newborns. *Obstet Gynecol.* 2002;100:1405–1412.

Boyer KM, Gotoff SP. Prevention of early onset neonatal group B streptococcal disease with selective intrapartum chemoprophylaxis. *N Engl J Med.* 1986;314:1665–1669.

Peterman T, Schillinger J, Blank S, et al. Syphilis testing algorithms using treponemal tests for initial screening—four laboratories, New York City, 2005-2006. *MMWR.* 2008;57(32):872–875.

Prenatal care. In: Cunningham FG, Leveno KJ, Bloom SL, Hauth JC, Rouse DJ, Spong CY, eds. *Williams Obstetrics.* 23rd ed. New York, NY: The McGraw-Hill Companies Inc; 2010:189–214.

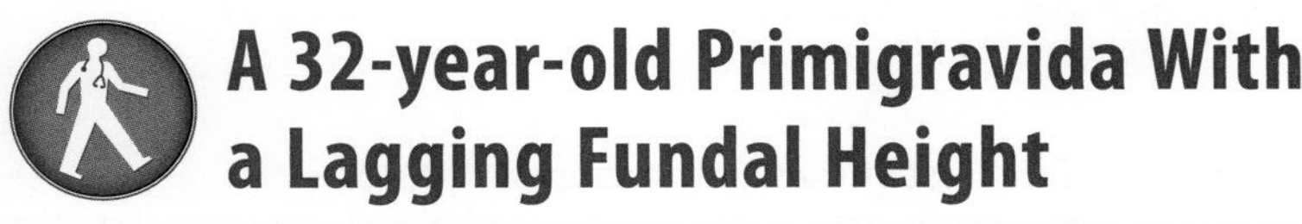

A 32-year-old Primigravida With a Lagging Fundal Height

Roxane Holt, MD

A 32-year-old G1P0 at 32 weeks comes to her scheduled clinic appointment. She does not have any medical problems, and her antepartum course has been uncomplicated. Fetal heart tones are in the 140s. Fundal height measures 28 cm.

1. How do you evaluate this patient?

Answer

1. This patient has been diagnosed with size less than dates by physical examination. The fundal height is much less than the gestational age. The fetus may be growth restricted. Ordering an obstetric ultrasound to evaluate fetal growth is appropriate.

CASE REVIEW

The routine clinic visit for the obstetric patient includes assessing maternal status by asking if she has had any complications such as leaking fluid, bleeding, contractions, or decreased fetal movement. The basic physical examination at each low-risk obstetric appointment after 20 weeks includes checking the weight and blood pressure of the patient, measuring fetal heart tones, and assessing fundal height. In this case, fundal height is lagging the gestational age of 32 weeks by 4 cm. This may represent intrauterine growth restriction (IUGR), or the recently preferred term of fetal growth restriction (FGR).

OBSTETRIC ULTRASOUND

Indications

There are multiple indications for the use of ultrasound during pregnancy. This chapter is not intended to cover every indication, but only the ones that will be most pertinent to the intern. Ultrasound during the first trimester can be used to determine the location of the pregnancy, confirm cardiac activity, evaluate vaginal bleeding and pelvic pain, estimate gestational age, determine number of fetuses, screen for aneuploidy, and evaluate for molar pregnancy (see Table 18-1). The first trimester ultrasound can be performed transabdominally or transvaginally. During the second and third trimesters, ultrasound can be used for some of the same indications as the first trimester, but it has additional uses as well

Table 18-1. Indications for First Trimester Ultrasound

Determine location of the pregnancy
Confirm cardiac motion
Evaluate vaginal bleeding
Evaluate pelvic pain
Estimate gestational age
Screen for aneuploidy
Guide for chorionic villus sampling
Evaluate for molar pregnancy

(see Table 18-2). Evaluation of fetal anatomy is best achieved during the mid-second trimester at 18 to 20 weeks. At this time a wide range of anomalies can be identified. If anomalies are identified, then ultrasound can be used to guide the needle for amniocentesis to evaluate for aneuploidy. Fetal presentation and growth can be evaluated. Amniotic fluid volume can be indirectly assessed, and the location of the placenta can be ascertained.

Table 18-2. Indications for Second and Third Trimester Ultrasounds

Determine location of the pregnancy
Confirm cardiac motion
Diagnose multiple gestations
Vaginal bleeding
Pelvic pain
Estimate gestational age
Evaluate for molar pregnancy
Evaluate anatomy
Determine placental location
Guide for amniocentesis
Determine fetal presentation
Assess growth
Determine amniotic fluid volume

Use of the Ultrasound

When evaluating your obstetric patient, it is important to consider if the patient needs an ultrasound. If she is presenting in the first trimester, ask if the patient has an unsure LMP, has vaginal bleeding or pelvic pain, or has a desire for early aneuploidy screening. If the answer is yes, then ordering a first trimester ultrasound is appropriate after the physical examination is performed. The physical examination should be performed before an ultrasound is requested to confirm that the patient is in fact in her first trimester. The first trimester ultrasound uses the gestational sac size or the crown–rump length of the fetus if it is present to establish the gestational age of the pregnancy. If the estimated gestational age is more than 7 days different from the LMP during the first trimester, then the ultrasound measurements should be used to determine estimated gestational age rather than the LMP.

During the second and third trimesters, ultrasound can also be used to estimate the gestational age of the pregnancy by making fetal measurements. During this time, 4 parameters are used to measure the fetus, which include the head circumference, biparietal diameter, abdominal circumference, and femur length. If the ultrasound-estimated gestational age is more than 10 days from the gestational age estimated by the LMP, then the ultrasound should be used to date the pregnancy. One should be cautious before redating a pregnancy by an ultrasound during the third trimester. The accuracy of the estimated due date is only ±3 to 4 weeks at this time. If a patient is 36 weeks on her third trimester ultrasound when she states she is 40 weeks, this could mean carrying the pregnancy post term when perhaps she has a growth-restricted or small fetus rather than a premature one. During the second and third trimester clinic visits, it is important to ask your patient if she has had vaginal bleeding. If there is vaginal bleeding, do not do a digital examination. If the placenta covers the cervix (placenta previa), digital examination could cause profuse bleeding. A speculum examination can safely be performed to assess the bleeding followed by ultrasound to evaluate for placental location. During the clinic visit, uterine growth can be assessed by pelvic examination before 18 weeks or by fundal height after 18 weeks. Fundal height in centimeters should be within 2 weeks of gestational age between 20 and 34 weeks. However, obesity can falsely increase the fundal height. In addition, FGR can be missed in one third of cases. If the fundal height is lagging as it is in our case presentation, then ordering an ultrasound for size less than dates is appropriate.

FGR is diagnosed when the estimated fetal weight by ultrasound is less than the 10th percentile for gestational age. Importantly 10% of neonates will be at or below the 10th percentile by weight. However, it is difficult to determine which fetuses are constitutionally small versus growth restricted. There is increased morbidity and adverse perinatal outcomes when fetuses measure less than the third percentile. When FGR is diagnosed by ultrasound, there are further tests that can be used to determine if the fetus is at risk for fetal death. Assessing the amniotic fluid volume by measuring the deepest pocket of fluid in 4 quadrants is defined as the amniotic fluid index. Oligohydramnios is present when an amniotic fluid index of less than 5 cm is found. Oligohydramnios in the setting of a fetal weight less than the 10th percentile increases the risk of fetal death. Umbilical artery Doppler velocimetry can also be used to evaluate growth-restricted fetuses. The Doppler effect or frequency shift during systole and diastole in the umbilical artery is proportional to the velocity of the blood flow in the umbilical artery. The placenta should be a low-resistance organ allowing blood to flow from the fetal umbilical arteries to the placenta. Placental resistance decreases as the pregnancy progresses and placental arterioles proliferate. When there is low resistance in the placenta, flow will be seen in the umbilical artery during systole and diastole. As placental arterioles pathologically decrease, the resistance in the placenta increases leading to a decrease in end-diastolic flow in the umbilical artery. This will cause the S/D ratio of the frequency shift during systole (S) divided by the frequency shift during diastole (D) to increase. These findings can progress to an absence of end-diastolic flow in the umbilical artery that may predict perinatal mortality. Most concerning is reversal of flow during diastole in the umbilical artery representing blood flow back toward the fetus. Both absent and reversed end-diastolic flows are associated with increased perinatal morbidity and mortality. Therefore, if a fetus has abnormal umbilical artery Dopplers at term, then delivery may be indicated. If the fetus is preterm, then the risks and benefits of preterm delivery must be weighed against the findings of the ultrasound to determine if delivery is indicated. In the case presented, an ultrasound for growth and amniotic fluid assessment would be appropriate with umbilical artery Dopplers then performed if the estimated fetal weight is less than the 10% for gestational age.

TIPS TO REMEMBER

- The physical examination is not replaced by the obstetric ultrasound.
- Indications for ultrasound can be found in Tables 18-1 and 18-2.
- Consider changing the estimated due date if the ultrasound differs by more than 7 days in the first trimester, or by more than 10 days in the early second trimester.
- When ordering an ultrasound, it is important to include the indication and LMP on the request. In addition, document any medical problems that the mother has on the request.
- When growth restriction is suspected by an estimated fetal weight less than the 10th percentile for gestational age, amniotic fluid assessment and umbilical artery Dopplers are important in evaluating the risk for perinatal morbidity and mortality.

COMPREHENSION QUESTIONS

1. The patient's LMP gives a gestational age of 8w1d, but ultrasound shows a crown–rump length with a gestational age of 6w3d. What should be done next?

   A. Continue using the LMP as the method to estimate the gestational age of the pregnancy.
   B. Change the gestational age of the pregnancy to match the gestational age determined by the ultrasound.
   C. Obtain a second trimester ultrasound to see if it matches her gestational age established by her LMP.
   D. Obtain serial ultrasounds to determine the gestational age of the fetus.

2. When FGR has been diagnosed on ultrasound, which of the following should be evaluated?

   A. Uterine artery Dopplers
   B. Middle cerebral artery Dopplers
   C. Umbilical artery Dopplers
   D. Umbilical vein Dopplers

3. The patient comes to her first obstetric clinic visit. Her pregnancy test is positive, and she tells you she is unsure when her last LMP was. What do you do next?

   A. Complete history and physical examination.
   B. Obtain fetal heart tones.
   C. Send her to the ultrasound suite for a dating ultrasound.
   D. Obtain initial obstetric labs.

Answers

1. **B.** The ultrasound-estimated gestational age is more than 7 days off from the gestational age estimated by her LMP. Therefore, the ultrasound should be used to establish the gestational age and estimated due date.

2. **C.** Umbilical artery Dopplers can be used to evaluate growth-restricted fetuses. Both absent and reversed end-diastolic flows are abnormal Doppler findings that indicate the fetus is at increased risk for perinatal morbidity and mortality.

3. **A.** A complete history and physical examination should be performed before an ultrasound is ordered. The physical examination can be used to determine if the patient is in the first or second trimester, and this can impact whether you request a first trimester scan or a second trimester scan for dating and anatomy evaluation.

SUGGESTED READINGS

American College of Obstetricians and Gynecologists. ACOG Practice Bulletin No. 134: fetal growth restriction. *Obstet Gynecol.* 2013;121(5):1122–1133.

American College of Obstetricians and Gynecologists. ACOG Practice Bulletin No. 101: ultrasonography in pregnancy. *Obstet Gynecol.* 2009;113(2 Pt 1):451–461.

Fetal growth disorders. In: Cunningham GF, Leveno KJ, Bloom SL, Hauth JC, Rouse DJ, Spong CY, eds. *Williams Obstetrics*. 23rd ed. New York, NY: The McGraw-Hill Companies Inc; 2010:842–858.

McIntire DD, Bloom SL, Casey BM, Leveno KJ. Birth weight in relation to morbidity and mortality among newborn infants. *N Engl J Med.* 1999;340:1234–1238.

Prenatal care. In: Cunningham GF, Leveno KJ, Bloom SL, Hauth JC, Rouse DJ, Spong CY, eds. *Williams Obstetrics*. 23rd ed. New York, NY: The McGraw-Hill Companies Inc; 2010:189–214.

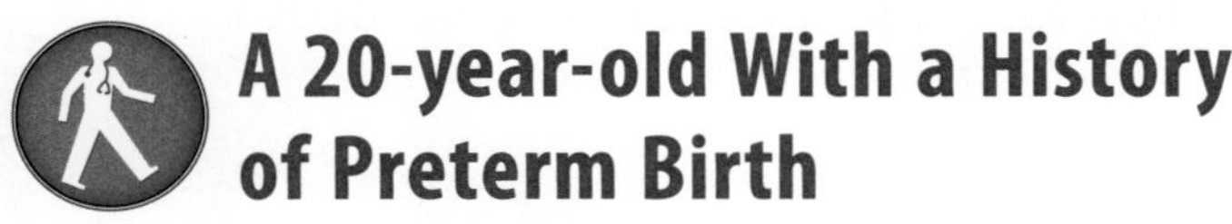

A 20-year-old With a History of Preterm Birth

Edward R. Yeomans, MD

A 20-year-old woman G3 P0202 presents to clinic at 16 weeks gestation by an 11-week ultrasound. Her past obstetric history is remarkable for 2 spontaneous preterm births (SPTBs), the first at 32 weeks and the second at 28 weeks. She states that in each pregnancy she just began to contract with gradually increasing pain and frequency. Membranes did not rupture until late in the labor course both times. Past medical and surgical history are negative. Her only medications are iron and vitamins. Both her babies required mechanical ventilation and extended NICU stays, but appear to be doing well now, having met appropriate developmental milestones. This young woman would like to know whether anything can be done to prevent another preterm birth.

1. How do you diagnose preterm labor?

2. Can anything be done to prevent preterm birth?

Answers

1. The diagnosis of preterm labor is frequently incorrect. More often it is overdiagnosed, but underdiagnosis can lead to the birth of an extremely preterm infant in a setting ill-equipped to deal with the problem. More than 20 years ago, Dr Creasy suggested some criteria for diagnosis pertaining to the cervix: ≥2 cm dilated, ≥80% effaced or changed to the same examiner, all in conjunction with uterine activity defined as 4 contractions in 20 minutes or 8 in an hour. However, if the patient is remote from term, she may not actually complain of contractions; instead, subtle or seemingly unrelated complaints such as back pain, menstrual cramps, pelvic pressure, or change in vaginal discharge may signal the onset of preterm labor. History and physical examination are important, as noted above, but there are other techniques in diagnosis of preterm labor (cervical length by ultrasound, fetal fibronectin, uterine activity monitoring) that will be discussed later in the chapter.

2. The current edition of *Williams Obstetrics* refers to prevention of preterm birth as an "elusive goal." Still, there are selected groups of women at risk for preterm birth for whom specific interventions may be beneficial. The patient in the case presentation has a documented history of preterm birth, and is therefore a candidate for progesterone therapy. Another small group of women with a diagnosis of incompetent cervix may benefit from placement of a cervical cerclage. Some investigators have suggested expanding this group to include women discovered to have a short cervix on ultrasound.

CASE REVIEW

In reviewing this woman's past obstetric history, a newcomer to the field might ask a reasonable question: was anything done to stop her preterm labor once it was diagnosed? A number of interventions including bed rest, hydration, sedation, and tocolytic (labor-inhibiting) drugs have been studied by multiple investigators. Unfortunately, at the present time, there are no effective treatment options. Preterm labor is probably the most important area of obstetric research in 2013. A history of preterm birth, like the patient in this scenario has, is the strongest historical predictive factor. The risk of recurrent preterm birth, even with treatment, in this case is likely 35% to 50%.

PRETERM LABOR/PRETERM BIRTH

In 2012, the American College of Obstetricians and Gynecologists issued 2 Practice Bulletins (see the section "Suggested Readings") on these important topics. The focus in this chapter will be on the management of preterm labor. However, for a broader understanding of the subject for beginners, preterm birth will be reviewed first. Preterm birth applies to any birth that occurs before 37 and 0/7 weeks (it is preferable to avoid such terminology as "the 37th week" or "37 completed weeks" and simply use the whole number and fraction as presented). The incidence of preterm birth currently stands at about 12%. It is by far the number 1 cause of neonatal mortality in the United States, but the financial and emotional burden of neonatal morbidity is enormous as well. Great advances in neonatal intensive care have improved outcomes and pushed the "threshold of viability" ever earlier: infants born at 23 weeks may now survive, but morbidity at that gestational age is very high. There are 3 antecedents of preterm birth: idiopathic preterm labor, preterm premature rupture of membranes (PPROM, covered in Chapter 20), and indicated preterm birth. The obstetric intern should ask detailed questions in a patient with a prior preterm birth to determine whether it was spontaneous (SPTB, which encompasses both idiopathic preterm birth and PPROM) or indicated. Preterm birth may be indicated for maternal, placental, or fetal reasons. Examples include severe preeclampsia, placenta previa, and severe fetal growth restriction. The subject of indicated preterm birth has been recently reviewed by Spong and colleagues, and will not be considered further here.

The patient in the scenario had idiopathic preterm labor in both of her previous pregnancies. Fewer than 10% of women with a clinical diagnosis of preterm labor actually deliver within 1 week, illustrating that the condition is frequently overdiagnosed. In fact, half of patients hospitalized for preterm labor are delivered at term. Although many centers employ fetal fibronectin testing (fetal fibronectin is a glycoprotein present in high concentration in amniotic fluid), and/or ultrasound measurement of cervical length to refine the diagnosis of preterm labor, the results have not been consistent. Currently, there is a push for routine transvaginal ultrasound measurement of cervical length to identify women at risk for preterm birth, but the limitations of such an approach are considerable.

Treatment of preterm labor is a source of frustration for practicing obstetricians. The desire to delay delivery for neonatal benefit is strong, but the benefit of many treatments (bed rest, hydration, sedation, pharmacologic tocolysis) is unproven and some treatments are potentially harmful to the mother. In the decades of the 1980s and 1990s, there were reports of maternal deaths resulting from administration of betamimetic agents to treat preterm labor. This is even more sobering when one considers that the effectiveness of such tocolysis is, at most, a 48-hour delay in delivery! Similarly, although antibiotics have been shown to prolong latency in women with PPROM, they have not been shown to prolong gestation or improve neonatal outcomes in preterm labor with intact membranes and should not be used for this indication.

There are 2 management strategies that have shown benefit for women with preterm labor. First, a single course of antenatal corticosteroids given to the mother results in reductions in neonatal mortality and morbidity. For example, corticosteroids reduce both the incidence and severity of respiratory distress syndrome (RDS). Second, magnesium sulfate given to the mother may provide protection against later development of cerebral palsy in the neonate. However, when a composite outcome of death and cerebral palsy was the end point in a large US study, magnesium sulfate did not prove beneficial.

Returning to the patient in the scenario, what can be done to prevent her from having another preterm birth? An important trial by Meis et al (see the section "Suggested Readings") evaluated the effect of 17-alpha-hydroxyprogesterone caproate administered intramuscularly weekly beginning at 16 to 20 weeks and continuing through 36 weeks compared with a group given placebo injections. All women enrolled in this trial had a history of previous SPTB. The control group had a recurrent preterm birth rate of 56%, whereas the treatment group had a rate of 37%. Although statistically and clinically significant, these results clearly indicate the high probability of recurrent preterm birth in this at-risk patient population. Whether other forms of progesterone therapy or other doses or routes of administration may produce similar or better results is actively being researched. The woman in this case should be offered weekly injections of 17-hydroxyprogesterone. The drug is expensive, but not compared with the high cost per day of stay in an NICU.

In summary, it is hoped that intensive research in preterm birth will produce advances in diagnosis, treatment, and prevention that will benefit women, babies, and obstetricians. In the interim, the proposed performance measure recommended by ACOG is to track the proportion of women with preterm labor <34 weeks who receive antenatal corticosteroid therapy.

TIPS TO REMEMBER

- For women who have a history of preterm birth, the intern should elicit the details of that birth: spontaneous or indicated, gestational age at birth, route of delivery, neonatal birth weight and complications, and current status of the infant.
- Women in preterm labor between 24 and 34 weeks should be given a course of betamethasone.
- Treatment with 17-hydroxyprogesterone should be offered to women with a history of SPTB.
- Pharmacologic tocolysis has not been shown to improve neonatal outcomes.

COMPREHENSION QUESTIONS

1. Which of the following is the strongest predictor of preterm labor?
   A. Uterine activity without cervical change
   B. History of prior preterm birth
   C. Cervical length of 2.5 cm by transabdominal ultrasound
   D. Copious white vaginal discharge

2. Which of the items listed below has proven to be effective in the treatment of preterm labor?
   A. Bed rest
   B. Hydration
   C. Sedation
   D. None of the above

3. Which of the following maternal interventions is most likely to reduce the incidence and severity of RDS in the preterm newborn?
   A. IV magnesium sulfate
   B. IV terbutaline
   C. IM betamethasone
   D. Endotracheal surfactant administration to the newborn

Answers

1. **B**. Every year many women in the United States are hospitalized and treated for preterm labor based solely on choice A—this is not indicated. To diagnose preterm labor (and it is a difficult diagnosis), there must be uterine activity and cervical change. Choice C is the lower limit of normal for cervical length and not a good predictor. Choice D is seen frequently in normal pregnancy.

2. **D**. In 2 different places in the chapter it is stated that each of the choices is *not* proven to be an effective therapy. Yet, just as in the answer to question 1 above,

these therapies continue to be recommended without supporting evidence to pregnant women presenting with either true or false preterm labor.

3. C. Choice A may be used for neuroprotection, but it has not been proven to be an effective tocolytic. It does not reduce the incidence of RDS. Choice B has unacceptable risk to the mother and should not be used. Choice D (read the question again!) is not a *maternal* intervention.

SUGGESTED READINGS

American College of Obstetricians and Gynecologists; Committee on Practice Bulletins—Obstetrics. ACOG Practice Bulletin No. 127: management of preterm labor. *Obstet Gynecol.* 2012;119:1308–1317.

Committee on Practice Bulletins—Obstetrics; The American College of Obstetricians and Gynecologists. Practice Bulletin No. 130: prediction and prevention of preterm birth. *Obstet Gynecol.* 2012;120:964–973.

Gonik B, Creasy RK. Preterm labor: its diagnosis and management. *Am J Obstet Gynecol.* 1986;154:3–8.

Meis PJ, Klebanoff M, Thom E, et al. Prevention of recurrent preterm delivery by 17 alpha-hydroxyprogesterone caproate. *N Engl J Med.* 2003;348:2379–2385.

Preterm birth. In: Cunningham GF, Leveno KJ, Bloom SL, Hauth JC, Rouse DJ, Spong CY, eds. *Williams Obstetrics.* 23rd ed. New York, NY: The McGraw-Hill Companies Inc; 2010:804–831.

Rouse DJ, Hirtz DG, Thom E, et al. A randomized, controlled trial of magnesium sulfate for the prevention of cerebral palsy. *N Engl J Med.* 2008;359:895–905.

Spong CY, Mercer BM, D'Alton M, et al. Timing of indicated late-preterm and early-term birth. *Obstet Gynecol.* 2011;118:323–333.

A 20-year-old G1 P0 at 28 Weeks Gestation Complaining of Leakage of Fluid

Edward R. Yeomans, MD

A young primigravida at 28 weeks by first trimester ultrasound presents to triage concerned that she may be leaking fluid vaginally. She is not able to quantify the amount and does not seem to be a reliable historian. Her pregnancy has so far been uncomplicated. The fetus is active and she has had no vaginal bleeding. She reports no uterine contractions.

1. **How do you diagnose ruptured membranes?**
2. **What is the appropriate management if the diagnosis of ruptured membranes is confirmed?**

Answers

1. Historically the diagnosis of ruptured membranes is made clinically, using several or all of the following tests: nitrazine, ferning, fluid in the posterior vaginal vault, and fluid coming directly from the cervical os either spontaneously or with Valsalva maneuver. The diagnosis in this fashion requires a sterile speculum examination (SSE). (If no test is positive, the student may see the shorthand notation, "SSE – x 4.") An ultrasound for assessment of amniotic fluid is also commonly performed. More recently, a few tests have been introduced that do not require a speculum examination. They rely on a swab of the vagina to detect a substance that is present in much higher concentrations in amniotic fluid than in either cervical or vaginal secretions. Placental alpha microglobulin-1 (PAMG-1) is one such substance that has been marketed as AmniSure. Compared with conventional testing, detection of PAMG-1 does not appear to offer additional accuracy.

2. If the diagnosis of ruptured membranes is confirmed, management depends on gestational age. In the case presented, at 28 weeks gestation, expectant management is recommended, but this involves more than simple watchful waiting. Antibiotics, most often ampicillin and either azithromycin or erythromycin, are administered with the intention of prolonging latency, defined as the time period between rupture of membranes (ROM) and onset of labor. A single course (2 doses) of betamethasone is given to enhance fetal lung maturity. Pharmacologic tocolysis is not recommended. Usually the patient is admitted to the hospital and placed on bed rest with either continuous or twice-daily electronic fetal monitoring. The recommended frequency of fetal monitoring,

as well as the type (nonstress test, biophysical profile, Doppler velocimetry, amniotic fluid index), is variable among obstetric centers. Once a week is a minimum interval.

CASE REVIEW

Surprisingly, the evidence base for managing preterm premature rupture of the membranes (PPROM) is not robust. The word preterm refers to gestational age less than 37 weeks, whereas premature in this context refers to ROM before the onset of labor. Term PROM or TPROM occurs more frequently than PPROM, and management is based on convincing evidence. Induction of labor with oxytocin immediately after diagnosis is recommended. The discussion that follows is limited to PPROM.

Once membranes rupture (and the use of the plural here refers to chorion and amnion which are fused from early in the second trimester), fetal and maternal risks increase, as will be seen in the next section. Let us assume that membranes were found to be ruptured in the case scenario. The patient was appropriately admitted, monitored, begun on latency antibiotics, and given a course of steroids.

PPROM

Diagnosis

The nitrazine test makes use of the normal vaginal pH of 4.5 to 5.5, at which the yellow nitrazine pH paper remains yellow. Amniotic fluid has a basic pH (7.4) and will turn the nitrazine paper a royal blue hue. However, other substances (blood, semen, cervical mucus) may also turn the paper blue, yielding falsely positive results. The ferning test or fern test refers to the pattern that amniotic fluid makes on a glass slide. Urine can accumulate in the vaginal vault and can be confused with amniotic fluid. The best test is seeing fluid coming directly from the cervical os.

Most of the time diagnosis is straightforward using the techniques presented above, but occasionally the findings as well as the history are equivocal. Sometimes repeating the examination after an hour with the patient recumbent will clarify the diagnosis. The importance of correct diagnosis cannot be overstated, because management depends on knowing that the membranes are in fact ruptured.

Risks

The risks of membrane rupture can be deduced from the combined functions of the membranes and amniotic fluid. Intact membranes and cervical mucus provide a barrier to ascending infection caused by vaginal bacteria. Following membrane rupture, bacteria can gain access to the uterine cavity and the fetus, creating chorioamnionitis and possible fetal infection. Infection may trigger the onset of labor, but even without infection PPROM is a significant contributor to preterm birth (see Chapter 19). When the membranes rupture, most or sometimes all of the amniotic fluid is lost. The fluid serves to cushion the umbilical cord, so the absence of fluid may lead to cord compression and variable decelerations on FHR monitoring. If membranes rupture very early in gestation (16-24 weeks), pulmonary hypoplasia is a risk.

Management

The management of PPROM is dependent on gestational age. At 34 to 37 weeks, most authorities would recommend either induction of labor with a vertex presentation or consideration of a cesarean delivery with either breech presentation or transverse lie. At 24 to 33(6/7) weeks, expectant management is usually indicated, but in current practice "expectant" is a more active process as detailed in the section "Case Review." Antibiotics are given to prolong latency, steroids are given to enhance lung maturity, and a program of fetal surveillance is initiated. The focus of daily inpatient rounds is on searching for evidence of labor, infection, or fetal compromise. At <24 weeks and particularly at <20 weeks, expectant management may still result in a favorable outcome, but fetal and maternal risks are increased. This time period was the subject of a recent detailed review of the literature.

TIPS TO REMEMBER

- Careful use of history, physical examination, lab tests, and ultrasound should lead to a correct diagnosis of ruptured membranes in the vast majority of cases.
- Between 24 and 34 weeks, antibiotic therapy to prolong latency is a proven intervention.
- An accurate knowledge of gestational age is important for management.
- If membranes rupture after 34 and 0/7 weeks, delivery is indicated.
- If membranes rupture before 24 weeks, detailed counseling on risks and benefits of various courses of action is required.

COMPREHENSION QUESTIONS

1. Which of the fluids listed below can cause a false-positive nitrazine test?
   A. Blood
   B. Semen
   C. Cervical mucus
   D. All of the above

2. Which of the following interventions is *not* recommended in the hospital management of PPROM?

A. Tocolytic therapy
B. Antenatal corticosteroids
C. Antibiotics
D. Weekly or more frequent fetal surveillance

3. Which of the following complications is most closely related to gestational age at the time of membrane rupture?

A. Infection
B. Fetal distress
C. Pulmonary hypoplasia
D. Fetal growth restriction

Answers

1. **D**. The nitrazine test is a pH test. The pH of urine is usually <6, and so is vaginal pH. Amniotic fluid has a pH of >7.0 so that is the basis of the test, but all the listed fluids may have a pH >7.0 also.

2. **A**. Tocolytic therapy is not recommended and, in fact, is of questionable benefit even in preterm labor with intact membranes. All of the other items are important adjuncts to expectant management of PPROM.

3. **C**. Pulmonary hypoplasia following ROM more often complicates PPROM at early gestational age (<24 weeks). Choices A and B are simply risks associated with PPROM, whereas choice D is not valid. When PPROM is managed expectantly, most fetuses continue to grow in utero.

SUGGESTED READINGS

ACOG Committee on Practice Bulletins—Obstetrics. ACOG Practice Bulletin No. 139: premature rupture of membranes. *Obstet Gynecol.* 2013;122(4):918–930.

Hannah ME, Ohlsson A, Farine D, et al. Induction of labor compared with expectant management for prelabor rupture of the membranes at term. *N Engl J Med.* 1996;334:1005–1010.

van der Ham DP, van Teeffelen ASP, Mol BWJ. Prelabour rupture of membranes: overview of diagnostic methods. *Curr Opin Obstet Gynecol.* 2012;24:408–412.

Waters TP, Mercer BM. The management of preterm premature rupture of the membranes near the limit of fetal liability. *Am J Obstet Gynecol.* 2009;201:230–240.

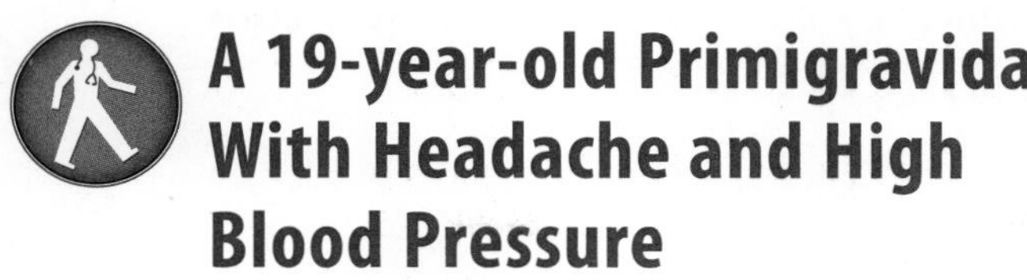

A 19-year-old Primigravida With Headache and High Blood Pressure

Edward R. Yeomans, MD

A 19-year-old G1 P0 presents at 38 weeks to triage complaining of severe headache for several hours. Her antepartum course and medical history are unremarkable. Blood pressure in the right arm in a sitting position is 170/110 and urine protein is 4+ on dipstick. Lungs are clear, fundal height is 31 cm, presentation is cephalic, and reflexes are brisk. Fetal heart rate is 150 beats/min.

1. What is your diagnosis?

2. What constitutes "immediate" management in this patient?

Answers

1. This patient has severe preeclampsia based on blood pressure, urine protein, and headache. In addition, because the fundal height is much less than gestational age, the fetus may be growth-restricted. Laboratory studies are needed to determine whether she may also have HELLP syndrome (a variant or complication of preeclampsia) (H, hemolysis; EL, elevated liver enzymes; LP, low platelet count).

2. There are 3 steps that comprise "immediate" management: IV magnesium sulfate to prevent seizures, IV medication to lower the blood pressure, and delivery of the infant, in this case by induction of labor and planned vaginal delivery.

CASE REVIEW

In most US teaching programs, interns are the first physicians to evaluate triage patients. As a practical matter, it would be appropriate for the intern to call for help from a senior resident and/or faculty, but let's assume that those individuals are currently performing a cesarean section. In the case presented, headache may be a harbinger of a seizure, so there is a need to act promptly. *All obstetric interns* should know how to administer magnesium sulfate and order medication to lower the blood pressure. The cervix should be checked, but oxytocin induction can be initiated as long as the presentation is cephalic and the fetal heart rate pattern is reassuring, even if the cervix is found to be closed. Further management is outlined below.

PREECLAMPSIA

Diagnosis

Preeclampsia is a clinical syndrome defined as hypertension (systolic pressure ≥140 mm Hg *or* diastolic pressure ≥90 mm Hg) that is first detected after 20 weeks gestation and accompanied by proteinuria of ≥1+ by dipstick or ≥300 mg/24 hours. It can be mild or severe (there is no moderate), but eclampsia (preeclampsia plus convulsion not attributable to an underlying seizure disorder) can occur without progression from mild-to-severe preeclampsia. Criteria for severe preeclampsia are listed in Table 21-1. It is evident from the criteria that many organ systems are affected by the disease process. The division of Table 21-1 into symptoms, signs, and labs parallels the responsibilities of the intern's history, physical examination, and laboratory studies. The assessment step in the patient presented should be conducted expeditiously (5-10 minutes, but no more than 15) due to the need to begin treatment.

It is commonly heard on clinical services that "preeclampsia labs" were sent, but preeclampsia is *not* a laboratory diagnosis. In contrast, HELLP syndrome, which some regard as a variant of preeclampsia, *is* a laboratory diagnosis. Hemolysis can be confirmed by an LDH >600 IU/L, a bilirubin >1.2 mg/dL, or an

Table 21-1. Indicators of Severe Preeclampsia

Symptoms
Headache
Visual disturbances
Epigastric or right upper quadrant pain
Signs
Diastolic blood pressure ≥110
Systolic blood pressure ≥160
Oliguria
Pulmonary edema
Fetal growth restriction
Lab abnormalities
Heavy proteinuria ≥3+ on dipstick or 5 g/24 h
Thrombocytopenia
Serum aminotransferase elevation
Increased serum creatinine

abnormal peripheral smear showing fragmentation of red cells. A value of AST >70 IU/L qualifies as an elevated liver enzyme and platelet count is most often less than 100,000/mm^3. Obviously there is overlap with some of the criteria for severe preeclampsia, but the management of HELLP syndrome and severe preeclampsia is the same at 37 weeks as in the case presented. There are, however, some women with HELLP syndrome whose clinical course may be particularly severe, involving complications such as pulmonary edema, acute kidney injury (formerly acute renal failure), and ruptured liver. The intern and all members of the team should remember that when low blood pressure occurs in a pregnant or recently postpartum woman with preeclampsia or HELLP syndrome, it almost never indicates resolution of the underlying disease. Instead, it may signify dangerous hypovolemia or intra-abdominal hemorrhage due to liver rupture.

Treatment

The emphasis in this chapter is on immediate management, as it should be for a book on resident readiness. A short section describing ongoing management of preeclamptic woman is also included.

Step 1: Prevent seizures with IV magnesium sulfate. After decades of debate, there is finally international agreement that magnesium sulfate is the drug of choice for the prevention and treatment of eclampsia. A loading dose of 6 g over 20 to 30 minutes, followed by a maintenance infusion of 2 g/h, should result in therapeutic magnesium levels in maternal blood 4 hours later. In contemporary practice, the magnesium comes premixed from the pharmacy, typically with 50 g in 500 mL. At such a concentration, the loading dose would require 60 cm^3 and the infusion pump should be set to deliver 20 cm^3/h. Some centers use a 4-g load and some use different concentrations, so interns and residents must familiarize themselves with local practice.

Step 2: Lower the blood pressure with IV medication. Committee Opinion #514 from ACOG states that an acute elevation in blood pressure to the level 170/110 seen in this sample case constitutes a hypertensive emergency if it persists for 15 minutes or more. Elevation of blood pressure to this degree may cause cerebral hemorrhage or infarction. The goal of treatment is to maintain blood pressure in the range of 140 to 160/90 to 100. Recommended agents include hydralazine (given as an IV bolus of 5-10 mg and repeated at 20-minute intervals until BP reaches the target level) or labetalol (an initial dose of 20 mg IV followed by 40 mg and then 80 mg 10 minutes apart until BP is controlled). A precipitous drop in maternal blood pressure may adversely affect the fetus. As a general rule when managing severe hypertension in a viable pregnancy, the lowest recommended dose for hydralazine and labetalol should be used first.

Step 3: Begin oxytocin induction and plan for vaginal delivery. Immediate cesarean delivery is not indicated for severe preeclampsia, eclampsia, or HELLP syndrome and may make matters worse. The dose of oxytocin is increased by amounts and intervals specified by local protocols. Experience has shown that at term, successful induction can be accomplished in 75% to 80% of women even if the cervix is unfavorable.

Steps 4 and 5: Avoid diuretics unless there is clinical evidence of pulmonary edema, in which case furosemide is the drug of choice. Carefully monitor total IV fluid to infuse 60 to 125 mL/h.

Ongoing Management

Induction of labor may take 24 to 36 hours, during which time the patient should be monitored for signs of magnesium toxicity. Clinically, this means checking for the presence of deep tendon reflexes (these may be absent at a magnesium level of 10 mg/dL), insuring that urine output is at least 100 mL/4 hours, and assessing respiratory rate. Urine output is important because more than 95% of magnesium is renally excreted. The level of serum creatinine should also be checked periodically and the magnesium infusion rate should be reduced if creatinine exceeds 1 mg/dL. These clinical checks are often supplemented by periodic assay of magnesium levels in maternal blood. Treatment of magnesium toxicity begins with an IV bolus of 10 mL of 10% calcium gluconate, but may require endotracheal intubation in very severe cases.

Electronic fetal heart rate monitoring is fairly standard and epidural anesthesia is not contraindicated. Close monitoring of the patient for hypotension and/or fetal heart rate abnormalities is especially important in the first hour following administration of an epidural anesthetic. Most often, magnesium is continued for 24 hours after delivery. The patient's recovery begins with delivery of the placenta. Despite decades of intensive research, the etiology of preeclampsia remains unknown. Therefore, management is still empirical, as outlined above.

TIPS TO REMEMBER

- Time is important—evaluate quickly and begin treatment promptly. Hypertensive disorders account for 16% of maternal deaths.
- Obstetricians use very few drugs in managing preeclampsia. The important ones are mentioned in the chapter. To get ready for residency, become very familiar with their pharmacology.
- Edema was dropped as a criterion for the diagnosis of preeclampsia more than a decade ago, but its presence, particularly if hands and face are involved, may still be useful. Rapid weight gain as term approaches may also be a useful sign.

- Hypervolemia of pregnancy is often reduced or even absent in severe preeclampsia or eclampsia. Normal or increased blood loss may lead to severe anemia, hypotension, and decreased renal perfusion, leading to acute kidney injury.
- Vasospasm is the key pathophysiologic event and can cause endothelial damage and capillary leak. Leaky capillaries in the pulmonary bed, along with increased hydrostatic pressure and decreased oncotic pressure, may result in pulmonary edema, a sign of severe preeclampsia (Table 21-1).

COMPREHENSION QUESTIONS

1. Which of the following statements is *true*?
   A. Immediate c-section is indicated following an eclamptic seizure.
   B. Epidural anesthesia is contraindicated in patients with severe preeclampsia.
   C. Urine output should be at least 100 mL/h to continue infusing magnesium sulfate.
   D. Eclampsia can occur in the absence of symptoms.

2. All of the following are clinical diagnostic criteria for severe preeclampsia, except which one?
   A. Pulmonary edema
   B. Right upper quadrant pain
   C. Headache
   D. Severe facial edema

3. If blood pressure is lowered too rapidly with either hydralazine or labetalol, which of the following is most likely to occur?
   A. Cerebral thrombosis
   B. Cerebral hemorrhage
   C. Angina
   D. Uteroplacental insufficiency

Answers

1. **D.** Eclampsia can occur in women with very mild preeclampsia. Symptoms, as noted in Table 21-1, signify severe preeclampsia, but do not precede all seizures. The other potential answers are specifically refuted in the chapter.

2. **D.** Although facial and hand edema may accompany severe preeclampsia, these have been removed as diagnostic criteria. The others listed are all clinical diagnostic criteria of severe preeclampsia.

3. **D**. Hypotension reduces blood flow to the uterine arteries and from there to the placenta, often manifesting as late decelerations on the fetal heart rate tracing. Thrombosis and hemorrhage in the brain are more likely to be seen with uncontrolled hypertension. A reduction in coronary blood flow sufficient to cause angina is highly unlikely.

SUGGESTED READINGS

Alexander JM, McIntire DD, Leveno KJ, Cunningham FG. Selective magnesium sulfate prophylaxis for the prevention of eclampsia in women with gestational hypertension. *Obstet Gynecol.* 2006; 108:826–832.

Committee on Obstetric Practice. Committee Opinion No. 514: emergent therapy for acute-onset, severe hypertension with preeclampsia or eclampsia. *Obstet Gynecol.* 2011;118:1465–1468.

Pregnancy hypertension. In: Cunningham GF, Leveno KJ, Bloom SL, Hauth JC, Rouse DJ, Spong CY, eds. *Williams Obstetrics.* 23rd ed. New York, NY: The McGraw-Hill Companies Inc; 2010:706–756.

Publications Committee, Society for Maternal-Fetal Medicine, Sibai BM. Evaluation and management of severe preeclampsia before 34 weeks' gestation. *Am J Obstet Gynecol.* 2011;205:191–198.

Seal SL, Ghosh D, Kamilya G, et al. Does route of delivery affect maternal and perinatal outcome in women with eclampsia? A randomized controlled pilot study. *Am J Obstet Gynecol.* 2012;206: 484.e1–484.e7.

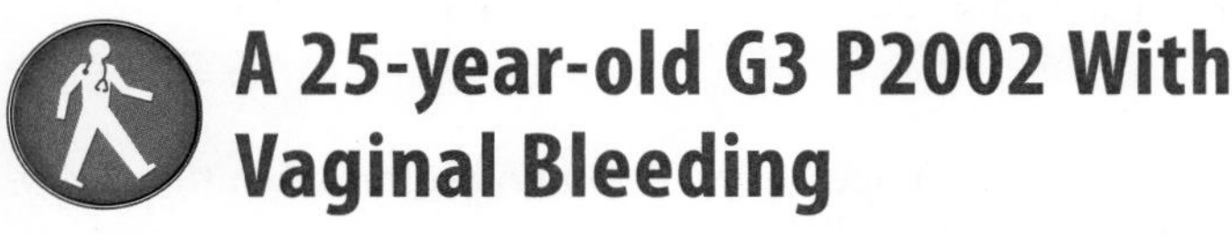

A 25-year-old G3 P2002 With Vaginal Bleeding

Fidelma B. Rigby, MD

A 25-year-old G3 P2002 at 28 weeks by LMP presents to triage with a chief complaint of vaginal bleeding. She has had no prenatal care. Her past obstetric history is significant for 2 prior cesarean sections due to premature labor with breech presentation. On examination, you notice that her jeans are soaked with blood. Her blood pressure (BP) is 80/50, pulse is 110 bpm, lungs are clear to auscultation, and fundal height is 28 cm. Sterile speculum examination shows blood clots in the vaginal vault, but no active bleeding from the cervix and no lesions on the cervix or in the vagina. The tocometer shows contractions every 10 minutes, and the fetal heart rate tracing is in the 150s with moderate variability.

1. What is in your differential diagnosis?

2. What do you need to do to narrow your differential diagnosis?

3. What constitutes immediate management?

Answers

1. There are many causes of vaginal bleeding in the antepartum period, but important elements in your differential diagnosis are preterm labor, placenta previa, and placental abruption.
2. Abdominal ultrasound should be performed prior to digital cervical examination in cases of vaginal bleeding in the second half of pregnancy in order to ascertain placental location and exclude previa.
3. Immediate management would consist of notification of your obstetric team including other residents, faculty and anesthesia, placement of 2 large-bore IVs, a Foley catheter, a complete blood count, and a type and crossmatch for 2 U of packed red blood cells.

CASE REVIEW

Most likely the intern would be the first person to evaluate this patient, and it is therefore important to realize that this patient is bleeding significantly (relatively low bp with increased pulse and blood-soaked jeans) and get the team involved quickly. Communicate with nursing and alert the operating room staff to the possibility that a cesarean delivery may need to be performed, so an operating room can be prepared. Blood work should be done immediately as noted above. In cases of placental abruption (especially in the presence of a fetal demise) or massive hemorrhage, disseminated intravascular coagulation (DIC) is a strong possibility.

Evaluate coagulation with a fibrinogen level, D-dimer, prothrombin time (PT), and partial thromboplastin time (PTT). Fibrinogen levels rise in pregnancy; any value below 300 mg/dL is abnormal and below 150 mg/dL is termed overt hypofibrinogenemia. Taping a red-top tube containing 2 to 3 cm^3 of blood to the wall and checking it to see the size of the clot that forms and persists will also help determine if the patient has DIC before the fibrinogen result is available. Obstetric interns should be aware of these initial steps. We will discuss more detailed management below.

ANTEPARTUM HEMORRHAGE

Diagnosis

The differential diagnosis should include placenta previa, placental abruption, vasa previa, uterine rupture, bleeding from rapid cervical dilation, vaginal/cervical trauma, masses, and finally supracervical bleeding of unknown etiology.

One of your first steps should be to try to quantitate how much bleeding has already occurred with a quick history and rough visual estimate. Realize that the patient's assessment of her bleeding can be misleading: some patients consider drops of blood in the toilet alarming, while others remain unconcerned despite significant blood loss.

Assess the patient's vitals, remembering that a healthy woman may maintain a relatively normal bp and heart rate until significant blood loss has occurred. A heart rate significantly above 100, especially with any drop in bp, should raise a red flag. While talking to her you should also be assessing the clothes she came in with—do they appear blood soaked or are there just a couple of spots of blood on a sanitary pad? Also, look directly at the perineum to determine if active bleeding is occurring. While doing this, you can be asking questions to confirm gestational age and antenatal complications: are there any prior ultrasounds that mention placenta previa? Does she have risk factors for placenta previa or abruption? (See Tables 22-1 and 22-2.)

Table 22-1. Risk Factors Associated With Placenta Previa

Prior cesarean delivery
Increased parity and maternal age
Tobacco use
Multiple gestation
Previous placenta previa
Prior uterine surgery

Table 22-2. Risk Factors Associated With Placental Abruption

Hypertension
Chronic
Preeclampsia
Cocaine-induced
Tobacco use
PPROM
Prior abruption

The purpose of the ultrasound is to look at the location of the placenta, and determine gestational age, fetal lie, number, and viability. Classically, placenta previa is associated with painless vaginal bleeding (unless intermittent contractions are occurring).

If placenta previa or vasa previa is not evident, then placental abruption should be your next concern. Abruption is a clinical diagnosis with supporting lab values. Ultrasound is *not* the best modality to diagnose abruption: initially the placenta simply appears thickened, and a hyperlucent area behind the placenta is a late (but important) finding. You should be highly suspicious for abruption if you have significant vaginal bleeding without evidence of previa, and the uterus is firm and tender to palpation. The uterine tocometer and fetal heart rate tracing should be inspected. The latter is the most sensitive sign of abruption, and may reveal late-appearing fetal heart rate decelerations. The tocometer may show an elevated uterine resting tone. Assess risk factors for abruption (see Table 22-2). The strongest associations with placental abruption are chronic hypertension, preeclampsia, or cocaine use. If you have ruled out previa (by ultrasound) and abruption (by physical examination and risk factors), then you should consider other diagnoses.

Vasa previa should be suspected when bright red vaginal bleeding occurs after rupture of membranes. It involves a velamentous cord insertion with the umbilical vessels traversing the cervical os. A succenturiate placental lobe, especially if near the cervical os, would increase the risk of vasa previa. Sometimes a sinusoidal fetal heart rate pattern, indicating fetal anemia, can be observed.

Uterine rupture should be suspected if you have acute loss of fetal station associated with a tearing sensation over the uterine scar and fetal bradycardia. This is a rare occurrence in an unscarred uterus. Any patient with a prior cesarean delivery undergoing a trial of labor should be watched carefully for this complication.

Attention should be turned to digital examination of the cervix if the above conditions have been ruled out. A speculum examination should be performed to assess the origin of the bleeding (vaginal/cervical/supracervical). Vaginal lesions/cervical or prolapsed uterine leiomyomas/trauma are rare sources of bleeding that can be visualized with speculum examination. If the bleeding is only supracervical, this should be described. Bleeding from rapid cervical dilation can be considered when all other sources have been ruled out and significant uterine contractions and cervical change are noted. This bleeding should be self-limited.

Treatment

Immediate cesarean delivery should be considered for a viable fetus when significant bleeding due to abruption is suspected. An exception would be a multiparous patient who is almost fully dilated with a normal fetal heart rate tracing, or in cases when a cesarean may cause harm (clinically unstable or coagulopathic patient). Immediate cesarean is indicated in cases of vasa previa and uterine rupture. Remember with abruption that the placenta has a 50% reserve capacity so that any sign of placental insufficiency (ie, late-appearing fetal heart rate decelerations) tells you that the placenta may already be compromised.

Decisions regarding optimal gestational age for delivery become more complicated when placenta previa is diagnosed during prenatal care, and the patient presents with a first episode of bleeding. Most often hospitalization is indicated, but outpatient management has been described. Also recall that placenta previa with a history of previous cesarean delivery (as in our patient) increases the risk of placenta accreta. Placenta accreta can be associated with massive blood loss and is a leading cause of cesarean hysterectomy.

Unexplained significant supracervical bleeding is often self-limited. However, these patients remain at risk for adverse outcomes, perhaps due to marginal placental separation. Close follow-up is recommended.

TIPS TO REMEMBER

- Do ABCs first! With severe hemorrhage 2 large-bore IVs, early upper level and anesthesia involvement, and calling for blood replacement can be lifesaving.
- Determine the gestational age and viability, and rule out previa expeditiously with ultrasound. Then look for evidence of placental abruption with physical examination and clinical presentation.
- Uterine rupture should be suspected in patients with a previous cesarean delivery and pain despite adequate regional anesthesia, and/or with loss of fetal station in light of fetal heart rate changes (late-appearing decelerations or bradycardia). Vasa previa should be suspected with bright red vaginal bleeding after membrane rupture accompanied by fetal bradycardia.
- If the above conditions are ruled out, a speculum examination should be performed to check for cervical and vaginal causes of bleeding.

COMPREHENSION QUESTIONS

1. A patient with placenta previa presents with copious vaginal bleeding and regular contractions. Of the following options, which is the best first step?
   A. Start a small-gauge peripheral IV and order a type and screen.
   B. Perform a quick bimanual examination to determine cervical dilation.
   C. Notify your upper level residents and anesthesia of the patient's presence.
   D. Wait for the clinic records before evaluating her to determine her gestational age.

2. A 35-year-old P2002 with a history of previous cesarean delivery has had a prolonged labor. She is quite irritable as she has persistent lower abdominal discomfort despite multiple attempts by anesthesia to dose her epidural. Her last cervical check was 5/50%/0 station 3 hours ago. You are called to her room for FHTs in the 60s. You note a moderate amount of vaginal bleeding during your cervical check that is 5/50%/–3 station. What should be done?
   A. Find the intern who did the last check to explain how to check station properly.
   B. Call upper levels and prepare for cesarean delivery.
   C. Increase her Pitocin as she has made no progress since her last check.
   D. Place an intrauterine pressure catheter (IUPC) to determine the strength of her contractions.

3. A 26-year-old patient at 30 weeks with placenta previa presents with contractions every 3 minutes. She states she was awakened from sleep by her contractions and about a half hour later her bleeding started. Your colleague has started intravenous magnesium sulfate in an attempt to decrease her contractions and for fetal neuroprotection at a rate of 1 g/h about 30 minutes ago. The nurse calls you to the room to let you know the contractions are still every 3 minutes and her bleeding is worse. You should do which of the following?
   A. Increase the rate of magnesium sulfate to 2 g/h.
   B. Stop the magnesium sulfate immediately.
   C. Reassure the nurse that an increase in bleeding can be seen and this should resolve soon.
   D. Perform a bimanual examination to assess cervical dilation.

Answers

1. **C.** You should notify your upper levels and anesthesia ASAP as she could experience life-threatening hemorrhage quickly. A single peripheral IV and type and screen are inadequate in this situation. Two large-bore IVs and crossmatch for at least 2 U are warranted. Bimanual examination is contraindicated with placenta previa.

2. **B**. The patient appears to have ruptured her uterus (vaginal bleeding, loss of fetal station, abdominal pain even with an epidural, and fetal heart rate deceleration). Increasing the Pitocin and placing an IUPC are not helpful in this setting.

3. **B**. Tocolytic use in the presence of a placenta previa that is bleeding must be done very cautiously and immediately discontinued if bleeding worsens.

SUGGESTED READINGS

American College of Obstetricians and Gynecologists. ACOG Practice Bulletin No. 4: prevention of RhD alloimmunization. *Obstet Gynecol.* 1999;93:17 [reaffirmed 2013].

Francois KE, Foley MR. Antepartum and post partum hemorrhage. In: Gabbe SG, Niebyl JR, Galan HL, et al, eds. *Obstetrics: Normal and Problem Pregnancies.* 6th ed. New York, NY: The McGraw-Hill Companies Inc; 2012:415–445.

Holmgren CM. Uterine rupture associated with VBAC. *Clin Obstet Gynecol.* 2012;55(4):978–987.

Obstetrical hemorrhage. In: Cunningham GF, Leveno KJ, Bloom SL, Hauth JC, Rouse DJ, Spong CY, eds. *Williams Obstetrics.* 23rd ed. New York, NY: The McGraw-Hill Companies Inc; 2010:757–803.

Watson WJ, Cefalo RC. Magnesium sulfate tocolysis in selected patients with symptomatic placenta previa. *Am J Perinatol.* 1990;7(3):251–253.

A 19-year-old Presents to Obstetric Triage, 38 Weeks Pregnant With Intermittent Abdominal Pain

Charlie C. Kilpatrick, MD

Ms R, a 19-year-old woman, presents to the obstetric triage area complaining of pain that began 45 minutes ago. The pain is not constant and is strong like a menstrual cramp. She also reports a mucus discharge after the pain started, but denies a big gush of fluid. She has had no vaginal bleeding, and has felt the baby kicking a lot. She previously had a miscarriage but no other obstetric history, and her prenatal care has been uneventful other than a UTI for which she was treated. She has no medical problems, has not had surgery, does not smoke or drink, and other than prenatal vitamins and iron, is not taking any medications. She has no allergies to medications. Her prenatal labs are normal, except for an iron-deficiency anemia, and her recent GBS screen is negative. The nurse has placed the uterine tocodynamometer (tocometer for short) and fetal Dopplers, and performed a dip urinalysis that is negative. The tocometer confirms that she is contracting about every 3 to 5 minutes, and the fetal heart rate tracing is in the 120s, has moderate variability, and there are accelerations present. On physical examination, she is in pain during the contractions but otherwise is feeling well without nausea or vomiting, the fundal height is 40 cm, and you palpate a contraction. By Leopold maneuvers the fetal head is the presenting part. You perform a sterile speculum examination that does not reveal pooling of amniotic fluid or any fluid coming from the cervix after Valsalva, and visually the cervix is dilated 2 cm. On sterile vaginal examination of the cervix, it is dilated to 2 cm, and is about 1 cm thick. You think that the head is at the level of the ischial spines.

1. What is in your differential diagnosis? What is most likely?

2. What is your next step?

Answers

1. The patient is likely in labor based on her symptoms (frequent, painful contractions), the tocometer readings (uterine contractions every 3-5 minutes), and your examination of the cervix (dilation, with effacement).
2. Your next step is to record your findings, present the information to your upper level resident/attending so that they may confirm your clinical findings, and then reexamine the patient in an hour to look for evidence of cervical change.

CASE REVIEW

Your examination is confirmed, and your plan to reexamine the cervix is affirmed. You perform a bedside ultrasound that confirms that the head is the presenting part. On your next examination, her SVE is 3/80%/0 station and you admit her for labor management and pain control. She elects to have an epidural. Later that evening, she delivers vaginally a healthy baby boy over a second-degree laceration that you repair under supervision.

OBSTETRIC TRIAGE

Diagnosis

As an intern at most obstetrics and gynecology residency programs in the United States, you will spend the majority of your time evaluating patients who present to obstetric triage. Typically, hospitals designate the obstetric triage area for pregnant patients beyond 20 weeks of gestation. Depending on where you train, obstetric triage may never empty, each examination room or bed uninhabited for only a brief moment while the next patient is moved in. Initially, you may tire of this responsibility, or begin to feel that this is "service over education," but once you finish the intern year and begin to evaluate patients throughout the hospital, you will long for the days of triage.

You will be the first clinician to evaluate patients in triage, and your main task is to perform a quick assessment of the situation to determine whether the patient is in labor (like the scenario above) or whether the situation is more serious. Even in cases of labor, the patient may need more urgent attention give the fetal heart rate tracing, bleeding, fetal number or presentation, or the stage of labor the patient is in. The examination begins with the determination of her gestational age, and asking the patient 4 simple questions: "Is the baby moving?" "Are you leaking fluid?" "Are you having any vaginal bleeding?" "Are you experiencing uterine contractions?" This may already be quite familiar to you after the clerkship.

Determination of the gestational age is important as almost all treatment decisions (and some of the actions you perform in triage) take this into account. The management of a patient with rupture of the membranes at term (delivery) is different than at 27 weeks of gestation (admission, intravenous antibiotics, and intramuscular steroids). If the patient had early prenatal care, it is likely that a first trimester ultrasound will provide you with a reliable gestational age. Often, patients will present with little or no prenatal care late in pregnancy, and the history, menstrual recall, and ultrasound will allow you to best estimate gestational age. (See Chapter 18 for more detail on gestational age estimation.)

Once you estimate gestational age, your attention should turn to the chief complaint, and finding answers to the 4 questions listed above (leaking fluid,

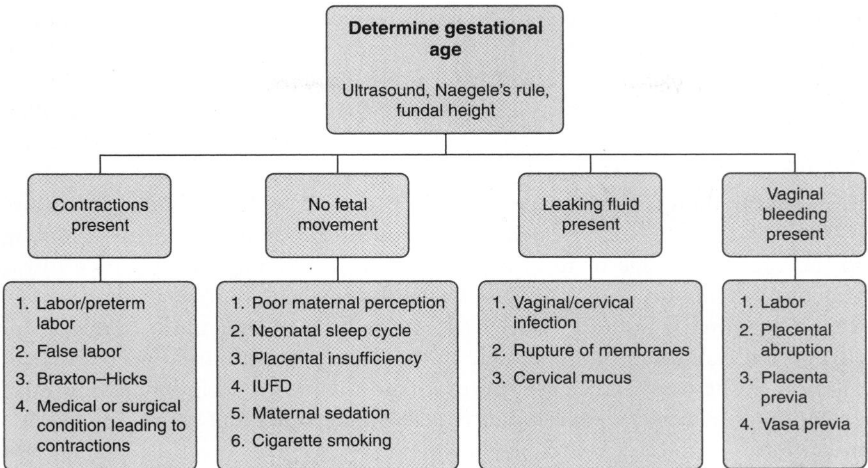

Figure 23-1. Obstetric triage algorithm.

vaginal bleeding, fetal movement, and contractions). Figure 23-1 is an algorithm that will help you begin to formulate a differential diagnosis based on gestational age, and the answers to these 4 questions.

Treatment

Treatment for the conditions that present to triage depends on the diagnosis. Always remember to elicit and address a patient's chief complaint. A patient determined to be in labor (regular painful contractions, cervical change) is usually admitted for pain control, and labor management. There may be times when the labor is very early in which pain medicine and observation may be preferable, and the patient may not always require admission. Preterm labor requires admission and is best managed in the hospital. For patients at term in labor, your history and physical examination should include the following obstetric details: cervical assessment with notation of time (dilation, effacement, station, position, and consistency), estimation of fetal weight (preferably in grams), fetal presentation (cephalic or breech), and fetal position (at ≥5 cm even with membranes intact). Documentation of the contraction pattern and fetal heart rate tracing is also necessary. Patients determined not to be in labor after repeat examination should be sent home with labor precautions and follow-up in the clinic.

The absence of fetal movement requires investigation with a nonstress test and ultrasound to assess amniotic fluid level. Sometimes maternal perception of movement is altered and ultrasound allows you to show the patient that the fetus is moving. A sudden complaint of decreased fetal movement should not be interpreted as lack of maternal perception and thorough assessment should be undertaken after consultation with your upper level resident or faculty. There is nothing more devastating than a fetal demise that occurs at term. You will often tire of evaluation for this chief complaint, but it can herald placental insufficiency, so a careful workup is necessary.

Leaking fluid requires a speculum examination with good light. If rupture of the membranes is confirmed on speculum examination (positive pooling in the vagina, leakage of fluid from the cervix with Valsalva, positive nitrazine and ferning test, positive placental alpha macroglobulin-1 protein assay), digital examination should be limited. Prior to 5 cm speculum examination and digital examination are similar in the accurate determination of cervical dilation. If the membranes are ruptured and the patient is in labor, minimize the number of cervical examinations performed to prevent ascending uterine infection.

Vaginal bleeding of any kind requires expeditious assessment. Even patients who are not yet in a triage room should "jump the line" in order to receive rapid assessment if they are bleeding. This is a condition when your first step should be communication with your upper level resident/faculty, as you begin assessment of the patient. While waiting for your upper level resident or faculty determine if the patient has placental abruption risk factors (hypertension, preeclampsia, smoking, cocaine use, abdominal trauma, premature rupture of membranes, prior abruption), scan the medical record (or ask the patient) for an ultrasound report that documents placentation, or perform abdominal ultrasound if she has had no prenatal care. You can examine the cervix once you are certain there is no evidence of placenta previa. Labor should not be identified as the cause until more serious conditions have been searched for. Immediate steps should include admission, fetal heart rate assessment, tocometer assessment, placement of 2 large-bore IVs, type and screen (or crossmatch), and determination of hemoglobin/hematocrit level. Vaginal bleeding in pregnancy trumps all in regard to the need for rapid assessment and communication with team members.

TIPS TO REMEMBER

- Labor is diagnosed with documentation of cervical change and regular painful contractions.
- Cervical dilation/effacement/station, fetal presentation, estimated fetal weight, position (if ≥5 cm), uterine activity, and fetal heart rate should be documented on every history and physical examination you perform for the diagnosis of labor.

- Decreased fetal movement always requires thorough and careful examination—do not attribute a sudden decrease in fetal movement to lack of maternal perception.
- Patients with confirmed rupture of membranes should have limited digital cervical examinations to prevent intrauterine infection.
- Vaginal bleeding in patients who present to triage requires rapid assessment, action, and team communication.

COMPREHENSION QUESTIONS

1. Ms R is a 24-year-old P3003 at 37.3 weeks with good dating criteria. You noticed her leaning against the wall on your way into triage and stopped to ask her if she was okay. She is complaining of contractions that began 4 hours ago, and is feeling pressure in her rectum. She denies vaginal bleeding and leaking fluid. What is the next best step?
   A. Cervical examination with notation of time
   B. Speculum examination
   C. Ultrasound to assess fetal movement
   D. Twenty minutes of fetal heart rate tracing prior to evaluation

2. Ms R is 7/C/–1 station and left occipitoanterior (LOA). You diagnose labor and admit her for management. Which of the following obstetric details is least important to document on your admitting history and physical examination?
   A. Fetal presentation
   B. Cervical dilation and effacement
   C. Estimated fetal weight
   D. Amniotic fluid volume determination

3. Ms C is 35 weeks gestation who presents complaining of brisk vaginal bleeding that began 30 minutes ago that she describes as a period. You are in the process of evaluating a patient in another room who may be in labor. Which of the following *would not* be the next best step that you could take in managing obstetric triage?
   A. Rapidly complete the history and physical examination you are working on and then turn your attention to Ms C.
   B. Communicate with your upper level team members and faculty that a patient with heavy vaginal bleeding is in triage.
   C. Scan the patient's medical record for an ultrasound report or perform abdominal ultrasound if she has no prenatal care.
   D. Request that the triage nurse place 2 large-bore IVs while you assess the cause of the patient's bleeding.

Answers

1. **A**. A parous patient leaning against the wall in pain and complaining of pressure in the rectum requires quick cervical assessment. Ultrasound may be necessary to document presentation, and a fetal heart rate evaluation should be performed, but the cervix should be examined first. Speculum examination, given the brief history, does not appear to be necessary.

2. **D**. Of the choices, assessment of amniotic fluid is least helpful in this situation.

3. **A**. Pregnant patients who present to obstetric triage (>20 weeks) complaining of bleeding like a period should "jump the line" and receive immediate evaluation. All of the other answer choices listed are appropriate and should be undertaken.

SUGGESTED READINGS

Oyelese Y, Ananth CV. Placental abruption. *Obstet Gynecol.* 2006;108(4):1005–1016.

Skornick-Rapaport A, Maslovitz S, Kupferminc M, Lessing JB, Many A. Proposed management for reduced fetal movements: five years' experience in one medical center. *J Matern Fetal Neonatal Med.* 2011;24(4):610–613.

van der Ham DP, van Teeffelen AS, Mol BW. Prelabour rupture of membranes: overview of diagnostic methods. *Curr Opin Obstet Gynecol.* 2012;24(6):408–412.

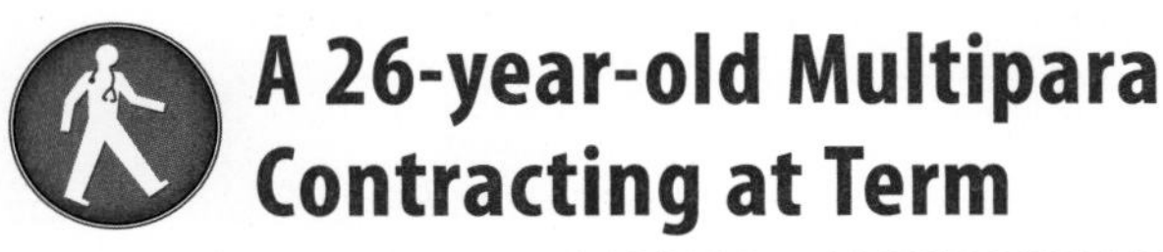

A 26-year-old Multipara Contracting at Term

Elizabeth Melendez, MD, FACOG

A 26-year-old G2P1 at 38 weeks gestation presents to triage with complaints of vaginal discharge that started last night. Her antepartum course has been unremarkable. Her past medical history is significant for 1 normal spontaneous vaginal delivery at term. The discharge is pink in color and clear in consistency. She reports lower abdominal pain that has been coming and going since last night. She denies any leakage of fluid or frank blood from her vagina. She reports good fetal movement. The patient is noted to be normotensive and in no acute distress. The fetal heart tones are reassuring. The tocodynamometer reveals irregular contractions every 6 to 8 minutes. The sterile speculum examination reveals a thin, mucousy discharge coming from the cervical os. The sterile vaginal examination reveals a cervix that is 3 to 4 cm dilated, 50% effaced, and station of −2 cm.

1. What is your diagnosis?

2. What constitutes "immediate" management in this patient?

Answers

1. This patient may be in early labor based on her complaints, cervical examination, and contraction pattern. However, false labor, especially in a parous woman, is also a possibility.
2. Continued observation with external fetal monitoring would be prudent management in this patient as she may remain in latent labor or enter active labor shortly. Especially important for interns is to discuss the case with an upper level resident or faculty supervisor before making a decision to either admit or discharge to home. A repeat vaginal examination is recommended after 1 hour of observation in triage.

CASE REVIEW

A cervical dilation of 3 to 4 cm used to be considered a reasonable threshold for the diagnosis of labor in most cases. However, recent work by Zhang et al has shown by analyzing contemporary patterns of spontaneous labor that 6 cm may be a more appropriate landmark for entering the active phase of labor. These investigators also showed that labor may take more than 6 hours to progress from 4 to 5 cm of cervical dilation. Time-honored concepts of labor management may no longer be pertinent for interns entering the practice of obstetrics, as will be discussed later in this chapter. The separation of labor from delivery in this textbook on resident readiness was purposeful. The emphasis for labor is on diagnosis and management, whereas Chapters 27 and 28 focus more on the procedural aspects. The case outlined in the preceding scenario introduces one of the gray areas that will confront all entering interns assigned to the triage area: is the patient in labor or not? In Ireland, the responsibility for making such an important diagnosis is assigned to the senior, most experienced midwife. In contrast, interns in the United States are often tasked to diagnose labor. The material that follows will aid students preparing to enter residency and those already in internship, but the necessary diagnostic skills can only be acquired through constant practice.

LABOR

Diagnosis

The initial encounter with a patient at term (37-42 weeks) presenting with complaints of vaginal discharge with blood and mucus (bloody show) and/or contractions should include a careful review of her prenatal record to identify complications during the antepartum period. The patient's blood pressure, temperature, pulse, and respiratory rate should be assessed and recorded. External fetal monitoring should be applied to assess the fetal heart rate and the quality and frequency of uterine contractions.

The definition of labor is increasing cervical dilation and effacement in the presence of uterine contractions. What complicates the diagnosis of labor is whether a "latent phase" of labor is clinically meaningful. Women who are admitted prior to active labor are subject to more physician interventions such as augmentation with oxytocin, amniotomy, and premature diagnosis of active phase arrest, potentially resulting in unnecessary cesarean delivery. Conversely, women who are less than 6 cm dilated, like the patient in this case, should not be discharged from triage based solely on their cervical dilation because that would risk having an unattended delivery outside the hospital. In the presence of normal maternal vital signs, intact fetal membranes, reassuring heart tones, and no indication for induction of labor (ie, prolonged pregnancy or other complications noted on prenatal record), women should be comprehensively assessed prior to deciding to admit for labor. In epidemiologic terms, interns should strive for high sensitivity (few false-negatives) and high specificity (few false-positives).

The physical examination should begin with vital signs, height, and weight. Examination of heart and lungs is obviously important; abdominal examination should be performed before vaginal examination. Components of the abdominal examination with obstetric significance include measurement of fundal height, finding fetal heart tones, estimating the fetal weight, and assessing presentation. Next, if warranted by the woman's history, a sterile speculum examination is performed to detect the presence of pooling of amniotic fluid in the posterior fornix or flowing from the cervix either spontaneously or with Valsalva maneuver.

A nitrazine test, in which the indicator paper turns blue in the presence of fluid with a pH greater than 6.5 (the pH of amniotic fluid is >7.0, whereas that of vaginal secretions is usually in the range of 4.5-5.5), may be helpful, but it may be falsely positive when blood, semen, or bacterial vaginosis is present. It may be falsely negative when fluid is scant. Finally, amniotic fluid crystallizes into a fernlike pattern when allowed to dry on a slide. The presence of ferning on microscopic examination may confirm the diagnosis of ruptured membranes. If membranes have ruptured, admission is indicated because the risk of intrauterine infection increases as the time interval between membrane rupture and delivery increases. Whether the fluid is clear or meconium-stained should be noted.

If membranes are intact, the cervix is assessed for:

1. Dilation: the diameter of the cervix as measured by the index and second fingers of the dominant hand in centimeters from 0 cm (closed cervix) to 10 cm (completely dilated).
2. Effacement: the length of the cervical canal ranging from 0% (no effacement; 3-4 cm in length) to 100% (complete thinning of the cervix; 0 cm in length).
3. Station: the relationship of the presenting fetal part to the ischial spines in centimeters. Zero station is at the level of the ischial spines. −5 to −1 station spans the distance between the pelvic inlet and the ischial spines, whereas +1 to +5 station encompasses the gap from the ischial spines to the pelvic floor. With intact membranes, the sterile speculum examination described above may be omitted and the cervix may be examined digitally. At that time, the adequacy of the maternal bony pelvis should be assessed.

Management

Once the decision is made to admit a patient in labor, her blood is collected to evaluate her hemoglobin, hematocrit, blood type, and antibody screen, as well as her syphilis, hepatitis B, HIV, and rubella immunity status. A urine specimen is tested for protein. A careful review of these results in addition to the prenatal record offers clues for any potential complications during the labor process. Maternal vital signs are checked at least every 4 hours. External fetal monitoring is used to evaluate fetal well-being and assess uterine contractions (for a more extensive discussion of electronic fetal monitoring the reader is referred to Chapter 26). Pelvic examinations are typically performed every 2 hours to assess the patient's progress. More frequent cervical examinations, especially after membrane rupture, may increase the risk of chorioamnionitis, and likely will not add clinically meaningful information.

Oral intake is restricted in the laboring patient for fear of aspiration pneumonitis, due to prolonged gastric emptying time. In uncomplicated cases, patients may be allowed sips of clear liquids. Most agree that an elective procedure (ie, scheduled cesarean section, postpartum bilateral tubal ligation) should be done only after the patient has fasted 6 to 8 hours. Because cesarean delivery may be indicated before such time has elapsed, solid foods are not usually permitted for the laboring patient. Intravenous infusion of a crystalloid solution (ie, lactated Ringer's with dextrose) is initiated at a rate of 125 mL/h to avoid dehydration in the fasting laboring patient.

The patient should be allowed to ambulate or sit in a chair if she so desires, as long as the fetal membranes are intact. She should also be provided with appropriate analgesia at her request. Patients who are culture-positive for group B *Streptococcus* are given chemoprophylaxis with IV penicillin for at least 4 hours prior to delivery to prevent neonatal infection.

A very important duty for the intern is documentation of labor progress. Progress notes should include an assessment of the woman's vital signs and general appearance, intensity and frequency of uterine contractions, and cervical examination. They should also include a description of fetal status including baseline heart rate, variability, and presence or absence of accelerations and decelerations (please see Chapter 26).

According to time-honored work on labor by Emanuel Friedman, the nullipara in active labor is expected to demonstrate a change in cervical dilation of at least 1.2 cm/h while the multipara should progress at a rate of at least 1.5 cm/h. When a laboring patient does not progress as expected, she is said to have a protraction disorder if there is slow change in cervical dilation, or an arrest disorder if there is no change in cervical dilation over a 2-hour period. These disorders may result from ineffective uterine contractions (power), malposition or excessive size of the fetus (passenger), or relative contraction of the maternal pelvis (passageway). These 3 terms in parentheses are often designated the 3 P's involved in the diagnosis of abnormal progress in labor. Oxytocin infusion may be initiated to augment spontaneous uterine contractions in the setting of an arrest or protraction disorder.

Amniotomy, or artificial rupturing of the fetal membranes, is often employed once active labor is diagnosed to accelerate contractions and shorten the length of labor. Amniotomy also provides information regarding the presence of meconium. Routine amniotomy has not been shown to significantly reduce the length of the first stage of labor. It has, however, been shown to increase the risk of cesarean delivery and the incidence of nonreassuring fetal heart tones.

In the setting of a protraction or arrest disorder, amniotomy may be performed and an intrauterine pressure catheter placed to assess uterine function. Various regimens for oxytocin infusion have been described, with the goal of reaching uterine activity of 200 to 250 Montevideo units. (A Montevideo unit is a quantity derived by adding the peak minus trough pressure in millimeters of mercury for all contractions in a 10-minute period. This quantitative assessment of contraction intensity is only valid when an intrauterine pressure transducer is in use.) A commonly used starting dose of oxytocin is 2 mU/min, increasing by 2 mU/min every 15 minutes to a maximum of 40 mU/min.

An arrest disorder necessitating cesarean delivery may be diagnosed after 4 hours of a sustained pattern of uterine activity greater than 200 Montevideo units or after 6 hours of oxytocin augmentation when the pattern cannot be achieved. These guidelines assume that the fetal heart rate is normal.

The second stage of labor begins when the cervix is completely dilated. At this point, the patient may begin to feel the urge to defecate, depending on her method of analgesia. She should be instructed to bear down as if straining with defecation. In the nullipara, this stage can last up to 3 hours. The multipara's second stage is most often shorter, ranging from 1 to 2 hours, but sometimes lasts only a few minutes. Progress should be assessed by pelvic examination every hour during the second stage. Additionally, the fetal heart rate tracing should be reviewed at 15-minute intervals. With effective pushing efforts, the fetal station should change by at least 1 cm each hour.

Once the perineum begins to bulge and/or the fetal scalp is visible at the introitus, the patient should be prepared for delivery. When delivery is not achieved after 2 to 3 hours of effective pushing in the second stage, an operative vaginal delivery may be considered.

TIPS TO REMEMBER

- A patient with intact fetal membranes should be admitted once active labor has been diagnosed.
- A patient with ruptured fetal membranes at term should be admitted for labor management regardless of cervical status.
- Labor progress is assessed every 2 hours in the first stage. The nullipara should progress at least 1.2 cm/h. The multipara should progress at least 1.5 cm/h.
- Protraction and arrest disorders may be managed with oxytocin administration.

COMPREHENSION QUESTIONS

1. The same 26-year-old G2P1 at term who presented earlier returns with complaints of leakage of fluid. A speculum examination reveals a small amount of clear discharge in the vaginal vault. Nitrazine paper turns blue when it comes in contact with the fluid, indicating a pH of 7. Another test that can help confirm the diagnosis is which of the following?

   A. Microscopic evaluation to detect ferning of the fluid
   B. Microscopic evaluation to detect clue cells
   C. Cervical examination to palpate amniotic sac
   D. Speculum examination to detect fetal hair

2. A cervical effacement of 75% corresponds to which of the following cervical lengths?

A. 4 cm
B. 3 cm
C. 2 cm
D. 1 cm

3. Which of the following changes in cervical dilation represents a protraction disorder for a nullipara in the active phase of labor?

A. 0.5 cm/h
B. 2 cm/h
C. 1.5 cm/h
D. 1.2 cm/h

Answers

1. **A**. Rupture of membranes can be evaluated by speculum examination looking for pooling of amniotic fluid, with nitrazine paper, and by microscopic evaluation to detect ferning.

2. **D**. The normal cervix has a length of 4 cm, or 0% effacement. Seventy-five percent effacement corresponds to a length of 1 cm, 50% to 2 cm, and 25% to 3 cm.

3. **A**. The nullipara in active labor is expected to demonstrate a change in cervical dilation of at least 1.2 cm/h while the multipara progresses at a rate of 1.5 cm/h.

SUGGESTED READINGS

American College of Obstetricians and Gynecologists Committee on Practice Bulletins—Obstetrics. ACOG Practice Bulletin No. 49, December 2003: dystocia and augmentation of labor. *Obstet Gynecol.* 2003;102:1445–1454.

Berghella V, Baxter JK, Chauhan SP. Evidence-based labor and delivery management. *Am J Obstet Gynecol.* 2008;199:445–454.

Committee on Obstetric Practice, American College of Obstetricians and Gynecologists. ACOG Committee Opinion No. 441: oral intake during labor. *Obstet Gynecol.* 2009;114:714.

Neilson JP. Amniotomy for shortening spontaneous labour. *Obstet Gynecol.* 2008;111(1):204–205.

Normal labor and delivery. In: Cunningham GF, Leveno KJ, Bloom SL, Hauth JC, Rouse DJ, Spong CY, eds. *Williams Obstetrics.* 23rd ed. New York, NY: The McGraw-Hill Companies Inc; 2010.

Zhang J, Landy HJ, Branch DW, et al. Contemporary patterns of spontaneous labor with normal neonatal outcomes. *Obstet Gynecol.* 2010;116:1281–1287.

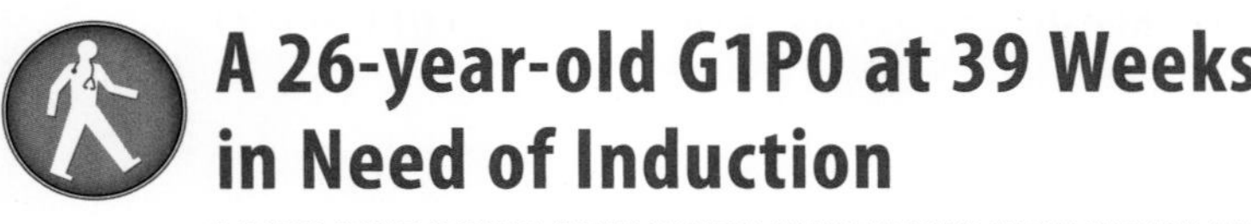

A 26-year-old G1P0 at 39 Weeks in Need of Induction

James Marshall Palmer, MD, MS

A 26-year-old G1P0 female at 39 weeks by 8-week ultrasound presents to triage. The patient is well known to your practice, and her pregnancy is only complicated by Rh-negative status, for which she was given RhoGAM appropriately in the third trimester. The patient reports having some contractions, denies any vaginal bleeding, denies any leakage of fluid, and reports the baby is moving as usual. Her initial blood pressure reading in triage is 149/91. She has had all normal blood pressures up until one blood pressure a week ago that was 140/90 at clinic. She denies any headache, visual changes, or right upper quadrant pain. Her serial blood pressures in triage show systolic blood pressures 140 to 150 over diastolic readings in the low 90s. There is no proteinuria and blood work shows no evidence of the hemolysis, elevated liver function, and low platelets (HELLP) syndrome. Her physical examination is unremarkable and her cervical examination is 1 cm dilated, 50% effaced, and −2 station. The cervix is in midposition with medium consistency, for a Bishop score of 5. Contractions are irregular on the tocometer and the fetal heart tones show a category I tracing with baseline in the 130s and moderate accelerations. She is group B *Streptococcus* negative on culture. You diagnose the patient with gestational hypertension and counsel her regarding induction of labor.

1. **What are your options for induction, what are the risks associated with each method, and how should the patient be counseled about these risks?**

Answer

1. Your options for induction include using prostaglandins such as Cervidil (dinoprostone) or Cytotec (misoprostol), oxytocin, amniotomy, or mechanical dilation using either a single- or double-balloon catheter. The risks associated with Cytotec and, to a lesser degree, Cervidil include uncontrolled stimulation of the uterus that could lead to tachysystole (greater than 5 contractions in 10 minutes) with nonreassuring fetal heart rate (FHR) tracing, which could lead to cesarean delivery. The risks of oxytocin also include tachysystole as well as the risks of volume overload and uterine atony after delivery. The risk of tachysystole with the single- or double-balloon catheter is less, but these balloon devices are often used in conjunction with oxytocin. In addition, the Foley balloon or double-balloon catheter is associated with greater discomfort during placement. Early amniotomy of first-time mothers carries possible risks of chorioamnionitis, possible need for amnioinfusion of fluid to resolve variable decelerations, and cord prolapse if the head is not engaged in the pelvis.

CASE REVIEW

After discussing the options with the patient and counseling her that she is at risk of requiring an emergent or nonemergent cesarean delivery for labor dystocia (abnormally progressing or arrested labor), you perform a brief bedside ultrasound to confirm vertex presentation as the head was not well engaged. You discuss the patient's history, vital signs, physical examination, lab findings, ultrasound findings, and your plan for induction with the obstetric resident team and attending physician. After reviewing the risks, benefits, and alternatives, you and the patient have decided on mechanical dilation using the single-balloon 60-mL Foley catheter. The catheter is placed under direct visualization with a speculum and the help of your upper level resident. The balloon is inflated with 60 mL of normal saline and taped to the patient's inner thigh. Oxytocin is started at 2 mIU/min and the patient begins to contract regularly. The Foley catheter falls out 6 hours later and the cervix is 5 cm dilated, 75% effaced, and −1 station. You continue oxytocin until she is completely dilated and effaced. Her second stage of labor lasts 90 minutes and she delivers a 7 lb 2 oz male infant with Apgar scores at 1 and 5 minutes of 9 and 9.

INDUCTION OF LABOR—IMPORTANT CONCEPTS FOR *DAY 1* ON LABOR AND DELIVERY

Diagnosis

Inducing labor in an obstetric setting refers to the practice of stimulating the uterus and bringing about contractions prior to spontaneous labor. Labor is defined as uterine contractions that produce cervical change. Inducing labor is usually undertaken when the benefits of delivery outweigh the risks associated with continuing pregnancy. The American College of Obstetricians and Gynecologists (ACOG) notes that 22% of all gravid women are induced for various indications. It is important to remember that the chances of successful vaginal delivery following an induction of labor are lower than if spontaneous labor occurs, especially induction of a nulliparous woman with an unfavorable cervix, where induction confers a 2-fold increased risk of cesarean delivery.

Cesarean delivery has increased over the last few decades, now comprising one third of all deliveries in the United States. The *Eunice Kennedy Shriver* National Institute of Child Health and Human Development (NICHD) has been a leader in advocating for hospitals to avoid elective induction of labor prior to 39 weeks, not only to reduce the number of cesarean deliveries but also to decrease NICU admissions and overall health care costs. To that end, it is important that each hospital system create a list of acceptable indications for induction of labor, that those indications are widely communicated, and that deviations from those indications are minimized.

The ACOG-recognized indications for induction of labor are not absolute, but they do provide a basic framework for obstetric practice. The commonly observed indications are as follows:

- Abruption of the placenta
- Chorioamnionitis
- Fetal demise
- Gestational hypertension
- Preeclampsia, eclampsia
- Premature rupture of membranes (PROM)
- Postterm pregnancy (greater than or equal to 41 weeks)
- Maternal medical conditions (diabetes mellitus, renal disease, chronic pulmonary disease, chronic hypertension, antiphospholipid syndrome)
- Fetal compromise (severe fetal growth restriction, alloimmunization, oligohydramnios)

Other possible indications for induction of labor that are acknowledged by ACOG include logistical reasons such as history of rapid labor, distance from hospital, and maternal psychosocial indications. Remember that with induction for logistical indications, the patient should be greater than 39 weeks gestation and have a favorable cervix.

The cervix must be thinned and dilated in order for vaginal delivery to occur. In 1964, Dr Bishop published findings using his scoring system of cervical dilation, effacement, station, consistency, and position. The Bishop score is the accepted way of communicating cervical "ripeness," but in essence was originally published to predict the likelihood of spontaneous labor in multiparous women. Using a scale of 0 to 13, a Bishop score greater than 8 generally confers the same likelihood of vaginal delivery with induction of labor as spontaneous labor and thus is an objective way of communicating that the cervix is "favorable" for induction. A Bishop score of 6 or less typically indicates an "unfavorable" cervix. Laughon et al published a "simplified Bishop score" (scale of 0-9) using only dilation, effacement, and station and found a similar predictive ability of successful induction as the original score, with any score of 5 or greater being indicative of a favorable cervix.

There are several contraindications to induction of labor that are important to remember. These include, but are not limited to:

- Vasa previa or complete placenta previa
- Transverse fetal lie
- Umbilical cord prolapse
- Previous classical cesarean delivery

- Active genital herpes infection
- Previous myomectomy entering the endometrial cavity

With an increasing number of cesarean deliveries over the past decade, induction of labor in cases of vaginal birth after cesarean (VBAC) is likely to become an important topic. Induction of labor with mechanical methods in these patients is reasonable and has received support from the Society of Obstetricians and Gynecologists of Canada and ACOG. There is a growing body of literature on the safety and efficacy of different induction methods in women with a prior cesarean, but in general, misoprostol is contraindicated in women undergoing VBAC due to a 15-fold increased risk of uterine rupture.

Treatment

Cervical ripening

As a first step in labor induction with an unfavorable cervix, some clinicians attempt to "ripen" the cervix. There are many different methods of cervical ripening, and there are insufficient data to suggest that any one type of cervical ripening agent is most effective.

The mechanical dilation method, specifically the Foley catheter single-balloon and the Cook Medical double-balloon catheter, has been shown in multiple studies to be an effective induction technique. The concept behind this method of induction is that an unfilled, deflated single- or double-balloon catheter is placed through the cervix, either manually or with ring forceps, above the internal cervical os. The balloon is then filled with 30 to 80 mL of fluid depending on hospital protocols and product specifications. The benefits of this technique include its low cost when compared with prostaglandins (a ring forceps roughly $3 for a Foley catheter compared with $175 for a Cervidil insert), its stability at room temperature, and the reduced risk of uterine tachysystole with or without nonreassuring FHR changes, which, if unresolved, requires cesarean delivery. One disadvantage is that if the cervix is closed or very posterior and high, it may be impossible to place in this situation. Mechanical dilation catheters should be used with caution, if at all, in the setting of marginal placenta previa, as the balloon may disrupt the edge of the placenta during placement, causing significant hemorrhage.

Dinoprostone (a PGE2 analog) is another well-studied ripening method that is commonly used across the United States. Two PGE2 preparations are commercially available: a gel available in a 2.5-mL syringe containing 0.5 mg of dinoprostone and a vaginal insert (Cervidil) containing 10 mg of dinoprostone. The vaginal insert has the advantage of being embedded on a wafer that can be removed with a string, and it releases prostaglandins at a slower rate (0.3 mg/h) than the gel. Compared with placebo or oxytocin alone, vaginal prostaglandins used for cervical ripening increase the likelihood of delivery within 24 hours. Another advantage is that Cervidil can be used in a patient with a closed cervix. However, Cervidil, when compared with mechanical dilation methods, is associated with a significant increase in the rate of uterine tachysystole with associated FHR changes (an approximate rate of 5%), and lavaging or flushing the vagina does not help in the resolution of this situation.

Misoprostol (Cytotec), a synthetic PGE1 analogue, can be administered intravaginally or orally, and is used for both cervical ripening and induction of labor. It currently is available in a 100-mcg (unscored) or a 200-mcg tablet, and can be broken to provide 25-mcg doses. It is the least expensive of the options, with 25 mcg costing roughly $0.25. The typical dose for induction of labor in the setting of a live fetus is 25 mcg vaginally every 3 to 6 hours. Careful monitoring of the contraction pattern is important prior to placing further doses as tachysystole is a very real risk with Cytotec.

Methods of induction

Oxytocin is the most commonly used method of labor induction and augmentation once cervical ripening has been achieved. It can be titrated, giving the provider a chance to control its dosing and administration, which is especially important in the setting of uterine tachysystole. Each hospital and institution should develop and implement its own protocol endorsing either a high-dose protocol, low-dose protocol, or both (both have been proven to be safe in systematic reviews). Water intoxication can occur with high concentrations of oxytocin infused with large quantities of hypotonic solutions, but in doses and fluids used in labor, this is extremely rare.

In the setting of PROM at term, it is recommended to initiate oxytocin if labor has not ensued at the time of presentation to labor and delivery. A meta-analysis that included 6814 women with PROM at term compared induction of labor with prostaglandins or oxytocin with expectant management. There was a significant reduction in the risk of women developing chorioamnionitis or endometritis and a reduced number of neonates requiring admission to the neonatal intensive care unit noted in the women who underwent induction of labor compared with expectant management.

Amniotomy is the act of rupturing the membranes artificially, usually with an amniohook, a sterile, plastic hook designed specifically for this purpose. It is recommended to use this technique in combination with oxytocin administration. There is little support for using amniotomy alone as an induction method. Potential complications of amniotomy include prolapse of the umbilical cord, chorioamnionitis, significant umbilical cord compression, and rupture of vasa previa. It is important to closely monitor the FHR tracing immediately before and after amniotomy. Despite a recent report in support of early amniotomy in nulliparous patients (amniotomy at 4 cm or less dilation), in which the authors showed a trend of increased rate of vaginal deliveries with no increase in complications, more research is needed before this becomes standard practice. Other methods of induction that are not recommended or are ineffective based on systematic reviews include nipple stimulation, sexual intercourse, ingestion of castor oil, and acupuncture.

Finally, it is very important to note that the progress of labor in women undergoing cervical ripening and induction of labor is likely to be very different from that of spontaneous labor. In an effort to prevent cesarean delivery in the setting of labor induction, it is important to define what is considered a failed induction. Even in spontaneous labor, but especially in induction of labor, recent reports show that in the United States the progress of labor from 4 to 6 cm may take up to 6 hours, which is a change from as little as 5 years ago. In order to curb the increasing cesarean rate and to prevent the first cesarean in patients undergoing induction, in the presence of reassuring maternal and fetal status, the diagnosis of arrest of labor should not be made until adequate time has elapsed. This includes *greater than 6 cm dilation with membrane rupture* and 4 or more hours of adequate contractions (eg, greater than 200 Montevideo units) or 6 hours or more if contractions are inadequate with no cervical change for first-stage arrest. For second-stage arrest, where the cervix is completely dilated, no progress (descent or rotation) of the fetal head for more than 4 hours in nulliparous women with an epidural, more than 3 hours in nulliparous women without an epidural, more than 3 hours in multiparous women with an epidural, and more than 2 hours in multiparous women without an epidural should be considered. A responsible Ob/Gyn, practicing in concert with ACOG standards, should avoid delivery for the indication of "arrest" before these time limits.

TIPS TO REMEMBER

- Induction of labor generally carries with it an increased risk of cesarean delivery, and, especially in an elective induction, this risk must be communicated to the patient.
- Labor induction should be performed only for medical indications; if done for nonmedical indications, the gestational age should be 39 weeks or more, and the cervix should be favorable (Bishop score more than 8), especially in the nulliparous patient.
- The diagnosis of failed induction should only be made after an adequate attempt. The literature contains several recommendations as to what constitutes an adequate attempt, but most would agree that membranes should be ruptured for at least 12 hours.
- The use of misoprostol in women with prior cesarean delivery or major uterine surgery has been associated with an increase in uterine rupture and, therefore, should be avoided in the third trimester.
- The Foley catheter is a reasonable and effective method for cervical ripening and inducing labor.

COMPREHENSION QUESTIONS

1. A 25-year-old nulliparous woman presents to labor and delivery triage at 39 weeks and 2 days of gestation with frequent uterine contractions for the past 4 hours. Her initial examination is 1 cm dilated and 50% effaced, with the fetus

at –3 station. The FHR tracing is category I with reassuring baseline and accelerations. After repeated examinations over the next 4 hours, her examination remains unchanged. The best next step in management is which of the following?

A. Placement of a Foley balloon catheter with low-dose oxytocin
B. Placement of Cervidil vaginal insert
C. Expectant management
D. Amniotomy with oxytocin

2. A 33-year-old gravida 2 para 1 with a previous low transverse cesarean delivery performed secondary to breech presentation with her first child presents to the office at 39 weeks of gestation for a prenatal visit. Her cervix is long, closed, and soft at –2 station. The patient would like to proceed with a trial of labor. The approach most likely to end in successful VBAC is which of the following?

A. Await spontaneous labor.
B. Begin cervical ripening with misoprostol.
C. Perform a repeat cesarean delivery.
D. Begin cervical ripening with a 60-mL Foley balloon.

3. A 19-year-old nulliparous woman at 39 weeks presents to labor and delivery reporting abdominal pain. She has received limited prenatal care and admits to using cocaine recently. She is mildly tachycardic and on the tocometer she is contracting every 1 to 2 minutes. On examination, there is a solid trickle of blood from the cervical os that is visually 2 cm dilated. Fetal heart tones are reassuring in the 130s, and maternal hemoglobin is 12 g/dL. What is the next step in management?

A. Placement of Foley catheter for induction of labor.
B. Expectant management.
C. Begin labor augmentation with oxytocin.
D. Perform an obstetric ultrasound.
E. Obtain patient consent and perform a cesarean delivery.

Answers

1. **C.** The patient is in the latent phase of labor. This phase is defined as the time from the onset of regular uterine contractions until active labor or roughly 4 cm dilation. The course of labor, particularly the relationship between the latent phase and the active phase of labor, has been described historically by the Friedman curve. The best choice in the case is expectant management to await active labor.

2. **A.** The number of VBAC candidates such as this one is increasing in the United States. It is acceptable to offer induction of labor to women undergoing trial of labor after cesarean, but the timing of this induction is difficult. It may be preferable to await spontaneous labor in such a patient than risk intervening and contributing to a uterine rupture or other complication. Misoprostol is contraindicated for induction of labor in any patient with a prior uterine scar. If induction

of labor were necessary either for medical indication or if the patient reached 41 weeks gestation, the Foley catheter would be preferable. Indeed, the Society of Obstetricians and Gynecologists of Canada has stated, "a Foley catheter may be safely used to ripen the cervix in a woman planning a trial of labor after cesarean section." It is the role of the physician to counsel and educate the patient about risks/benefits/alternatives and allow the patient to share in decision making.

3. **D**. This patient has a classic presentation of a placental abruption. In this setting more information is needed and an ultrasound to confirm position of the fetus and location of the placenta is important before further management decisions are made. The ultrasound is not likely to show evidence of an abruption, as this modality has not been shown to reliably detect abruption. Induction of labor is likely not necessary in this setting as the abruption has already set this process in motion. The patient is hemodynamically stable and the fetus may tolerate a significant abruption for some time before uteroplacental insufficiency becomes obvious. It would be appropriate to obtain informed consent in this setting, as this situation can deteriorate rapidly in the setting of excessive blood loss, but abruption is not an absolute indication for cesarean. If the bleeding stopped and contractions decreased, a Foley catheter and/or oxytocin may become appropriate assuming there is no evidence of previa on ultrasound.

SUGGESTED READINGS

ACOG Committee on Practice Bulletins—Obstetrics. ACOG Practice Bulletin No. 107: induction of labor. *Obstet Gynecol.* 2009;114(2 pt 1):386–397.

Dare MR, Middleton P, Crowther CA, Flenady VJ, Varatharaju B. Planned early birth versus expectant management (waiting) for prelabour rupture of membranes at term (37 weeks or more). *Cochrane Database Syst Rev.* 2006;(1):CD005302.

Delaney S, Shaffer BL, Cheng YW, et al. Labor induction with a Foley balloon inflated to 30 mL compared with 60 mL: a randomized controlled trial. *Obstet Gynecol.* 2010;115(6):1239–1245.

Harper LM, Cahill AG, Boslaugh S, et al. Association of induction of labor and uterine rupture in women attempting vaginal birth after cesarean: a survival analysis. *Am J Obstet Gynecol.* 2012; 206(1): 51.e1–51.e5.

Laughon SK, Zhang J, Troendle J, Sun L, Reddy UM. Using a simplified Bishop score to predict vaginal delivery. *Obstet Gynecol.* 2011;117(4):805–811.

Levey KA, Arslan AA, Funai EF. Extra-amniotic saline infusion increases cesarean risk versus other induction methods and spontaneous labor. *Am J Perinatol.* 2006;23(7):435–438.

Macones GA, Cahill A, Stamilio DM, Odibo AO. The efficacy of early amniotomy in nulliparous labor induction: a randomized controlled trial. *Am J Obstet Gynecol.* 2012;207(5):403.e1–403.e5.

Salim R, Zafran N, Nachum Z, Garmi G, Kraiem N, Shalev E. Single-balloon compared with double-balloon catheters for induction of labor: a randomized controlled trial. *Obstet Gynecol.* 2011;118(1):79–86.

Spong CY, Berghella V, Wenstrom KD, Mercer BM, Saade GR. Preventing the first cesarean delivery: summary of a joint Eunice Kennedy Shriver National Institute of Child Health and Human Development, Society for Maternal-Fetal Medicine, and American College of Obstetricians and Gynecologists Workshop. *Obstet Gynecol.* 2012;120(5):1181–1193.

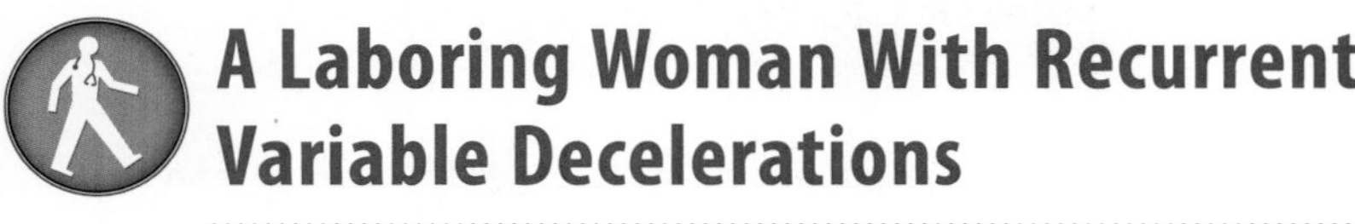

A Laboring Woman With Recurrent Variable Decelerations

Edward R. Yeomans, MD

An 18-year-old primigravida at 40 weeks gestation was admitted through triage with a diagnosis of spontaneous rupture of membranes. Her cervix was 5 cm dilated, fully effaced, and the fetal head was at 0 station. External fetal heart rate (FHR) monitoring and tocodynamometry revealed a baseline FHR of 145 beats/min (bpm), moderate baseline variability, no accelerations, recurrent variable decelerations, and no obvious trend after 30 minutes of monitoring. Contractions were occurring every 3 minutes and lasting 60 seconds.

1. **What is your diagnosis (ie, how do you interpret the electronic monitoring data and in what category would you classify this FHR tracing)?**
2. **What is your management plan?**

Answers

1. The patient in this scenario has a Category II strip. In order to give a more complete verbal description of your interpretation, you will need to familiarize yourself with some definitions. Some of these definitions are straightforward and must simply be memorized. Others are somewhat vague and broad. For example, in a 3-tiered classification system, Category II includes all FHR tracings not included in Category I or III.
2. Precise recommendations for managing Category II FHR strips are elusive. Compression of the umbilical cord is a frequent cause of variable decelerations, especially after rupture of membranes. A vaginal examination to rule out cord prolapse is recommended, as is maternal repositioning. If the variable decelerations are not resolved, amnioinfusion (instillation of fluid via a small catheter into the uterine cavity) is a potential intervention, but in actual clinical practice is employed relatively infrequently.

CASE REVIEW

An important take-home point for the fourth-year student or intern is learning to present a FHR tracing. An excellent presentation requires that 6 points be addressed:

1. What is the baseline heart rate? This rate is rounded to the nearest 5 bpm and read in the interval between contractions. The baseline must persist for a minimum of 2 minutes in any 10-minute segment. Normal baseline FHR is between 110 and 160 bpm. The baseline in this case is normal.

2. What is the variability? Variability is a feature of the baseline and is quantitated as the amplitude of peak to trough in bpm. There are 4 descriptions of variability:

    - Absent: amplitude range undetectable
    - Minimal: ≤5 bpm
    - Moderate: 6 to 25 bpm
    - Marked: >25 bpm

    The moderate variability noted in this scenario, combined with a normal baseline rate, is very reassuring and almost always signifies the absence of fetal acidosis.

3. Accelerations—a visually apparent increase in FHR of 15 bpm or greater, lasting for ≥15 seconds. If the acceleration lasts from 2 to 10 minutes, it is described as prolonged. If it lasts more than 10 minutes, it is classified as a baseline change. Although absent in the case presented, accelerations are an important indicator of fetal well-being. When no spontaneous accelerations are present, they may be stimulated either vibroacoustically or by digital scalp massage.
4. Decelerations—a visually apparent decrease in heart rate of 15 bpm or greater, lasting for ≥15 seconds. It is not acceptable to say that "decelerations are present." The type of deceleration must be described as early, late, or variable. The decelerations in the case presented are variable. This designation implies that the decelerations are variable in shape, timing, duration, and amplitude. The modifier "recurrent" means that decelerations occur with ≥50% of uterine contractions. Amplitude is likely to be an important feature of variable decelerations, but is not addressed in the current classification system.
5. Trend or pattern—FHR tracings are dynamic and often change quickly. In the case presented, there was no change during 30 minutes of observation. A good rule of thumb for the novice when asked to interpret an FHR tracing is to begin by quickly reviewing the preceding 30 to 60 minutes of strip.
6. Uterine activity—the so-called bottom line. This very important feature of the tracing may involve either external or internal contraction monitoring. In the case above, external monitoring was in use, so only frequency and duration can be determined. Quantitation of strength or amplitude of contractions requires the placement of an intrauterine pressure catheter (IUPC).

To summarize, the patient in the case above requires close observation, but minimal intervention. The medical student and beginning resident reading this chapter would do well to bear in mind that such a prescription—observe without intervening—is appropriate in many different scenarios in obstetrics. It is important for the beginner to keep his or her superiors informed regarding abnormalities that occur in the FHR tracing.

ELECTRONIC FHR MONITORING

Electronic FHR monitoring is impossible to reduce to a short chapter. In fact, it is the title of a highly recommended textbook, the last edition of which was published before the 3-tiered classification was adopted.

A reasonable question that might be asked by someone embarking on the study of this topic might be: "How much useful information can one get from monitoring a single vital sign (heart rate)?" The answer to that question is the focus of this chapter.

The goal of intrapartum electronic fetal monitoring is to assess the adequacy of fetal oxygenation during labor. Although baseline rate is an important feature of the FHR tracing, other features are the key to assessing oxygenation. An adequately oxygenated fetus relies on aerobic metabolism. When oxygen is inadequate, the fetus shifts to anaerobic metabolism and generates lactic acid, producing a metabolic acidosis. Two important features of the FHR baseline, accelerations and moderate variability, reliably indicate the *absence* of metabolic acidosis in the fetus. It is the presence of these 2 features, coupled with a normal baseline rate and without late or variable decelerations, that defines a Category I strip.

Category III requires *absent* variability and 1 of the following: recurrent variable decelerations, recurrent late decelerations, or fetal bradycardia. (Sinusoidal patterns are also included in Category III, but such patterns are infrequent and will not be considered further here. The interested reader is referred to the reference Freeman et al, 2003 for details.) If intrauterine resuscitative measures such as oxygen administration, maternal repositioning, correction of hypotension, and stopping oxytocin fail to resolve a Category III tracing, delivery is probably indicated.

Between the extremes of Category I and III is Category II; this category accounts for the majority of FHR tracings encountered in clinical practice. Recall that the fetus in the case presentation had a Category II tracing. These tracings require evaluation, continued surveillance, initiation of resuscitative measures when indicated, and reevaluation.

Interpretation of FHR tracings depends heavily on the clinical scenario, for example, early Stage 1 labor or pushing in Stage 2. Term fetuses typically have more reserve than preterm fetuses and are better able to tolerate brief interruptions in oxygen delivery. Interpreting FHR tracings is a highly visual skill and requires the beginner to have a thorough understanding of the various definitions highlighted at the beginning of this chapter and detailed in the reference American College of Obstetricians and Gynecologists (2009). Only when the interpretation is accurate is it appropriate to move on to management. Figure 26-1A to C are snapshots of

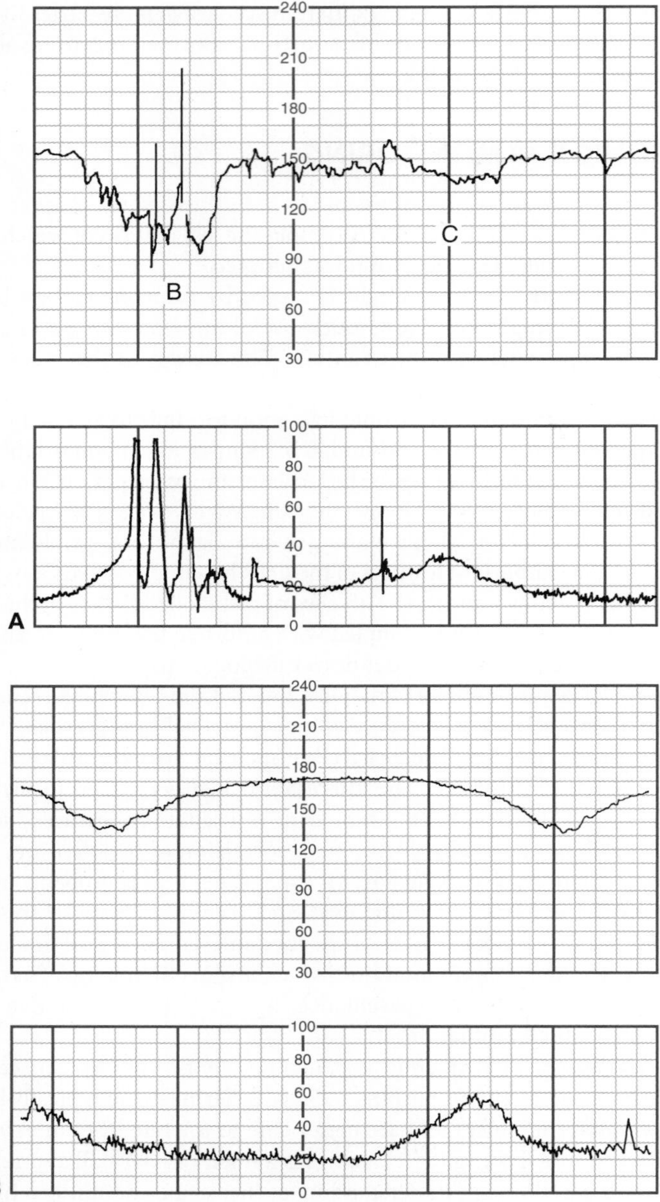

Figure 26-1. Types of decelerations. (A) Early deceleration: gradual onset (>30 seconds from onset to nadir), timed with contraction. (B) Late decelerations: gradual onset, but shifted to the right of the contractions. (C) Variable decelerations: abrupt onset (less than 30 seconds from onset to nadir).

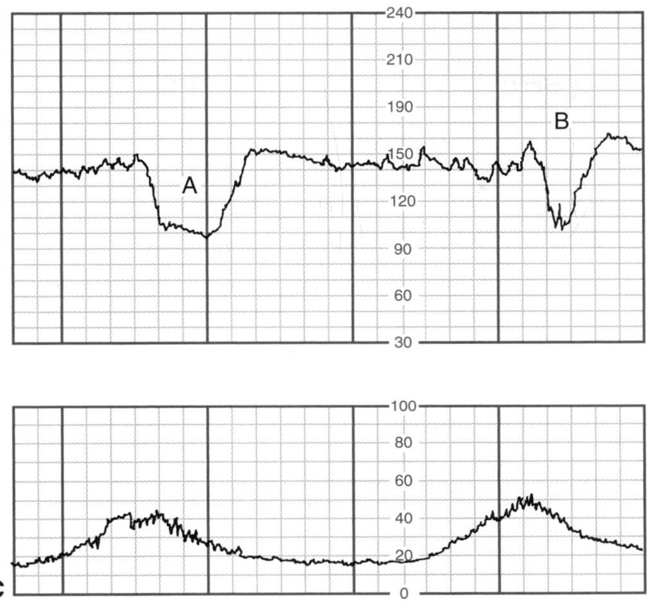

Figure 26-1. (*Continued*)

the 3 types of deceleration (early, variable, and late). All 3 types of these decelerations rely on their associations with contractions, and are therefore termed periodic changes in the FHR.

Uterine contractions are recorded below the FHR pattern and this information regarding uterine activity has been referred to in the literature as the "bottom line." The units on the uterine activity scale are millimeters of mercury, but recall from the section "Case Review" that amplitude can only be quantified when an IUPC is in use.

It is appropriate to conclude this brief overview of electronic fetal monitoring with a perspective on the use of this technology in clinical obstetrics. Such a perspective was provided in a recent editorial entitled *Electronic Fetal Monitoring—The Debate Goes On and On and On*. The author of that editorial concludes (and I agree) that EFM has resulted in an increase in the rate of cesarean and operative vaginal deliveries, but no decrease in perinatal mortality, neonatal seizures, or the risk of cerebral palsy. Despite those facts, the entity of EFM is "entrenched" in American obstetrics and leads to my advice to the beginner: strive to become thoroughly familiar with the principles of electronic fetal monitoring before or shortly after beginning obstetric residency and make a concerted effort to keep up with this dynamic field throughout the course of your training and subsequent clinical practice.

TIPS TO REMEMBER

- Definitions are important. These should be memorized in order to correctly "speak the language."
- Learn and use the proper format for presenting FHR tracings: baseline rate, variability, accelerations, decelerations, trend, and uterine contractions.
- Practice classifying FHR tracings into 1 of 3 categories.
- Understand the options for intrauterine resuscitation.
- Keep your superiors informed regarding abnormal FHR tracings.

COMPREHENSION QUESTIONS

1. You are managing the labor of a primigravid woman who is being monitored electronically. She is receiving oxytocin intravenously and you note 3 consecutive late decelerations. What should you do?

   A. Turn off the oxytocin.
   B. Turn the patient on her side.
   C. Notify your upper level resident.
   D. All of the above.

2. Shortly after artificial rupture of membranes, the FHR tracing shows new-onset variable decelerations. Which of the choices listed below is the best immediate step?

   A. Turn off the oxytocin.
   B. Stop the epidural infusion.
   C. Perform a digital vaginal examination.
   D. Begin an amnioinfusion.

3. Which of the following is an observed benefit of electronic fetal monitoring?

   A. A reduction in the cesarean delivery rate
   B. A decrease in perinatal mortality
   C. A decline in the frequency of cerebral palsy
   D. None of the above

Answers

1. **D.** All of the listed actions are appropriate. Intrauterine resuscitation encompasses 6 possible interventions: oxygen administration, repositioning, increasing IV fluids, stopping oxytocin, amnioinfusion, and, rarely, administration of a tocolytic drug.

2. **C.** The purpose of a digital vaginal examination is to rule out cord prolapse. The remaining choices are wrong only because they are not the best immediate step.

3. **D.** Despite its limitations, electronic fetal monitoring is likely here to stay. Choice A is wrong because EFM has contributed to an increase in cesarean delivery. Choices B and C were outcomes that were hoped for when the technology was introduced, but neither has materialized.

SUGGESTED READINGS

American College of Obstetricians and Gynecologists. ACOG Practice Bulletin No. 106: intrapartum fetal heart rate monitoring: nomenclature, interpretation, and general management principles. *Obstet Gynecol.* 2009;114:192–202.

American College of Obstetricians and Gynecologists. Practice Bulletin No. 116: management of intrapartum fetal heart rate tracings. *Obstet Gynecol.* 2010;116:1232–1240.

Antepartum fetal monitoring. In: Freeman RK, Garite TJ, Nageotte MP, eds. *Fetal Heart Rate Monitoring.* 3rd ed. Philadelphia, PA: Lippincott Williams & Wilkins; 2003:181–202.

Miller DA, Miller LA. Electronic fetal heart rate monitoring: applying principles of patient safety. *Am J Obstet Gynecol.* 2012;206:278–283.

Resnik R. Electronic fetal monitoring: the debate goes on and on and on. *Obstet Gynecol.* 2013;121: 917–918.

Ross MG, Jessie M, Amaya K, et al. Correlation of arterial fetal base deficit and lactate changes with severity of variable heart rate decelerations in the near-term ovine fetus. *Am J Obstet Gynecol.* 2013; 208:285.e1–285.e6.

A 30-year-old P3003 at 38.2 Weeks With Contractions and Feeling Pressure

Lydia D. Nightingale, MD, FACOG

You are currently in triage and a 30-year-old G4 P3003 with an IUP at 38.2 weeks gestation presents with complaints of a 2-hour history of painful uterine contractions occurring every 3 minutes and rectal pressure. She denies loss of fluid and vaginal bleeding, and reports regular fetal movement. A review of the records shows an uncomplicated prenatal course with routine care. She had a dating ultrasound at 18 weeks that was consistent with her LMP. GBS culture at 36 weeks was positive, and her cervix at that time was 2 cm dilated.

In triage, her blood pressure is 120/70 and she is afebrile. A vertex fetus is noted on both Leopold maneuvers and sterile vaginal examination (SVE). SVE shows the cervix to be 7 cm dilated, 80% effaced, and the vertex is at 0 station. Uterine contractions are occurring every 2 to 4 minutes, and the fetal heart rate baseline is 140 with moderate variability, accelerations, and variable decelerations with contractions.

1. **What is the next best step in the management of this patient?**
2. **What other physical examination finding on SVE is needed to complete the assessment of this patient?**

Answers

1. The patient is in labor, and given her parity and SVE needs to be admitted to a labor room quickly. As the intern in triage, your job will be to ensure that deliveries take place in labor rooms and not triage! The complaint of rectal pressure is an indication that the fetus is low enough in the pelvis to cause compression of the rectum, and the variable decelerations with contractions support this.
2. The finding missing from the SVE is the position of the fetus. Always challenge yourself to record the fetal position once cervical dilation reaches 5 cm or greater. Determining fetal position is a skill, and like any other skill, requires continued practice and constant alertness. Fetal position must be known prior to application of forceps, and aids in determining how you place your hands on the fetal head at the time of delivery.

CASE REVIEW

You communicate to your upper level that the patient is parous and in labor, and you move her to a labor room quickly. You return to triage, but you are called back to the labor room immediately as the patient is pushing. You gown and glove rapidly and deliver a healthy baby girl, followed by placental delivery. The patient's blood loss is normal and you offer congratulations to mother and father and then it's back to triage. The night has just begun!

NORMAL VAGINAL DELIVERY

Diagnosis and Treatment

As a patient progresses through labor, she may begin to feel an urge to push as she nears the second stage. The fetal head may begin to mold to accommodate the passage through the pelvis. When molding occurs, the parietal bones will overlap and the overriding sutures make evaluation of fetal position more difficult. This is another reason why assessment of position on admission is so important. Caput succedaneum is fetal scalp edema that develops due to pressure on the cervix. Both molding and caput can lead to errors in determining fetal station. The leading portion of the fetal head is thought to be at or below the spines, but the biparietal diameter (BPD) is still at the level of the pelvic inlet or above.

If the fetal station is high when the second stage begins, the patient can "labor down" to allow the fetus to descend in the pelvis prior to pushing. Indications to start pushing immediately at time of full dilation include intra-amniotic infection and fetal intolerance of labor, as well as maternal preference. An optimal pushing position is unclear; however, many women in the United States deliver in the dorsal lithotomy position. As long as the fetal tracing is reassuring, primiparous patients can be allowed to push in the second stage of labor for up to 2 hours without an epidural and 3 hours with an epidural. In a multiparous patient, these times are 1 and 2 hours, respectively.

Options for pain relief include narcotics, epidural, spinal, combined spinal–epidural, and local anesthesia with or without a pudendal block. Patients should be provided with the risks and benefits of each type of pain relief and allowed to choose which method they prefer.

The responsibility of the provider at the time of delivery is to reduce maternal injury in the form of genital tract lacerations and to prevent birth trauma to the infant. There is no consensus on how to prevent perineal injury. Episiotomy can facilitate delivery of the fetal head by enlarging the vaginal outlet, and is indicated in situations of fetal distress or in planning for an operative delivery, but its routine use is discouraged. As the fetal vertex is crowning, efforts should be made to keep the head in a flexed position to decrease the diameter that is presented to the vaginal outlet, and control the rate of delivery.

After delivery of the fetal head, restitution will occur and the shoulders may be aligned in an AP diameter. Evaluation for a nuchal cord should be undertaken, and if present, can sometimes be reduced over the fetal head. If it is too tight to accommodate this maneuver, then the nuchal cord can be clamped and transected at the neck or the fetus can be delivered by slipping the cord over the fetal shoulders. Once the head is delivered, it is grasped with 2 hands and gentle downward traction is placed until the anterior shoulder is visualized under the pubic arch, indicating it has cleared the symphysis pubis. Once the anterior shoulder can be seen, visual attention is directed to the perineal body, while elevating the fetal head to deliver the posterior shoulder. This is likely the most important part of the delivery, and great attention and control must be used to decrease trauma to the perineal body. You may need to kneel down on 1 knee if you are standing in order to get low enough to visualize the perineal body. Once the baby is delivered, the cord is then clamped in 2 places and transected between. Most often the cord is clamped within the first minute of life. It is unclear if there is clinical benefit from routine use of delayed cord clamping. The baby can be placed skin-to-skin after delivery if the mother desires; this has been shown to assist in neonatal transitioning. If meconium is present or there are other neonatal concerns, the baby should be handed off to another health care provider for assessment and interventions if necessary.

Cord blood is collected for neonatal type and screen, and potentially to test for other abnormalities. This is collected either from the cord before delivering the placenta or from vessels on the fetal surface of the placenta after its expulsion. If a cord gas is collected, it should be taken from the umbilical artery by a needle and syringe.

The third stage of labor is the interval from the birth of the baby to the expulsion of the placenta. On average, the third stage is 5 to 7 minutes, and is considered abnormal after 30 minutes. The major complications that can occur during the third stage of labor are hemorrhage, retained products of conception, cord avulsion, and uterine inversion. Signs of placental separation include cord lengthening, a sudden gush of blood, and the uterus rising in an anterior/cephalic direction as it becomes more firm and globular. Gentle traction on the cord using the dominant hand is used to deliver the placenta. To avoid uterine inversion, which is associated with severe hemorrhage and hypovolemic shock, suprapubic pressure with the nondominant hand is applied simultaneously. Take care not to pull too hard or avulse the cord—in other words, "Don't be the jerk on the cord!" Manual extraction of the placenta should be undertaken if the placenta is not delivered within 30 minutes. Inspect the placenta after delivery to ensure it is intact, count the number of fetal vessels, and note the umbilical cord insertion site.

Once the placenta is delivered, it is indicated to massage the uterus externally to ensure that it becomes firm. If bleeding persists or the uterus remains boggy, additional measures should be undertaken to control bleeding. Average blood loss for a vaginal delivery is 500 cm^3, and postpartum hemorrhage is defined as blood loss of greater than 500 cm^3. Inspect for lacerations of the birth canal, and those that are bleeding should be repaired with an absorbable suture on a tapered needle.

TIPS TO REMEMBER

- Episiotomies should not be performed routinely, but rather reserved for obstetric indications.
- Practitioners should be skilled in repair of surgical and spontaneous obstetric lacerations.
- After delivery of the placenta, it should be examined to ensure it is intact and the number of vessels in the cord should be verified.

COMPREHENSION QUESTIONS

1. Which of the items listed below is most susceptible to errors in ascertainment when caput and molding are present?

   A. Presentation
   B. Dilation
   C. Effacement
   D. Station

2. What is the net effect of epidural anesthesia for both nulliparous and parous women on the suggested limits for pushing in the second stage of labor?

   A. No effect compared with those without an epidural
   B. Increases the limit of pushing time by 1 hour
   C. Accelerates progress in the second stage because catecholamine release is blunted
   D. None of the above

3. What is the biggest risk of hastening the delivery of the placenta by traction on the umbilical cord?

   A. Uterine rupture
   B. Avulsion of the cord
   C. Uterine inversion
   D. Premature separation of the placenta

Answers

1. **D.** Even without caput and molding, station is the most difficult element to determine for the beginner due to the normal architecture of the bony pelvis. Caput and molding contribute to elongation of the fetal head and make palpation of the leading part an inaccurate indicator of station.

2. **B.** Epidurals prolong the duration of both the first and second stages of labor. The addition of 1 hour to the upper limit of pushing time was somewhat arbitrarily adopted by ACOG.

3. C. Uterine inversion is a relatively rare complication of the third stage of labor, occurring with a frequency of about 1:2500. It is often accompanied by brisk bleeding. Avulsion can result from cord traction, but is nowhere near as serious as inversion. A & D are simply distractors.

SUGGESTED READINGS

APGO Clinical Skills Curriculum. Vaginal delivery. <http://www.apgo.org/elearn/clinical_skills_curriculum/HTML/delivery-learningoutcomes.html>.

Normal labor and delivery. In: Cunningham FG, Leveno KJ, Bloom SL, Hauth JC, Rouse DJ, Spong CY, eds. *Williams Obstetrics*. 23rd ed. New York: McGraw-Hill; 2010.

DeCherney AH, Nathan L. *Current Obstetric & Gynecologic Diagnosis & Treatment*. 9th ed. New York: McGraw-Hill; 2003.

Evans AT. *Manual of Obstetrics*. 7th ed. Philadelphia: Lippincott Williams & Wilkins; 2007.

Gibbs RS, Karlan BY, Haney AF, Nygaard I. *Danforth's Obstetrics and Gynecology*. 10th ed. Philadelphia: Lippincott Williams & Wilkins; 2008.

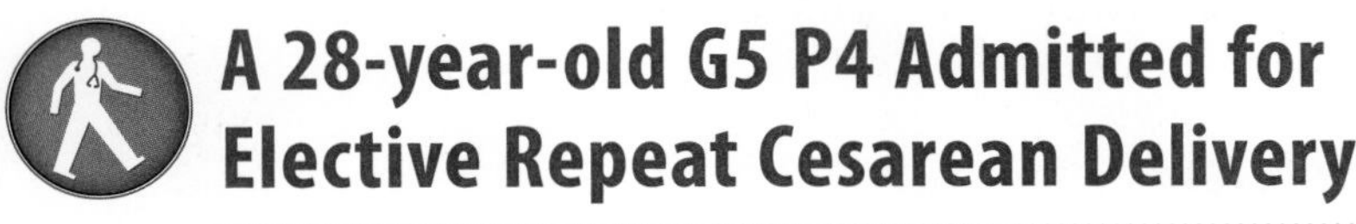

A 28-year-old G5 P4 Admitted for Elective Repeat Cesarean Delivery

Edward R. Yeomans, MD

A 28-year-old woman G5 P4004 is admitted to labor and delivery for repeat cesarean delivery and bilateral tubal ligation. Her gestational age is 39 weeks, confirmed by an ultrasound done at 8 weeks. Her history is remarkable for 4 term cesarean deliveries. The first was for arrest of descent in the second stage of labor and all the others were elective repeat cesareans at term. The pregnancy has been uncomplicated and a third trimester ultrasound revealed a posterior fundal placenta with no previa. The woman requests permanent sterilization.

1. What dating criteria must be present to schedule elective cesarean delivery?

2. What are the important risks associated with multiple cesarean deliveries?

Answers

1. The American College of Obstetricians and Gynecologists has stipulated that elective cesarean delivery ought not to be performed before 39 and 0/7 weeks gestation. Dating criteria include:

   - Fetal heart sounds documented for 30 weeks by Doppler.
   - Thirty-six weeks have elapsed from a positive urine or serum pregnancy test.
   - A sonographic measurement of crown–rump length between 6 and 11 weeks putting a patient at ≥39 weeks estimated gestational age.
   - History and physical examination along with 12- to 20-week ultrasound measurements supports a gestational age ≥39 weeks.

   If none of these criteria are met, there are only 2 options: await spontaneous labor or document fetal lung maturity by amniocentesis. Elective delivery at 37 to 38 weeks is associated with significant neonatal morbidity.

2. In general, the risks associated with multiple cesarean deliveries have been underemphasized in the obstetric literature. These risks include the life-threatening consequences of placenta accreta and uterine rupture, along with placenta previa, blood transfusion, injury to bowel or bladder, hysterectomy, and admission to an ICU. Because maternal mortality is increasing in the United States and the increased rate of cesarean delivery is 1 of 4 or 5 major contributors (others include advanced maternal age, obesity, and chronic medical conditions complicating pregnancy) to that increase, recent reports have focused on preventing the first cesarean delivery.

CASE REVIEW

The patient in our scenario is at 39 weeks by a reliable dating criterion (crown–rump length measurement at 8 weeks gestation). Therefore, it is appropriate to proceed with elective repeat cesarean delivery. There is no placenta previa or evidence for accreta, which should reduce, but not eliminate, the risk associated with this, her fifth cesarean section. She has chosen to undergo bilateral tubal ligation for permanent sterilization. Two concerning questions are prompted by the case presentation: at what station and fetal position did her labor arrest in her first pregnancy (ie, was operative vaginal delivery an option?) and was she offered a trial of labor after cesarean (TOLAC) in pregnancy number 2?

CESAREAN DELIVERY

In this book on resident readiness, very few chapters have provided any historical background. However, in regard to cesarean delivery, a little history review will help the student to understand how we got to where we are today. In 1876, Porro reported a case of cesarean delivery, after which the uterine fundus was excised and the cervical stump drained through the anterior abdominal wall. The patient survived only for a short time after the procedure. Four years later, Sanger reported what was later called a "classical" hysterotomy. He incised the uterus vertically extending superiorly well into the thick, contractile portion of the organ and after delivery he repaired the uterus with sutures. In 1912, Kronig suggested a "low" vertical hysterotomy, staying out of the contractile portion. A few years later, in 1921, Kerr reported a low transverse incision in the uterus for cesarean delivery and that is still by far the most common technique used today. In Kerr's time, there were no antibiotics, blood transfusion was not safe, and anesthetic practices were rudimentary! By 1950, 1 group of investigators reported 1000 cesarean deliveries without a maternal death. Another report in 1980 detailed 10,000 cesareans without a maternal death. Clearly the safety of cesarean delivery had remarkably improved. In 1970, the cesarean delivery rate in the United States was about 5%. Today, >40 years later, it is close to 33%. The author (and several other groups cited in the section "Suggested Readings") believes this rate to be too high.

Cesarean section has evolved into the most frequent abdominal surgery performed in the United States today. Four indications account for the majority of cesarean deliveries: repeat cesarean, dystocia (abnormal labor), nonreassuring fetal status, and malpresentation (mainly breech). The woman in the case presentation falls into the first category, but her very first cesarean was performed for dystocia. Some suggested measures to lower the incidence of cesarean for dystocia include using 6 cm as the cutoff for diagnosing active labor, allowing adequate time for the second stage of labor, and encouraging operative vaginal delivery when appropriate (whether this was indicated in the woman in her first pregnancy done for arrest of descent is not known).

Only uncommonly in July are first-year residents the primary surgeon at cesarean delivery, but they are often entrusted with preoperative preparation and postoperative care. All women undergoing elective cesarean delivery should be verified to be at least 39 weeks gestation by the criteria outlined above. Women undergoing either primary or repeat cesarean should receive prophylactic antibiotics (commonly cefazolin) prior to skin incision. A preoperative evaluation by anesthesia personnel is standard. Consideration should be given to prevention of venous thromboembolism, particularly in obese gravidas. Once the woman has been prepped and draped, the right-handed surgeon typically stands on the patient's right, the first assistant on the left, and the second assistant to the first assistant's left. The scrub tech stands to the right of the surgeon.

The various steps in cesarean delivery have been the subject of intense research and are listed in Table 28-1. Reading about the procedure in a standard

Table 28-1. Steps in Cesarean Section

Step	Comment
1. Skin incision	Usually Pfannenstiel, less often subumbilical midline. Check scar for repeat operations
2. Carry incision through subcutaneous tissue to rectus fascia	Camper's—loose Connective Tissue Scarpa's—dense Connective Tissue Extend laterally bluntly
3. Incise fascia near midline; extend sharply laterally if Pfannenstiel	Don't cut the rectus muscle
4. Undermine fascia sharply and bluntly superiorly and inferiorly Separate rectus muscles bluntly	Watch for perforating vessels
5. Enter peritoneum superiorly, bluntly or sharply and expand the opening bluntly	Use caution, especially with repeat c-sections—the bladder may be injured
6. Create a bladder flap bluntly for primary c-section, sharply for repeat c-section	This not a necessary step—sometimes can be safely omitted
7. Incise uterus, most often low transverse, but sometimes vertically Don't cut the baby! Enter the uterine cavity cautiously	Significant fetal lacerations have been caused by unnecessary speed in this step

(*continued*)

Table 28-1. Steps in Cesarean Section (*Continued*)

Step	Comment
8. Deliver the baby! Elevate the head (or breech) into the incision before asking for fundal pressure	Have forceps available for use at cesarean delivery for either high or low heads
9. Deliver the placenta Cord traction is preferred, but manual extraction is *not* contraindicated	Start infusing oxytocin before the placenta is delivered
10. Repair the hysterotomy in 1 or sometimes 2 layers with the uterus outside or inside the abdomen	Reach over the suture strand with your forceps to facilitate locking
11. Insure hemostasis; irrigate and, if exteriorized, replace the uterus	Be alert for atony and use compression, uterotonic drugs, and surgical measures as indicated
12. Some close the bladder flap and anterior peritoneum; others do not	Studies in the literature are conflicting
13. Close fascia, ± subcutaneous tissue and skin	Subcuticular closure may be preferable to staples

textbook will familiarize the student with details of the sequence of events. In most programs today, residents will be the primary surgeons on hundreds of c-sections and skill and speed should improve rapidly with practice. The important principles of postoperative care of the c-section patient include close monitoring of vital signs, urine output, uterine tone, and vaginal bleeding. Over the first few days the wound should be inspected for signs of infection, serous drainage, or separation. Ambulation is encouraged and diet is advanced early in the postoperative course. The patient is usually discharged from the hospital on postoperative day 3 or 4.

A very important reference for the beginning intern is the paper by Spong and colleagues cited in the section "Suggested Readings." The best way to limit the number of women with multiple cesarean deliveries is to prevent the first one. In the United States, more than 90% of women delivered by cesarean in the first pregnancy will be delivered by cesarean in the second and subsequent pregnancies. This fact has contributed to the alarming increase in incidence of placenta accreta, increta, and percreta. Large centers in the United States have assembled special teams to deal with the potential torrential hemorrhage that often accompanies these complications.

ACOG in 2010 updated their vaginal birth after cesarean (VBAC) guidelines and introduced the term TOLAC to describe an attempt at VBAC. From 1996 to the present, the VBAC rate has declined steadily and it is hoped that encouragement from the specialty society in the form of these new guidelines may reverse that trend.

In summary, residents entering the field of obstetrics and gynecology will quickly master the technique of cesarean delivery. Whether they will be given the knowledge and tools to reduce the rate of this overused method of delivery is a matter of speculation.

TIPS TO REMEMBER

- To schedule an elective c-section, it is important to ensure that the patient is at least 39 weeks gestation by reliable dating criteria.
- Maternal morbidity is greatly increased in women with multiple cesarean deliveries.
- Because of the second bullet above, it is very important to try to prevent the *first* cesarean delivery.
- Repeat cesareans are the leading contributors to the overall c-section rate in the United States today.
- Dystocia is the leading indication for primary cesarean section.

COMPREHENSION QUESTIONS

1. Maternal mortality is increasing in the United States today. Which of the following is *not* a leading contributor to that increase?

    A. Advanced maternal age
    B. Increase in the c-section rate
    C. Epidural anesthesia
    D. Obesity

2. Which of the following dating criteria can be used without any supporting evidence to schedule an elective c-section at 39 weeks?

    A. Crown–rump length measurement between 6 and 11 weeks
    B. Ultrasound at 18 weeks
    C. Genetic amniocentesis
    D. None of the above

3. Regarding technique for cesarean delivery, which step listed below is at the discretion of the surgeon?

A. Creation of a bladder flap
B. Closure of the anterior peritoneum
C. Skin closure with either subcuticular suturing or staples
D. All of the above

Answers

1. C. Although there are a number of complications associated with epidural anesthesia, it is not one of the leading contributors to maternal mortality. The other 3 choices are, along with an increase in pregnancies in women with medical complications.

2. A. The measurement of crown–rump length between 6 and 11 weeks gives an estimate of gestational age that is accurate to within 4 days. That accuracy allows it to be a "stand-alone" criterion. Ultrasound at 18 weeks requires supportive findings on history and physical examination. Genetic amniocentesis is completely separate from amniocentesis for lung maturity.

3. D. Despite abundant research on cesarean delivery technique, all of the listed choices allow for operator preference. Some very recent evidence suggests that suturing the skin may have advantages over stapling, but staples are still being used all over the country.

SUGGESTED READINGS

Boyle A, Reddy UM, Landy HJ, Huang CC, Driggers RW, Laughon SK. Primary cesarean delivery in the United States. *Obstet Gynecol.* 2013;122:33–40.

Ong S. *Guidelines for Perinatal Care.* 6th ed. Elk Grove, IL: American Academy of Pediatrics, The American College of Obstetricians and Gynecologists; 2007:160.

Silver RM, Landon MB, Rouse DJ, et al. Maternal morbidity associated with multiple repeat cesarean deliveries. *Obstet Gynecol.* 2006;107:1226–1232.

Spong CY, Berghella V, Wenstrom KD, Mercer BM, Saade GR. Preventing the first cesarean delivery: summary of a joint Eunice Kennedy Shriver National Institute of Child Health and Human Development, Society for Maternal-Fetal Medicine, and American College of Obstetricians and Gynecologists Workshop. *Obstet Gynecol.* 2012;120:1181–1193.

Tita ATN, Landon MB, Spong CY, et al. Timing of elective repeat cesarean delivery at term and neonatal outcomes. *N Engl J Med.* 2009;360:110–120.

Zhang J, Troendle J, Reddy UM, et al. Contemporary cesarean delivery practice in the United States. *Am J Obstet Gynecol.* 2010;203:326.e1–326.e10.

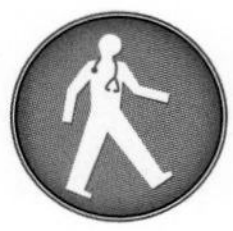

An 18-year-old Primigravida Pushing for 3 Hours

Edward R. Yeomans, MD

An 18-year-old gravida 1 was admitted for induction of labor for mild preeclampsia at 39 weeks. Her initial 24 hours with intact membranes was notable only for 100% effacement. She started the induction at 2 cm dilated and 50% effaced. Membranes were artificially ruptured at 2 cm and internal monitors were placed. She progressed slowly but steadily at 1 cm/h to complete dilation and she has been pushing for the past 3 hours. The fetal head is in right occiput posterior position and visible with contractions, but not between. The estimated fetal weight is 7.5 lb (3400 g). There is moderate caput. The patient is 4 ft 10 in tall, her pregnant weight is 60 kg, and the perineal body is firm, muscular, and short. The bony pelvis was assessed to be gynecoid earlier in labor.

1. Should you cut an episiotomy?

2. If you decide to do so, what type would you cut and how can you minimize the risk of deep perineal lacerations (third- or fourth-degree extensions)?

Answers

1. The author recommends cutting an episiotomy in this patient, but there is no clear right or wrong answer to the question. Clinical judgment is involved and you will spend years, even decades, refining yours. Prior to cutting an episiotomy, manual rotation of the fetal head to an occiput anterior position should be attempted.

2. The best choice would be a mediolateral (the British call it posterolateral) episiotomy, either right or left depending on the dominant hand of the operator. This choice would be less likely than a midline episiotomy to result in damage to the external or internal anal sphincter or to produce a tear in the rectal mucosa. There are a number of technical "fine points" that may reduce the incidence of severe lacerations. Briefly they include using the nondominant hand to maintain flexion (assuming that the position is now occiput anterior) and slow the egress of the head, perineal support with the dominant hand trying to secure the fetal chin (together these maneuvers are referred to as the modified Ritgen maneuver), asking the patient to push with less than maximal effort (sometimes in the interval between contractions), and paying special attention to maternal position during delivery.

CASE REVIEW

This case was selected as a "perfect storm" of risk factors for complications either without or with an episiotomy. Prominent among the risk factors are nulliparity, occiput posterior position, small maternal stature, long first and second stages of labor, and a short perineal body. The resolution of the case was a successful manual rotation to occiput anterior, a right mediolateral episiotomy without extension, a controlled delivery of the fetal head and shoulders, and an anatomically correct repair of the episiotomy. Both mother and baby were discharged on hospital day 2, doing well. The subject of episiotomy and repair will be briefly reviewed below, but for more detail the reader is referred to the section "Suggested Readings" (particularly the reference Episiotomy, 1995).

EPISIOTOMY

An outline of the discussion that follows should make it easy for the student and beginning intern to grasp some key concepts. This section begins with a review of the frequency of episiotomy and the 2 commonly used types. The advantages and disadvantages of each type are presented next. The third section lists some factors other than just the cutting of the episiotomy itself that may influence outcome, and repair of both types. Finally, immediate- and long-term complications are briefly presented. The management of early repair of episiotomy breakdowns is beyond the scope of this chapter.

Frequency

At the beginning of the 20th century (1903-1925) the 2 leading figures in American obstetrics were diametrically opposed in their views on episiotomy. DeLee favored episiotomy prophylactically or routinely, while Williams thought it was rarely necessary. One hundred years later, Murphy and colleagues conducted a small randomized trial to examine the merits of routine versus restrictive use of episiotomy at operative vaginal delivery. They found no conclusive evidence to support either policy. For normal vaginal delivery a maximum episiotomy rate of 30% has been suggested, but many centers perform the procedure much less frequently. The concept of routine episiotomy should be abandoned, but conversely never cutting an episiotomy is equally indefensible. Only with increasing experience will you know when one is necessary.

The only 2 types of episiotomy for which an intern is responsible are midline and mediolateral. That said, most interns in the United States will never cut or repair a mediolateral episiotomy due to the long-standing preference for midline episiotomy in this country. This contrasts with experience in the United Kingdom and continental Europe, where almost all episiotomies are mediolateral. Both incisions are most often made with scissors and start at the same location: at the 6 o'clock position on the vaginal introitus. The midline is cut vertically down to, but not through, the external anal sphincter, whereas the mediolateral is cut at a 45° angle to avoid the sphincter (see Figure 29-1). When a midline extends, there is invariably damage to the external sphincter. The author and

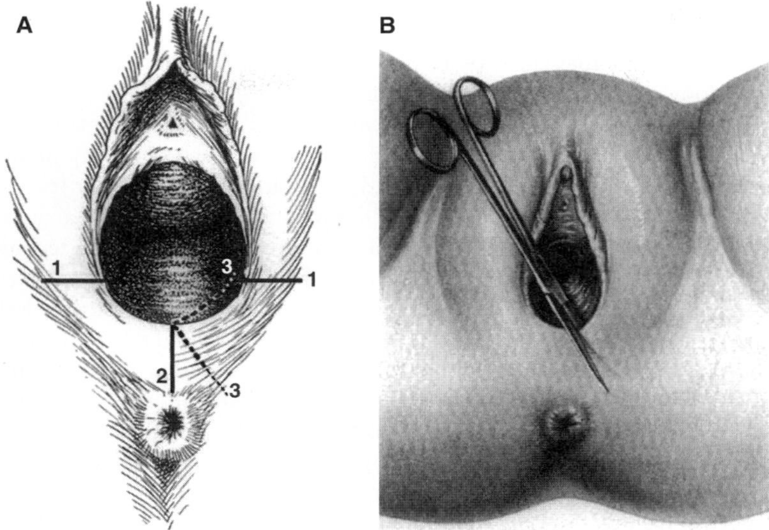

Figure 29-1. Midline versus mediolateral episiotomy positions. (A) Number 2 shows the direction for a midline episiotomy and number 3 for a mediolateral. In the United States, number 1 should not be used. (B) The figure shows the proper direction for a left mediolateral episiotomy. (Reproduced, with permission, from DeLee JB, Greenhill JP. *Principles and Practice of Obstetrics*. Philadelphia, PA: WB Saunders Company; 1947:244–245 [chapter 16].)

several groups of investigators prefer to reserve the term "third-degree" extension for cases where the entire thickness of the external sphincter is severed. A fourth-degree extension additionally involves a variable-length tear of the anterior rectal mucosa.

Advantages and Disadvantages of Each Type

The advantages of a midline episiotomy are the following: easy to cut, easy to repair, heals well, causes little discomfort, associated with less blood loss, and is rarely complicated by later dyspareunia. Its 1 disadvantage probably outweighs all of its advantages: it predisposes to third- and fourth-degree extensions, which in turn may result in fecal incontinence later in life. The salient advantage of mediolateral episiotomy is that it is less frequently associated with tears of either the sphincter or the rectum or both. It creates more room for the fetal head, especially in forceps deliveries. However, repair is difficult, pain is increased, blood loss is greater, and healing is sometimes faulty.

Technical Pointers

It is naïve to think that the type of episiotomy is the dominant factor leading to lacerations of the sphincter and rectum. Hals and colleagues reported on a 4-pronged initiative to reduce the incidence of anal sphincter tears. The study was conducted in Norway, where performance of almost exclusively mediolateral episiotomy is the norm. They reduced the incidence of sphincter tears from 4%-5% to 1%-2% by returning to some older practices that had been abandoned over time: delivery of the fetal head with a 2-handed, modified Ritgen technique, interdiction of active pushing during delivery of the head, pushing the perineal ring under the infant's chin, and positioning the woman in such a way that the operator can observe the perineum during delivery. One could add to their initiatives the crucial importance of having the operator adjust the woman's position in stirrups (if stirrups are used) so that the legs are not hyperabducted and the hips not overly flexed. It has become common to exhort the woman to push as hard as she can as the head is delivering and compound that by pushing in McRoberts position. Too little attention has been paid to maternal position and expulsive effort as they relate to episiotomy extensions.

Repair of both types of episiotomy in a manner that restores anatomy and minimizes postoperative discomfort should be assigned to the intern but directly supervised by senior residents or faculty until the intern has demonstrated proficiency. Fine sutures of absorbable material with knots that are approximated and not tightened excessively will help to minimize postoperative discomfort. In both types of episiotomy closing the deep layers is more important than "embroidery" of the superficial layers. Standard obstetric textbooks illustrate and describe the steps, but the fact is that repair technique is learned from resident or faculty instructors. This is especially true of third- and fourth-degree repairs. Still, there are a few suggestions that will assist in these more complicated repairs. Make sure you have good lighting and good exposure. This may require moving the patient to an operating room. Ensure that anesthesia is adequate. Irrigate liberally with normal saline to help identify the internal anal sphincter. Approximate the torn ends of the external anal sphincter with simple interrupted sutures using the PISA acronym: posterior, inferior, superior, anterior. Lastly, copy and read carefully the article in the reference DeLancey et al (1997).

Immediate and Long-term Complications

Immediate complications of episiotomy include blood loss, pain, infection, and hematoma formation. If there is evidence of serious infection, the episiotomy should be taken down and debrided of suture material, clot, and nonviable tissue. Necrotizing soft tissue infection can progress to death if not treated aggressively.

Long-term consequences include rectovaginal fistula formation and episiotomy breakdown (if diagnosed in a timely manner, this can be dealt with by early repair); ultimately faulty repair may contribute to later development of anal incontinence of gas, liquid stool, or solid stool. This problem is embarrassing to patients and they may suffer silently for years.

TIPS TO REMEMBER

- Study the anatomy of the perineum and pelvic floor carefully.
- Cut episiotomies when indicated to gain experience with repair.
- Use repair of lacerations and episiotomies to develop your instrument handling and knot-tying skills.
- Ask for instruction and feedback.
- Position the patient for delivery yourself.
- Know your limitations—ask for help if uncertain about how to proceed.
- If possible, rotate to occiput anterior before delivery.

COMPREHENSION QUESTIONS

1. In performing the modified Ritgen maneuver, which of the steps listed below is correct?

    A. Place your dominant hand on the fetal occiput.
    B. Cut an episiotomy before attempting to grasp the fetal chin.
    C. Use the dominant hand to secure the fetal chin through the maternal soft tissue posterior to the rectum.
    D. Take the patient out of stirrups before delivering the head.

2. Which of the following is an advantage of midline episiotomy?

    A. Ease of repair
    B. Less blood loss
    C. Better healing
    D. All of the above

3. In attempting to prevent a perineal laceration with a midline episiotomy, which of the listed suggestions is potentially harmful?

    A. Have the patient stop pushing as the head is crowning.
    B. Place the patient in McRoberts position for delivery of the head.
    C. Make sure the legs are not abducted.
    D. Cut a mediolateral episiotomy.

Answers

1. **C**. A is wrong because it should be the nondominant hand. B is wrong because an episiotomy is not necessary prior to reaching for the chin. D is not a bad idea, but has nothing to do with the Ritgen maneuver.

2. **D**. All of the choices are accepted as advantages, but one must bear in mind that injury to the sphincter and rectum is a big disadvantage.

3. **B**. McRoberts position was introduced for the management of shoulder dystocia, not normal delivery. Hyperflexion of the thighs on the maternal abdomen may stretch the perineum and cause extensions, especially with midline episiotomies.

SUGGESTED READINGS

DeLancey J, Toglia MR, Perucchini D. Internal and external anal sphincter anatomy as it relates to midline obstetric lacerations. *Obstet Gynecol.* 1997;90:924–932.

Episiotomy. In: Gilstrap LC, Cunningham FG, Van Dorsten JP, eds. *Operative Obstetrics.* 2nd ed. New York, NY: The McGraw-Hill Companies Inc; 1995:63–88.

Greenberg JA, Lieberman E, Cohen AP, Ecker JL. Randomized comparison of chronic versus fast-absorbing polyglactin 910 for postpartum perineal repair. *Obstet Gynecol.* 2004;103:1308–1313.

Hals E, Oian P, Pirhonen T, et al. A multicenter interventional program to reduce the incidence of anal sphincter tears. *Obstet Gynecol.* 2010;116:901–908.

Kalis V, Laine K, de Leeuw JW, et al. Classification of episiotomy: towards a standardisation of terminology. *BJOG.* 2012;119:522–526.

Murphy DJ, Macleod M, Bahl R, et al. A randomized controlled trial of routine versus restrictive use of episiotomy at operative vaginal delivery: a multicenter pilot study. *BJOG.* 2008;115:1695–1703.

Stedenfeldt S, Pirhonen J, Blix E, et al. Episiotomy characteristics and risks for anal sphincter injuries: a case–control study. *BJOG.* 2012;119:724–730.

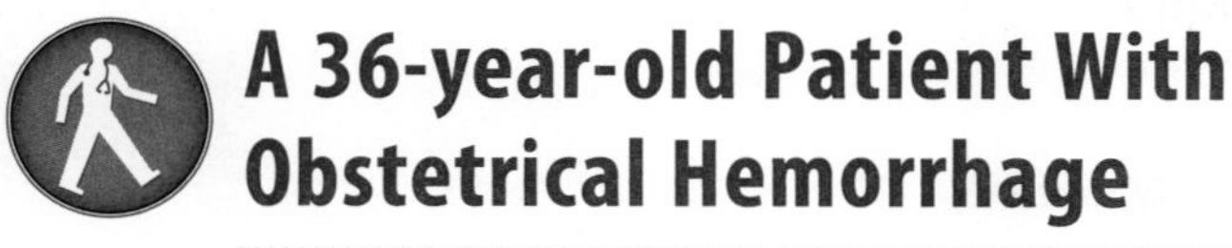

A 36-year-old Patient With Obstetrical Hemorrhage

Alita K. Loveless, MD

A 36-year-old G8 P5-0-3-5 was induced at 40 weeks and 2 days gestation for preeclampsia. Oxytocin was used for induction of labor, which lasted for approximately 20 hours, and during which time the maximum oxytocin rate was 40 mU/min. A healthy, 4035-g male infant was delivered an hour ago. The patient was treated with magnesium sulfate for seizure prophylaxis during induction and labor, and is currently in the second hour of her magnesium recovery. You are called by the nurse to evaluate the patient due to a large amount of vaginal bleeding, and you arrive to the room to find the pad beneath her completely soaked, with continued brisk flow from the vagina. Her blood pressure is 100/60 and pulse rate is 98.

1. What is your diagnosis?

2. What constitutes "immediate management" in this patient?

Answers

1. This patient has postpartum hemorrhage. She had several identifiable risk factors that should have heightened a good resident's alertness for the possibility of such an event in the immediate postpartum period.
2. Call for help. Call for blood products. Determine and correct the cause of the bleeding. Correct coagulopathy if present.

CASE REVIEW

The first sentence of the chapter "Obstetrical hemorrhage" in *Williams Obstetrics* reads, "Obstetrics is bloody business." As a specialty, obstetrics encounters large-volume blood loss on par with that of trauma surgery, on an only slightly less frequent basis. It is one of the most common emergencies interns will encounter, and one that they should begin residency mentally prepared to handle on day 1. Having a good working knowledge of the principles and treatment of obstetrical hemorrhage will equip an intern with the information necessary to manage an emergency until help and other team members arrive, and could potentially save a patient's life. In any textbook, the obstetrical hemorrhage chapter is one of the most important and should be read and put to memory *prior* to starting internship. This chapter in no way encompasses every important aspect and is meant to include only highlights.

OBSTETRICAL HEMORRHAGE

Diagnosis

Obstetrical hemorrhage can be categorized as antepartum or postpartum. Antepartum hemorrhage is most commonly caused by placental abruption or placenta previa (see Chapter 22). The above case, however, focuses on hemorrhage in the postpartum period. Postpartum hemorrhage is further classified as immediate (within the first 24 hours after delivery) or late (after the first 24 hours). Delayed postpartum hemorrhage is a third and separate entity. Late and delayed hemorrhages are not considered here.

In cases of postpartum hemorrhage, emphasis should be placed on stabilizing the patient, and then determining the etiology. The most common causes are as follows: uterine atony, retained placenta, defects in coagulation, uterine inversion, subinvolution of the placental site, retained products of conception, infection, and inherited coagulation defects. In most scenarios, skilled residents are assimilating information about many aspects of the emergency, albeit somewhat unconsciously. On entering the room, an upper-level resident would remember that the patient had multiple risk factors for postpartum hemorrhage: advanced age, high parity, delivery of a large infant from an overdistended uterus, induction of a lengthy labor on a rather high dose of oxytocin, and treatment for preeclampsia with magnesium sulfate. Although these may seem like the "perfect storm" of hemorrhage-inciting characteristics, management of such patients is common in labor and delivery. A more complete list of risk factors for postpartum hemorrhage is provided in Table 30-1.

Table 30-1. Risk Factors for Postpartum Hemorrhage

Prolonged labor
Augmented labor
Rapid labor
History of postpartum hemorrhage
Episiotomy, especially mediolateral
Preeclampsia
Overdistended uterus (macrosomia, twins, hydramnios)
Operative delivery
Asian or Hispanic ethnicity
Chorioamnionitis

Reproduced, with permission, from American College of Obstetricians and Gynecologists. *Postpartum Hemorrhage.* ACOG Practice Bulletin 76. Washington, DC: ACOG; 2006.

Treatment

Postpartum hemorrhage should be treated with the urgency of a trauma or code. The "ABCs" of resuscitation—airway, breathing, and circulation—are readily applicable to obstetrical emergencies.

Step 1: Call for help. This includes upper level residents and faculty, additional nursing staff, and anesthesiologists. Remember to communicate with all team members!

Step 2: Call for 2 U of O negative (universal donor) blood. Many hospitals have a massive transfusion protocol that can be initiated. Investigate the process at your institution and know where the blood bank is located. An intern who can run to the blood bank to procure uncrossmatched blood can be invaluable. Keep in mind when reading these steps that most of them occur simultaneously in well-orchestrated hemorrhage management.

Step 3: Monitor vital signs closely—blood pressure, pulse, and oxygen saturation—and immediately place an additional large-bore IV catheter. Remember that baseline labs and blood crossmatch can be drawn and sent STAT at the time of the IV placement. While these tasks are being performed, a Foley catheter should be placed to monitor urine output. The other important reason for Foley placement is to ensure adequate bladder drainage. If the bladder is full, the uterus will not contract adequately, and if the patient had epidural anesthesia, she is at a higher risk of retaining urine. In the example, the patient may already have a Foley in place due to magnesium recovery management, but never assume—always check. Crystalloid fluid should be hung immediately, until blood is available for transfusion.

Step 4: Determine and correct the cause of hemorrhage. Examine the uterus—is it contracted or atonic? Atony is a leading cause of postpartum hemorrhage. If the cavity has filled with blood and clot, or contains retained placental fragments, it will not contract adequately. A thorough bimanual examination should be performed, during which time *all* clots and products of conception should manually be removed from the cavity if necessary. Exploration of the uterine cavity should be performed by an experienced member of the team. If the cavity is empty and the uterus is well contracted, but bleeding has persisted, the suspicion for a genitourinary tract laceration should be high. A thorough examination to rule out vaginal or cervical laceration should be performed. Occasionally, this requires adequate positioning and exposure that only an operating room and its associated lighting and instrumentation can provide. Less frequent causes of hemorrhage should be kept in mind as possibilities to exclude and are listed in Table 30-1.

Table 30-2. Medical Management of Postpartum Hemorrhage

Drug	Dose/Route	Frequency	Comment
Oxytocin (Pitocin)	IV: 10-40 U in 1 L normal saline or lactated Ringer's solution IM: 10 U	Continuous	Avoid undiluted rapid IV infusion, which causes hypotension
Methylergonovine (Methergine)	IM: 0.2 mg	Every 2-4 h	Avoid if patient is hypertensive
15-Methyl $PGF_{2\alpha}$ (Carboprost) (Hemabate)	IM: 0.25 mg	Every 15-90 min, 8 doses maximum	Avoid in asthmatic patients; relative contraindication if hepatic, renal, and cardiac disease. Diarrhea, fever, tachycardia can occur
Dinoprostone (Prostin E_2)	Suppository: vaginal or rectal 20 mg	Every 2 h	Avoid if patient is hypotensive. Fever is common. Stored frozen, it must be thawed to room temperature
Misoprostol (Cytotec, PGE_1)	800-1000 mcg rectally		

From Obstetrical hemorrhage. In: Cunningham GF, Leveno KJ, Bloom SL, Hauth JC, Rouse DJ, Spong CY, eds. *Williams Obstetrics*. 23rd ed. New York, NY: The McGraw-Hill Companies, Inc; 2010 [chapter 35].

CONTROLLING HEMORRHAGE

If the uterus is empty, but atonic, *bimanual compression* is the first and most important step in decreasing blood loss. This technique is vitally important and all interns should be familiar with how to perform it.

While compression is being performed, *uterotonics* should be used. Several common medications and their dosages are listed in Table 30-2. It cannot be overemphasized that adequate blood volume must be present in order to circulate these medications—*early* transfusion of O negative blood in cases of ongoing blood loss is essential!

Surgical intervention and tamponade are reserved for cases when compression and uterotonic medications fail. Several types of uterine compression sutures

Table 30-3. Tamponade Techniques for Postpartum Hemorrhage

Technique	Comment
Uterine tamponade	
• Packing	4-in gauze; can soak in 5000 U of thrombin in 5 mL of sterile saline
• Foley catheter	Insert 1 or more bulbs; instill 60-80 mL of saline
• Sengstaken-Blakemore tube	
• SOS Bakri tamponade balloon	Insert balloon; instill 300-500 mL of saline

Reproduced, with permission, from American College of Obstetricians and Gynecologists. *Postpartum Hemorrhage*. ACOG Practice Bulletin 76. Washington, DC: ACOG; 2006.

and techniques for tamponade (ie, the Bakri balloon) have been described in the literature and residents should become familiar with all of them (see Tables 30-3 and 30-4).

ONGOING MANAGEMENT

Serial labs to monitor hematocrit should be drawn every 4 to 6 hours. Patients will often require additional transfusions after resolution of the hemorrhage. Urine output and creatinine should be monitored to rule out acute kidney injury due to hypotension. Frequent examinations should be performed to assess the fundus and ensure a continued state of contraction.

Table 30-4. Surgical Management of Postpartum Hemorrhage

Technique	Comment
Uterine curettage	Can be hazardous if placenta accreta
Uterine artery ligation	Bilateral; can also ligate utero-ovarian vessels
B-Lynch suture	
Internal iliac artery ligation	Less successful than earlier thought; difficult technique; generally reserved for practitioners experienced in the procedure
Repair of uterine rupture	
Hysterectomy	

Adapted, with permission, from American College of Obstetricians and Gynecologists. *Postpartum Hemorrhage*. ACOG Practice Bulletin 76. Washington, DC: ACOG; 2006.

TIPS TO REMEMBER

- *Atony, atony, atony!* Know how to manage it!
- Know where your blood bank is located and be familiar with how long it takes to process a type and screen versus type and cross at your institution!
- In cases of coagulopathy, which can develop rapidly in the face of massive blood loss, keep in mind that blood products such as FFP need 30 minutes to thaw. If there is concern for the possibility of DIC, or blood loss is torrential and constant, ask the blood bank to thaw necessary components as early in the event as possible.
- Preeclamptic women do not have the normal degree of pregnancy-induced blood volume expansion, and the more severe the disease, the less the expansion. They often do not tolerate blood loss as well as normotensive women. Therefore, efforts to resuscitate the patient must happen more urgently.
- Read the obstetrical hemorrhage chapter in several textbooks prior to internship and memorize them!

COMPREHENSION QUESTIONS

1. If the above scenario occurred in a patient who had the additional complication of a recent asthma exacerbation severe enough to require a 2-day hospitalization and treatment with a steroid taper, methylergonovine (Methergine) would be the uterotonic medication of choice after oxytocin. True or false?

2. If the infant in the example had been delivered with the assistance of forceps, which of the following would probably rank highest on the list of potential causes of postpartum hemorrhage?

   A. Uterine inversion
   B. Retained products of conception
   C. An inherited coagulation defect
   D. Cervical laceration

3. One of the fastest and most efficient ways to control postpartum hemorrhage is which of the following?

   A. B-Lynch suture
   B. Bimanual uterine compression
   C. Uterine packing
   D. Bakri balloon tamponade

Answers

1. **True**. It is important to remember that most contraindications to medication use are relative. In most cases, Methergine would be avoided in preeclamptic or

otherwise hypertensive patients. However, this patient was relatively *hypo*tensive secondary to hemorrhage. If she had recently been treated for an asthma exacerbation severe enough to require hospitalization and treatment with a steroid taper, the risks of possible bronchospasm and respiratory distress if treated with the alternative uterotonic medication Hemabate outweigh the smaller risk of hypertension associated with Methergine.

2. **D**. Forceps-assisted deliveries are occasionally associated with lacerations high in the vaginal vault or involving the cervix. These areas should always be inspected, especially in the face of continued bleeding with a firmly contracted uterus. Uterine inversion would have been noted early in the thorough examination of the genitourinary tract and is not associated with the use of forceps. Retained products of conception can cause bleeding, but bleeding is not specific for forceps use. Bleeding due to inherited bleeding defects usually occurs later and is not associated with forceps delivery.

3. **B**. Bimanual compression of the uterus between a fist in the anterior vaginal fornix and an abdominal hand on the posterior aspect of the uterus should be the first maneuver used to reduce blood loss while additional resuscitative measures are being taken. This is often sufficiently effective to stop the hemorrhage completely. Uterine packing, Bakri balloon tamponade, and surgical placement of a B-Lynch suture are considered last resorts if compression and medications fail.

SUGGESTED READINGS

Al-Zirqi I, Vangen S, Forsen L, Stray-Pedersen B. Prevalence and risk factors of severe obstetric haemorrhage. *BJOG*. 2008;115:1265–1272.

American College of Obstetricians and Gynecologists. *Postpartum Hemorrhage*. ACOG Practice Bulletin 76. Washington, DC: ACOG; 2006.

Obstetrical hemorrhage. In: Cunningham GF, Leveno KJ, Bloom SL, Hauth JC, Rouse DJ, Spong CY, eds. *Williams Obstetrics*. 23rd ed. New York, NY: The McGraw-Hill Companies Inc; 2010 [chapter 35].

Sosa CG, Althabe F, Belizan JM, Buekens P. Risk factors for postpartum hemorrhage in vaginal deliveries in a Latin-American population. *Obstet Gynecol*. 2009;113:1313–1319.

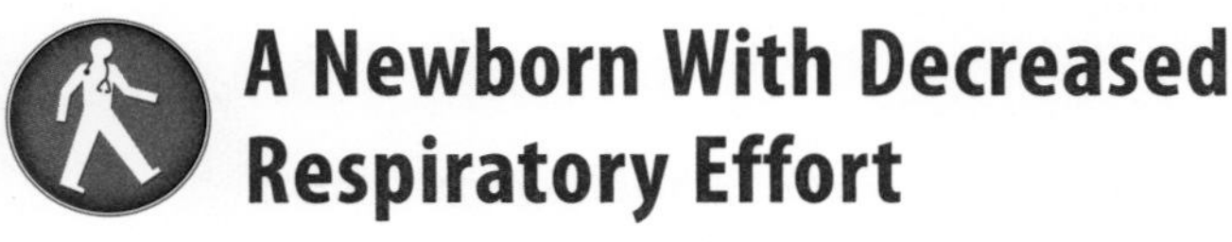

A Newborn With Decreased Respiratory Effort

Thomas A. Bowman, MD, MBA

A 20-year-old primiparous woman at 33 weeks gestation is undergoing induction of labor due to severe preeclampsia and is on magnesium for seizure prophylaxis. During the labor course there are episodes where the fetus demonstrates nonrepetitive late-appearing decelerations, but otherwise the fetal heart rate tracing is reassuring. You are called to deliver the neonate that you perform without difficulty. After delivery, the baby has gasping, ineffective respiratory effort.

The neonatal resuscitation team is unavailable, and the mother is being attended by the senior resident. You are asked to assist the baby.

1. What are the first steps in neonatal resuscitation?

2. If bag-mask positive-pressure ventilation (PPV) is not effective, what corrective steps are recommended prior to initiating chest compressions?

Answers

1. If a newborn is not breathing or crying, the first steps in resuscitation are to dry and stimulate the baby, to open the airway by placing the baby in the sniffing position, and to warm the baby using a radiant warmer, chemical warming mattress, and/or warm blankets. The sniffing position involves flexion of the neck on the body, and extension of the head on the neck.

2. PPV using a mask and bag or t-piece resuscitator is indicated if the initial resuscitation steps are not successful in establishing spontaneous respirations and a heart rate >100 beats per minute. If PPV is unsuccessful, the Neonatal Resuscitation Program (NRP) recommends a series of corrective steps aimed at confirming adequate ventilation prior to proceeding with chest compressions. The steps are organized using the mnemonic "MR. SOPA" (see Table 31-1).

CASE REVIEW

In the case above, the baby has respiratory insufficiency at delivery. The precise etiology is not clear. The differential diagnosis is broad and includes drug exposure (either illicit drug exposure or medications for medical management), placental insufficiency, prematurity, persistent pulmonary hypertension of the newborn, infection (early onset neonatal sepsis or congenital pneumonia), and delayed clearance of fetal lung fluid (FLF), termed transient tachypnea of the newborn (TTN).

Prompt action by skilled delivery attendants who can rapidly recognize and stabilize a baby failing transition from fetal to neonatal status may avoid potential catastrophe. Ideally, at every delivery there should be one person who is

Table 31-1. NRP Recommendations for Corrective Steps to Confirm Adequate PPV

	Actions
M	Adjust **mask** to confirm a good seal on the face
R	**Reposition** airway by adjusting head to "sniffing" position
S	**Suction** mouth and nose of secretions if present
O	**Open** the mouth and move jaw forward
P	Increase **pressure** to achieve chest rise
A	Consider alternate **airway** (endotracheal tube or laryngeal mask airway)

immediately available to tend to the newborn as his or her sole responsibility and who is capable of providing PPV. Delivery at 33 weeks gestation, as in this case, is a high-risk delivery and a team trained in neonatal resuscitation should be present to attend to the baby at the time of delivery. That team should include at least one person trained to fully resuscitate newborns and skilled in airway management including intubation, along with at least one assistant with skills in neonatal resuscitation. As you begin your OB-GYN training you will become certified in neonatal resuscitation. In addition to personnel, the delivery room should have the appropriate equipment available for the resuscitation.

Teamwork and communication between the obstetrical team and the neonatal resuscitation team, as well as within the resuscitation team, are crucial to achieving optimal neonatal outcomes.

DELIVERY ROOM CARE OF THE NEWBORN

Everyone who regularly attends deliveries should have a basic understanding of neonatal transition and the appropriate steps of neonatal resuscitation.

Neonatal Transition

Major changes in blood flow and pressure occur following delivery in both the pulmonary and systemic circulation. The pulmonary vascular resistance falls significantly following ventilation of the lungs and establishing gas-filled functional residual capacity (FRC). The pulmonary vasculature also responds to the vasodilatory effects of oxygen that further decreases pulmonary vascular resistance. The systemic vascular resistance increases considerably when the umbilical cord is clamped removing the very low resistance placenta from the circuit. The net effect is elevated left-sided and lower right-sided pressures, functionally closing the foramen ovale, and dramatically increasing pulmonary blood flow.

During gestation, the lungs are filled with FLF, and are held at a volume that approximates FRC (not "collapsed"). The FLF is actively excreted into the alveolar space and eventually out of the trachea and contributes to amniotic fluid. During labor, the FLF excretion halts, the process is reversed, and the fluid is actively reabsorbed into the lung tissue. The majority of FLF is cleared from the alveolar space by active reabsorption into the tissue rather than mechanical forces of delivery squeezing fluid out of the trachea.

Basics of Neonatal Resuscitation

Unlike adult cardiorespiratory failure, the cause for neonatal cases is almost always respiratory failure. Therefore, a focus on establishing or restoring adequate alveolar ventilation is key to resuscitation of the newborn.

The initial steps in resuscitation are to dry and stimulate the baby, and to position the baby such that the airway is open. Drying the baby provides tactile stimulation, but also helps decrease evaporative heat loss and avoids hypothermia. Additional techniques to stimulate a baby to breathe are tapping the soles of the feet or rubbing the baby's back. Overly aggressive tactile stimulation may cause harm and be counterproductive. Positioning the baby in the sniffing position aligns the airway to avoid inadvertent occlusion of it. Both flexion and hyperextension may narrow or occlude the airway, and should be avoided. Suctioning the airway may result in bradycardia during resuscitation, and should only be done for babies who have an obstructed airway or who need PPV. If the baby does not respond within several seconds of tactile stimulation, it is unlikely that additional stimulation will result in the onset of breathing. The baby would be best served by proceeding with PPV.

PPV is the single most effective way to improve the baby's outcome. Frequently, the progression to more invasive interventions (chest compressions and medications) can be avoided by adequate PPV. This focus on PPV led to the inclusion of additional steps in NRP evaluating PPV prior to proceeding with chest compressions during resuscitation. These corrective steps are organized in the mnemonic "MR. SOPA." Following each corrective step, the resuscitation team should evaluate for response. The first sign of response to intervention is a rise in heart rate, followed by a return of respiratory effort.

Thermoregulation

Newborn babies lose heat faster than adults for several reasons. They have a larger head to body ratio, a larger body surface area to body mass ratio, and they are wet, allowing for more evaporative heat loss. Premature newborns are at additional risk for hypothermia due to less subcutaneous fat, thin skin allowing more evaporative heat loss, and limited metabolic response to hypothermia. Lower admission temperatures to the NICU have been associated with worse neonatal outcomes including mortality in low-birth-weight infants.

To combat heat loss at delivery, normally transitioning babies should be placed skin-to-skin on the mother's chest. This also facilitates bonding and early breast-feeding success. Babies who need resuscitation or stabilization at delivery should be placed on a servo-controlled radiant warmer, dried, and the wet linens should be removed. Babies <29 weeks gestation should be placed on chemical warming mattresses and covered with polyethylene wrap. The World Health Organization and NRP recommend the ambient temperature of the delivery room should be 25°C (77°F) for preterm deliveries. Care should be taken to avoid hyperthermia particularly in the setting of hypoxic ischemic encephalopathy.

Oxygen

Delivery of supplemental oxygen can be lifesaving in a compromised newborn. However, the timing of oxygen delivery and what fraction of inspired oxygen (FiO_2) is indicated have been the focus of much research. In the fetus, aortic oxygen saturations are approximately 60% to 65%, which is sufficient for growth and development, thanks largely to the oxygen affinity of fetal hemoglobin. Healthy term newborns take approximately 10 minutes to make the transition from an SpO_2 of 60% at birth to an SpO_2 of >90%.

Asphyxiated term newborns resuscitated with an initial FiO_2 of 21% as compared with those resuscitated with an initial FiO_2 of 100% had a lower mortality rate and a shorter time to first spontaneous breathing effort. NRP recommends that resuscitation of newborns at term begins with 21% oxygen, but has the ability to titrate as needed up to 100% FiO_2. Preterm infants are more susceptible to the oxidative stress of excess supplemental O_2, but also are more likely to require some amount of supplemental oxygen. Therefore, it is recommended that resuscitation of preterm newborns start with a FiO_2 >21% and <100%. A common practice is to begin near 40%, but this varies between institutions.

Resuscitators cannot reliably assess percent hemoglobin saturation based on assessment of skin color or cyanosis; therefore, it is recommended that pulse oximetry be utilized if PPV or supplemental oxygen is being administered. The FiO_2 should be adjusted to age-specific goals using an oxygen blender. The targets for pulse oximetry are based on healthy term infant transition. The target at 1 minute after delivery is 60% to 65%, then increases by 5% each minute for the first 5 minutes to a goal of 80% to 85% at 5 minutes of age, and then increases more slowly to a 10-minute goal of 85% to 95%.

TIPS TO REMEMBER

- Assess risk prior to delivery and be prepared with personnel and equipment.
- First steps in resuscitation—dry, stimulate, and position with open airway.
- If no response to the initial steps, effective PPV is the key to successful resuscitation.

- If no improvement with PPV, use "MR. SOPA" mnemonic to confirm effective PPV.
- Remember to provide adequate thermoregulation.
- If providing PPV or supplemental O_2, use a pulse oximeter attached to the right wrist or hand. Adjust FiO_2 to reach age-specific SpO_2 targets.

COMPREHENSION QUESTIONS

1. What is the most effective next step in delivery room resuscitation if the baby does not respond to drying, stimulation, or being placed in the sniffing position?
   A. Chest compressions
   B. Positive-pressure ventilation
   C. Volume expansion
   D. Sodium bicarbonate administration

2. At what age would a term infant be expected to have pulse oximetry reading on the right wrist of >90% at the earliest?
   A. 1 minute
   B. 5 minutes
   C. 10 minutes
   D. 15 minutes

3. What is the first physiologic parameter that indicates recovery following adequate resuscitation?
   A. Respiratory rate
   B. Heart rate
   C. Pulse oximetry
   D. Blood pressure

Answers

1. **B**. Effective ventilation is the single most effective step in neonatal resuscitation. Chest compressions are required in <1% of resuscitations. Volume expansion should be used judiciously because overaggressive fluid replacement may overload an already poorly functioning heart. The utility of sodium bicarbonate infusion during resuscitation is a source of debate and has no proven clinical benefit.

2. **C**. At birth SpO_2 is approximately 60% and in term healthy newborns it can take approximately 10 minutes to achieve hemoglobin saturations of 90%.

3. **B**. Rise in heart rate is the first sign of response to interventions. Spontaneous respiratory effort is the second most clinically useful indicator of effective

resuscitation. Blood pressure is not routinely monitored during resuscitation. Pulse oximetry is a useful parameter to follow response to resuscitation but has technological limitations and is slower to respond.

SUGGESTED READINGS

Carlton DP. Regulation of liquid secretion and absorption by the fetal and neonatal lung. In: Polin RA, Fox WW, Abman SH, eds. *Fetal and Neonatal Physiology*. 4th ed. Philadelphia, PA: Elsevier Saunders; 2011:907–919.

Davis PG, Tan A, O'Donnell CP, Schulze A. Resuscitation of newborn infants with 100% oxygen or air: a systematic review and meta-analysis. *Lancet*. 2004;364(9442):1329–1333.

Kattwinkel J. *Textbook of Neonatal Resuscitation*. 6th ed. Elk Grove Village: American Academy of Pediatrics; 2011.

Kattwinkel J, Perlman J. The neonatal resuscitation program: the evidence evaluation process and anticipating edition 6. *NeoReviews*. 2010;11(12):e673.

Laptook AR, Salhab W, Bhaskar B. Admission temperature of low birth weight infants: predictors and associated morbidities. *Pediatrics*. 2007;119(3):e643–e649.

A 28-year-old G5 P2123 Postoperative Day Number 2 From a Cesarean Delivery

Charlie C. Kilpatrick, MD

Ms R is a 28-year-old woman who had a cesarean delivery and tubal ligation 2 days ago for fetal intolerance of labor at term. She is ambulating, tolerating a regular diet, and emptying her bladder completely. Her pain is well controlled on oral pain medication. Her bleeding is decreasing, the baby is doing well, and she is bottle-feeding the infant.

1. **What other postoperative milestones must Ms R reach in order to be discharged home?**
2. **What other postpartum items should be reviewed prior to her discharge home?**

Answers

1. After any obstetric/gynecologic surgery your patient should demonstrate that she can tolerate liquids or a regular diet, pain is well controlled, she can ambulate, and completely empty her bladder. Ms R has demonstrated all of these, and is thus ready to be discharged home.
2. Postpartum items that should be addressed (after vaginal or abdominal delivery) can be remembered easily by thinking of the *B*'s. The patient should be queried as to whether she is *b*reast- or *b*ottle-feeding, the amount of *b*leeding, the *b*irth control method she would like, whether she has any postpartum *b*lues, and how the *b*aby is doing (Table 32-1). In our scenario, we did not discuss whether she has symptoms consistent with postpartum blues.

CASE REVIEW

Ms R says that she has been doing well, although she has much more pain after the cesarean than she did after her other vaginal deliveries. You ask her whether she is having any crying spells, mood swings, or anxiety, all common symptoms of postpartum blues. She is not. You explain that postpartum blues are common for the first 2 weeks after delivery, but if they persist after this time she should be evaluated. She feels ready to go home. You prepare her discharge paperwork and schedule her for a follow-up appointment in a week to evaluate her incision (which was closed with a subcuticular suture). Last night one of your fellow colleagues completed a circumcision on her son. She is also given a pediatric follow-up appointment.

Table 32-1. Postpartum B's

Baby
Birth control method
Bleeding
Blues
Breast- or bottle-feeding

In a week you see her in the clinic, inspect the wound that is healing well without evidence of disruption or infection, and review her pathology report from the tubal ligation that reveals bilateral complete cross-sections of fallopian tube segments. She has no complaints and is doing well with help at home to care for her newborn. She is to follow up with you 1 more time for the 6-week postpartum check. She arrives for this visit and is doing well. She has not resumed vaginal intercourse yet and would like to. You perform a pelvic examination that reveals that the uterus has decreased in size, or involuted. You wish her well and advise her to return to clinic in a year for her annual examination.

POSTPARTUM CARE

As a fourth-year intern, you should be well versed on routine postpartum and postoperative care. On visiting rotations or during your "sub-I" your performance in managing routine postpartum care will be watched closely, and it is a real opportunity for you to shine. First, keep the ultimate goal in mind: expeditious and efficient transition from the postpartum/postoperative state to home. In order to get home your patient should be able to ambulate, tolerate a regular diet, void, and have adequate pain control. All of your physical examination findings, assessments, and plans should keep this goal in mind; otherwise you may get lost in the details. Let's begin with the postpartum orders (see Tables 32-2 and 32-3 for a summary).

The patient needs transfer to the postpartum floor from the labor and delivery suite or operating room. If the delivery was uncomplicated, you will likely transfer the patient to a low-risk postpartum floor. If the patient experienced a complication, such as hemorrhage, or requires a higher acuity of care, you may need to admit her to a high-risk unit. Your program/hospital will likely have guidelines as to who does and does not need greater supervised care. Once you have determined where to transfer the patient, ensure that you include the patient's diagnosis. For example, status post cesarean delivery and tubal ligation would be appropriate in the above case. Keep in mind as well that rounding on the patient and documenting your findings are just 2 elements of the expectations you must

Table 32-2. Routine Postpartum Orders

Immediate Postpartum Orders
Admit to either low risk or high risk
Diagnosis
Condition of the patient
Vitals, routine or specify interval
Allergies
Activity
Nursing orders
Diet
IV fluids
Medications (verify, pain, nausea, med Hx)
Labs

meet. In most programs you will be required to orally communicate your findings to other team members and faculty. So, make sure you know the indication for the procedure that your patient received. At many programs "board checkout" or "postpartum rounds" is an opportunity to review and assess the patients who were cared for overnight. It is always correct to say "I don't know" when the details of

Table 32-3. Routine Postoperative Orders

POD #1
Advance diet as tolerated
Encourage ambulation and inspirex use
If ambulating, d/c Foley
Tolerating diet—d/c PCA, heplock IV
Begin oral pain medication
POD #2
When fully ambulatory, d/c SCDs
Lactation consultant
Communicate with pediatrics
Discharge planning

a patient escape you, but the indication for a cesarean or rationale for induction is not something you want to get in the habit of not knowing.

The *condition* of all of your patients on the postpartum unit will be stable; otherwise they will likely be admitted to an ICU. Think how often you would like your patient's *vital signs* recorded. Routine vital signs are recorded every 8 hours. Recent hemorrhage is a condition in which you would want more frequent vital signs. List the *activity* level (bed rest, ad lib, etc) and any known drug or other *allergies*. Specify activities that you would like *nursing* to carry out and any parameters for which you need to be notified. For example, after postpartum hemorrhage or for patients to whom you are administering magnesium sulfate, you would like to know that they are producing urine (indicating renal perfusion). A common order is to be notified if the urine output is $<30\ cm^3/h$. The *diet* you would like your patient to have, as well as her *IV fluids* (type of fluids and rate of infusion), should be specified. *Medications* for the patient will consist most likely of pain medicine (patient-controlled analgesia [PCA], or oral pain medicine), and agents that address gastrointestinal dysfunction. Your patient may also require antibiotics or medication appropriate for any underlying medical problems. Also, each time your patient is transferred to/from a floor the medications and dosages she is taking have to be reviewed and verified. Medication administration error can cause serious patient harm, and in order to decrease these adverse events this safeguard was put into place. You will need to go through the same activity at the time of patient discharge. The last item to specify is *laboratory* values to be drawn. There are no "routine daily labs" that are required. In fact, a postpartum/postoperative hematocrit has proven to be of little value, except in cases of excessive hemorrhage. Ensure that HIV, RPR, HBsAg, and rubella status were performed on admission. Also, if the patient is Rh negative, check the infant's blood type to determine the need for RhoGAM administration.

Postoperatively on rounds, keeping in mind your goal of getting the patient safely home. You'll want to advance your patient's diet as tolerated. There is no need to wait for passing flatus or determining the type of diet based on the presence or absence of bowel sounds. Auscultation for bowel sounds and documentation of this in your note, especially in light of nausea or abdominal distension, is reasonable. Some patients may be more nauseated than others, so this will need to be individualized; but once they can tolerate liquids or a regular diet, you can discontinue any IV pain medication, have the nurse heplock their IVs, and begin them on oral pain medication.

Getting the patient out of bed and ambulating is another important milestone. Until the patient is ambulating well, encourage inspirex use to lessen the chance of postoperative hypoxemia and avoid atelectasis. Continue sequential compression devices (SCDs) until fully ambulatory to decrease the risk of postoperative venous thromboembolism (VTE). The risk of VTE is at its greatest postpartum (higher after cesarean than vaginal delivery), up to 80 times higher than in the nonpregnant state. The obese patient is especially at risk for hypoxemia and VTE. Be sure to listen to your patient's lungs, noting decreased breath sounds, and inspect her lower extremities for evidence of swelling. The first time out of bed your patient may need help, especially while taking pain medicine that can be sedating, so request nursing assistance the first time out or provide assistance yourself. Falls in the hospital are another source of preventable errors that can cause major patient harm. You want to ensure that the patient is capable, has the necessary strength, and is not sedated prior to suggesting she get out of bed. Once she is able to ambulate, most patients will want the Foley catheter out. Foley catheter drainage postoperatively is performed due to pain, regional anesthesia, and in cases where there was extensive bladder manipulation or hemorrhage. With the Foley out you can determine if she is adequately emptying her bladder by asking her if she feels that it is completely empty. On physical examination a distended bladder will push the uterus up higher into the abdomen, and you will record a fundal height above the umbilicus. The patient will also complain of abdominal pain, unless the regional anesthesia has not worn off. Once she is fully ambulatory, the need for SCDs to decrease postoperative VTE diminishes. Last, make sure her pain is well controlled on oral pain medication, and confirm absence of tenderness on physical examination. Palpate the abdomen and incision site to assess her pain level. The location of the incision (Pfannenstiel, or midline vertical) and any signs of erythema, drainage, or tenderness should be documented and presented on rounds. A transverse incision that runs parallel to the lines of the skin does not require as much strength to remain closed; so if clips were used to close the skin, these may be removed on POD #2 or 3 prior to discharge. Vertical incisions require more strength and are usually left in place for a week, and can be evaluated in clinic.

While ensuring that your patient reaches her postoperative milestones, make sure to follow up on your B's. Is her bleeding, or lochia, decreasing? Inspection of the perineum, a peripad count, and communication with nursing will allow you to quickly assess her bleeding. Communicate with the nursery to assess the infant, or visit the nursery yourself, especially if there was a difficult delivery. You will appear uncaring if there was an adverse event overnight and you were unaware of it. Make sure you have taken the time to discuss birth control options, and that you are encouraging breast-feeding. She may need a lactation consultant if she is experiencing difficulty. Reviewing, documenting, and presenting the *B*'s in a succinct fashion while on rounds will facilitate the care of your patient, and allow you to shine on the rotation.

TIPS TO REMEMBER

- Familiarize yourself with postpartum and postoperative order sets.
- Address the *B*'s on all patients after vaginal or abdominal delivery.
- Your goal is to get your patient ambulating, tolerating a regular diet, voiding, and with adequate pain control. Once she reaches these milestones, you can begin discharge planning.

COMPREHENSION QUESTIONS

1. Ms T underwent a cesarean delivery due to arrest of active phase last night, and at the time of delivery experienced a postpartum hemorrhage. You are rounding on her this morning. Which of the following is not necessary for you to review prior to performing her physical examination and presentation at AM rounds this morning?

   A. Hematocrit value documentation
   B. Urine output since surgery
   C. GBS status
   D. Status of the infant

2. You examine Ms T and note that she is afebrile, but tachycardic in the 100s. On examination her lungs are clear, the fundus is at the level of the umbilicus and firm, she has positive bowel sounds on auscultation, her incision is covered with tape (which is dry), and her extremities are hard to assess because she has SCDs on. What other physical examination item should be performed?

   A. Inspection of the perineum to look for evidence of bleeding
   B. Breast examination
   C. Removal of the tape to look for evidence of wound infection
   D. Speculum examination of the cervix

3. You speak with her and let her know that the infant did well in the nursery overnight. She lets you know that her pain is well controlled, and does not feel nauseated, but tired. She would like to see the baby, and is planning on breastfeeding. You are entering orders for her care. Which of the below best describes the sequence of orders for advancing her diet?

   A. Discontinue her PCA; begin clear liquids; once passing flatus, advance to regular diet.
   B. Start clear liquids; when tolerating, discontinue PCA, and once passing flatus, advance to regular diet.
   C. Begin a regular diet as tolerated.
   D. Discontinue her PCA and begin oral pain medicine; advance to a regular diet if pain is controlled.

Answers

1. **C**. At this time her GBS status is irrelevant. Given that she had a postpartum hemorrhage, a hematocrit value after surgery will give you another estimate of her blood loss at the time of delivery and may suggest the need for transfusion. Her urine output allows you to gauge renal perfusion, and is another indirect evaluation of blood loss and current blood volume. Always check on the infant!

2. **A**. Inspection of the perineum to look for ongoing bleeding or bleeding that happened during the night (present on the peripad) will allow you to visually

document that the postpartum bleeding is decreasing appropriately. Infection of the incision is not going to develop this rapidly after delivery, speculum examination of the cervix is excessive and not necessary, and a breast examination isn't routinely indicated postpartum unless pain/complications arise.

3. **C**. Begin a regular diet as tolerated! There is no need to await flatus, or bowel sounds, and beginning oral pain medication prior to a regular diet will make her nauseated. If she is not nauseated, and does not appear distended, the diet can be started as soon as it is tolerated.

SUGGESTED READINGS

American Academy of Pediatrics, American College of Obstetricians and Gynecologists. *Guidelines for Perinatal Care*. 7th ed. Elk Grove Village, IL/Washington, DC: AAP/American College of Obstetricians and Gynecologists; 2012.

Petersen LA, Lindner DS, Kleiber CM, Zimmerman MB, Hinton AT, Yankowitz J. Factors that predict low hematocrit levels in the postpartum patient after vaginal delivery. *Am J Obstet Gynecol*. 2002;186(4):737.

SUGGESTED READINGS

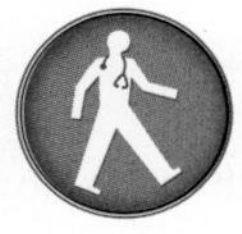

A 27-year-old With Fever 1 Day After Cesarean Delivery

Kristen R. Uquillas, MD and
Abigail Ford Winkel, MD

A 27-year-old P1 on postoperative day number 1 after primary cesarean section due to arrest of descent is febrile to 101.6°F, with a BP 100/60, HR 98, RR 18, and SpO_2 98% RA. The patient initially presented with a chief complaint of leaking fluid at term, and was admitted with rupture of membranes (negative group B *Streptococcus* screen). After 10 hours of Pitocin augmentation, and numerous cervical examinations to document her labor course, she progressed to the second stage. She pushed for 2 hours and with no change in station over the past hour was diagnosed with an arrest of descent and delivered abdominally under regional anesthesia. Prior to the cesarean delivery, she was given cefazolin 1 g intravenously within an hour of skin incision.

1. What is your differential diagnosis? What is most likely?

2. What is your workup?

Answers

1. The patient has postpartum fever. Differential diagnosis includes the following: endomyometritis (metritis), wound infection, mastitis, upper urinary tract infection, atelectasis, pneumonia, deep vein thrombosis, and septic pelvic thrombophlebitis (SPT). Metritis is the most common etiology of postpartum fever and also likely in this scenario given this patient's risk factors: cesarean delivery, numerous cervical examinations, prolonged rupture of membranes, and duration of labor.

2. The first step in the workup of postpartum fever includes a full assessment of the patient's symptoms. The next step includes a focused physical examination, looking for fundal tenderness and foul-smelling lochia. A careful examination of the breast, lungs, abdomen, pelvis, and lower extremities should be performed. Laboratory work may include a complete blood count with differential, urinalysis, and blood cultures.

CASE REVIEW

In your assessment of the patient in the vignette above you find out that she is complaining of abdominal pain, despite use of her patient-controlled analgesia (PCA) device. This morning the Foley catheter was discontinued and she voided without pain. She got out of bed this morning with assistance, walked to the bathroom, and tolerated a regular diet for breakfast. On examination she is in no distress, lungs are clear to auscultation, and her breasts are enlarged but not tender. She has positive bowel sounds with tenderness noted at the umbilicus but is without peritoneal signs. A speculum examination reveals lochia that is normal in quantity, and a bimanual examination confirms uterine tenderness. Her extremity examination is within normal limits with no cords or swelling noted. You diagnose metritis, begin IV antibiotics, and within 48 hours she has defervesced and her clinical examination is normal. She is discharged to home on postoperative day number 4.

POSTPARTUM FEVER

Etiology

Postpartum fever is defined by an oral temperature of greater than 38.0°C (100.4°F) occurring on any 2 of the first 10 days postpartum (exclusive of the first 24 hours), or a single oral temperature of 38.7°C (101.6°F) in the first 24 hours. The timing of postpartum fever can provide clues for diagnosis. The mnemonic "7 W's" represents common causes of fever in the postpartum state, and is summarized in Table 33-1. Additional causes of postpartum fever include perineal cellulitis, retained placenta, and SPT.

Most cases of metritis are polymicrobial, a mixture of aerobic and anaerobic organisms that colonize the bowel and vagina (ie, *Bacteroides*, *Clostridium*, *Escherichia coli*, and gram-positive cocci). Factors that increase the risk for metritis are cesarean delivery, prolonged duration of labor, premature rupture of membranes, use of internal monitoring devices, preexisting pelvic infection including bacterial vaginosis, retained placental fragments, operative or traumatic delivery, diabetes, poor nutritional status, and obesity. Cesarean delivery has a 20- to 30-fold relative risk of postpartum metritis compared with vaginal delivery. This increased predisposition may be due to tissue necrosis, postoperative fluid collection, and/or the presence of bacteria in surgically traumatized tissue.

Diagnosis

The diagnosis of postpartum fever is usually arrived at clinically. Therefore, it is important to evaluate the patient's history and course of the delivery. Pertinent positives include chills, dysuria, flank pain, erythema and drainage from the surgical or episiotomy site, respiratory symptoms, abdominal pain, foul-smelling lochia, and breast engorgement.

Patients with metritis will have fundal tenderness and sometimes foul-smelling lochia. Wound or episiotomy infections are characterized by erythema, edema, tenderness, and discharge from the site. Mastitis presents with tender,

Table 33-1. "7 W's" of Postpartum Fever

"W"	Refers to	Diagnosis	Onset After Delivery	Treatment
Womb	Uterus	Metritis	24-48 h	Antibiotics
Weaning	Breast	Engorgement, mastitis, abscess	24-48 h or longer	Empty breast, antibiotics, incision and drainage
Wind	Respiratory system	Atelectasis, pneumonia	24-48 h or longer	Incentive spirometry, antibiotics
Water	Upper urinary tract	Pyelonephritis	3-5 days	Antibiotics
Walking	Thromboembolism	DVT, PE	4-6 days	Anticoagulation
Wound	Surgical site	Infection, seroma	5-7 days	Debridement, antibiotics
Wonder drugs	Medications	Allergic reaction	Varies	Discontinue agent, supportive therapy

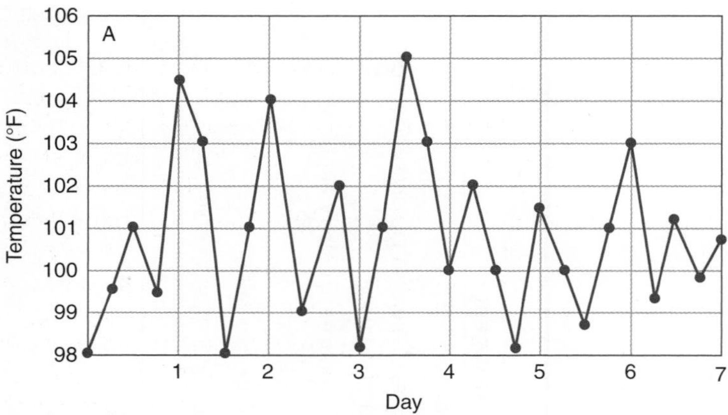

Figure 33-1. "Picket fence" fever of septic pelvic thrombophlebitis.

engorged, and erythematous breasts (infection is generally unilateral). Upper urinary tract infections often present with costovertebral angle tenderness on examination. Patients with respiratory tract infections may have tachypnea, rales, or crackles, while SPT usually has no physical examination findings other than fever. The diagnosis of SPT should be considered in anyone who continues to be febrile despite appropriately dosed antimicrobial therapy, and is characterized by a classic "picket fence"–shaped fever curve (Figure 33-1).

Laboratory studies to consider include the following: CBC, urinalysis, urine culture and sensitivities, wound cultures, and blood cultures (if sepsis is suspected). Radiologic studies may also be useful in patients with an atypical clinical picture or for the patient diagnosed with metritis who has failed to respond to antibiotics.

Prevention

Postpartum fever and sepsis are among the leading causes of preventable maternal morbidity and mortality in both developed and undeveloped countries. Hand hygiene is the most important component of infection control, and hand washing should be performed for 15 to 30 seconds prior to and between every clinical encounter. Antimicrobial prophylaxis is recommended for all cesarean deliveries unless the patient is already receiving appropriate antibiotics (eg, for chorioamnionitis), and should be administered within 60 minutes of the start of the cesarean delivery. Intravaginal application of antiseptics such as chlorhexidine and iodine before delivery may be effective to reduce infection. Postoperatively, incentive spirometer use and early ambulation are encouraged to decrease hypoxia and respiratory complications.

Treatment

Empiric treatment for metritis is broad spectrum, commonly gentamicin and clindamycin. Gentamicin provides coverage for gram-negative organisms and clindamycin covers gram-positive and anaerobic organisms. Second- or third-generation cephalosporins in combination with metronidazole are another option. A response to the initial antibiotic regimen should be evident within 24 to 48 hours. Intravenous antibiotics are generally continued until the patient is clinically improved and afebrile for 24 to 48 hours.

Wound infections following cesarean delivery are usually caused by skin flora, although the prevalence of methicillin-resistant *Staphylococcus aureus* (MRSA) is increasing in postoperative soft tissue infections. The wound must be opened and debrided in such cases. Sometimes it is necessary to perform wound debridement in the operating room to facilitate visualization, allow for adequate pain control, and ensure the entire wound is probed for pockets of purulence. Fascial integrity must be confirmed by probing the fascial closure line. Fascial dehiscence is associated with high morbidity, and if discovered constitutes a surgical emergency. The decision on closure of the wound should be based on daily inspection of the granulation tissue present and clinical improvement on appropriate antibiotics. Wound seromas may also lead to febrile morbidity, but once the wound is opened the fever usually subsides quickly. Episiotomy site infection is rare, and these should also be opened and debrided accordingly. Mastitis is treated with a penicillinase-resistant antibiotic in addition to local care such as ice packs, anti-inflammatory medications (eg, ibuprofen), and breast support. Breast-feeding should be continued unless an abscess develops.

Gastrointestinal organisms cause the majority of upper urinary tract infections during the postpartum period. A 3-day course of antibiotics is usually sufficient for uncomplicated infections.

SPT can be treated with broad-spectrum antibiotics for 7 to 10 days, but some authorities recommend anticoagulation with heparin as well.

TIPS TO REMEMBER

- The key to determining the etiology of postpartum fever is to fully evaluate the patient's history and course of the delivery, completely assess the patient's symptoms, and perform a focused physical examination.
- A single temperature elevation less than 38.4°C (101°F) in the first 24 hours does not constitute postpartum fever, but physical examination and continuing observation of the patient's vital signs is recommended.
- The timing of the postpartum fever can provide important clues for narrowing your differential diagnosis. Endometritis commonly occurs in the first 48 hours after delivery. Remember the mnemonic "7 W's"—womb, weaning, wind, water, walking, wound, and wonder drugs.

- Metritis is a common cause of postpartum fever. It is generally polymicrobial and is most often treated with gentamicin and clindamycin.
- Prompt evaluation and treatment of a postpartum fever is crucial in preventing complications of untreated infection such as pneumonia, pelvic abscess, sepsis, and septic shock.

COMPREHENSION QUESTIONS

1. A 32-year-old P2012 undergoes a planned repeat cesarean delivery. Her past medical history is significant for type 2 diabetes and obesity. She has an uncomplicated postoperative course and is discharged home on postoperative day 3 with pain well controlled, ambulating, voiding, tolerating regular diet, and breast-feeding exclusively. She returns to her obstetrician's office on postoperative day 7 complaining of abdominal pain and discharge from the incision. She is also complaining of mild bilateral breast pain and fullness and is unable to breast-feed on a regular schedule. Her examination is significant for mild breast engorgement and incisional erythema, induration, warmth, and tenderness to palpation. What is the most likely source of infection in this scenario?

    A. Endometritis
    B. Surgical wound infection
    C. Mastitis
    D. Urinary tract infection

2. A 39-year-old P3013 is postpartum day number 4 from a spontaneous vaginal delivery of a healthy female infant. The delivery was uncomplicated, but on postpartum day 2 she was noted to spike a fever to 101.2°F and exhibited uterine tenderness on examination. She was started on intravenous antibiotics for postpartum metritis. After 48 hours of treatment, the patient denies uterine tenderness and her WBC count is $12{,}000/\text{mm}^3$. Nevertheless, she continues to spike intermittent fevers.

    What is the next best step?

    A. Send urine for culture
    B. Broaden antibiotic coverage
    C. Obtain CT scan of the abdomen/pelvis
    D. Perform PA and lateral chest x-ray

3. In a patient with a history of anaphylaxis after exposure to sulfa drugs, which of the following antibiotics is recommended for postpartum metritis?

    A. Vancomycin
    B. Trimethoprim–sulfamethoxazole
    C. Penicillin G
    D. Gentamicin and clindamycin

Answers

1. **B.** Surgical wound infection is most likely based on the patient's risk factors (cesarean delivery, diabetes, obesity) and time since delivery (7 days). Mastitis is unlikely as the patient has no other physical findings on breast examination besides engorgement.

2. **C.** Suspect SPT when postpartum fever continues despite adequately dosed broad-spectrum antibiotic therapy. SPT often has no pathognomonic physical examination or laboratory findings. Imaging studies, CT scan or MRI, are used to confirm the diagnosis, and should be considered when there is no clinical improvement after antibiotic treatment for 48 to 72 hours.

3. **D.** Intravenous gentamicin and clindamycin are the first-line treatment for postpartum metritis. Both antibiotics may be used in a patient with an allergic reaction to sulfa drugs.

SUGGESTED READINGS

Hamadeh G, Dedmon C, Mozley PD. Postpartum fever. *Am Fam Physician.* 1995;52(2):531–538.

Maharaj D. Puerperal pyrexia: a review. Part I. *Obstet Gynecol Surv.* 2007;62(6):393–399.

Maharaj D. Puerperal pyrexia: a review. Part II. *Obstet Gynecol Surv.* 2007;62(6):400–406.

van Dillen J, Zwart J, Schutte J, van Roosmalen J. Maternal sepsis: epidemiology, etiology and outcome. *Curr Opin Infect Dis.* 2010;23(3):249–254.

Wong AW, Rosh AJ. Postpartum infections. Emedicine Medscape reference. <http://emedicine.medscape.com/article/796892-overview>; 2012.

SUGGESTED READINGS

A 22-year-old With Breast Pain 3 Days After a Vaginal Delivery

Roxane Holt, MD

A 22-year-old G1P1001 presents to triage and complains of pain and swelling in both breasts, and a low-grade fever 3 days after her vaginal delivery. She states she had a mild fever when the nurse checked her temperature in triage. She is breast-feeding, but is not sure that she is doing it right, and is tearful when she relates this information. She looks tired and frustrated. Her BP is 100/60, pulse 95, RR 16, and temperature 38°C.

1. What is your differential diagnosis?

2. What is your management?

Answers

1. This patient has breast engorgement based on her history. The differential diagnosis for breast pain includes breast engorgement, mastitis, breast abscess, galactocele, fissures of the nipple, and gigantomastia. Mastitis sometimes occurs at the end of the first week, but more commonly during the third to fourth weeks postpartum, and can be complicated by the development of an abscess. A localized area of erythema, and warmth, accompanied by tachycardia, and fever indicates mastitis. Identification of a fluctuant mass with these symptoms indicates an abscess. An obstructed milk duct causes a galactocele, which is an accumulation of milk in 1 or more mammary lobes. A galactocele can cause pain and may present as a mass without the infectious symptoms of an abscess. Fissures are common and will be identified as cracks on the nipple, which can be quite painful. Gigantomastia is a rare proliferation and overgrowth of the breast tissue that can occur during and after pregnancy.

2. It is important to acknowledge the difficulty of breast-feeding and encourage the patient to continue. Management of engorgement includes regular breast-feeding of the baby and the use of oral analgesics such as acetaminophen or ibuprofen. In addition, a lactation consultation may be of benefit to the patient. Lactation suppressants are not recommended. A tight-fitting brassiere such as a sports bra and ice packs can be used as well.

CASE REVIEW

You expand on the patient's history and find out she has not been breast-feeding regularly, as she is exhausted and has very little energy. She is frustrated and is not sure she is doing it right, and the infant doesn't seem to stay on the breast well. Her temperature is mildly elevated, with normal vital signs, and on visual examination of the breasts they are enlarged and appear similar in size. There is no erythema or areas of infection. On palpation the breasts are warm, tender, and without any signs of fluctuance. The axillae are not painful or enlarged. She is engorged.

You reassure her that breast-feeding is difficult, painful, and exhausting, and emphasize the many benefits of breast-feeding over bottle-feeding for her and the infant. You order a lactation consultant to come by and see her, prescribe Tylenol for fever and pain, and recommend ice packs and a better-fitting bra for her breasts.

BREAST-FEEDING

Diagnosis

Breast-feeding can be challenging, as the skill is new to both the mother and neonate. Increasing the knowledge about breast-feeding that a mother has prior to birth can help increase the duration of breast-feeding. Initially, there is not a large amount of milk that is expressed from the breast, which can be distressing for the new mother. It is helpful to remind the mother that the baby's stomach is very small. There is only a little colostrum secreted during the first day after delivery. During the second day after birth, the colostrum will begin to be secreted in small amounts. Colostrum has minerals, amino acids, and proteins along with IgA in it. Colostrum is present for 5 days and converts to mature milk during the following 4 weeks. A woman can produce up to 600 mL of milk daily. Mature milk contains amino acids, fatty acids, proteins, and vitamins. Importantly, both colostrum and milk do not contain vitamin K and are deficient in vitamin D, requiring these to be supplemented in exclusively breastfed infants.

Breast-feeding is preferred over bottle-feeding for neonates and infants. The American College of Obstetricians and Gynecologists recommends exclusive breast-feeding for the first 6 months of an infant's life except for vitamins, minerals, and medications. Breast-feeding provides numerous maternal and infant benefits. Maternal benefits include increased postpartum weight loss, partial protection against pregnancy, and decreased breast and ovarian cancer risk. Neonatal benefits include decreased acute illnesses (respiratory infections, otitis media), decreased incidence of obesity, and decreased childhood cancer (leukemia and lymphoma). The IgA present in breast milk confers neonatal immunity. Intelligence scores are also shown to be higher in breastfed infants.

Due to the benefits the mother–child dyad receives from breast-feeding, there are programs and goals to increase breast-feeding. The UNICEF-WHO Baby Friendly Hospital Initiative (BFHI) was developed as an international program based on the WHO "Ten Steps to Successful Breastfeeding" in order to increase the number of mothers who exclusively breast-feed as well as the duration that they breast-feed (Box 34-1). The United States has a Healthy People 2020 goal

Box 34-1. Ten Steps to Successful Breast-feeding

Every facility providing maternity services and care for newborn infants should:

1. Have a written breast-feeding policy that is routinely communicated to all health care staff.
2. Train all health care staff in skills necessary to implement this policy.
3. Inform all pregnant women about the benefits and management of breast-feeding.
4. Help mothers initiate breast-feeding within 1 hour of birth.
5. Show mothers how to breast-feed, and how to maintain lactation even if they should be separated from their infants.
6. Give newborn infants no food or drink other than breast milk, unless medically indicated.
7. Practice rooming-in—that is, allow mothers and infants to remain together—24 hours a day.
8. Encourage breast-feeding on demand.
9. Give no artificial teats or pacifiers (also called dummies or soothers) to breast-feeding infants.
10. Foster the establishment of breast-feeding support groups and refer mothers to them on discharge from the hospital or clinic.

of 81.9% ever-breastfed infants, which is an increase from 76.9% in 2009. Most women are able to breast-feed, and there are few contraindications. These include several active infections (HIV, HSV, tuberculosis, and varicella), breast cancer treatment, maternal substance abuse, and galactosemia in the infant. Skin-to-skin positioning of the baby immediately after birth facilitates bonding of the mother and neonate, as well as breast-feeding soon after birth. During the first few weeks of life, there should be 8 to 12 feedings a day that can be on demand from the neonate. The neonate shows hunger by increased alertness and activity, sucking motions or mouthing, and later crying. Over time, these feeds may be decreased to 8 per day when breast-feeding is well established.

When women do not breast-feed regularly during the first days postpartum, choose not to breast-feed, or have a contraindication to breast-feeding, engorgement of the breasts can occur. Women who do not breast-feed may encounter milk leakage 1 to 3 days postpartum, and the engorgement begins between 1 and 4 days postpartum with a peak on days 3 to 5. However, some women can have pain that lasts up to 14 days. Breast engorgement can be accompanied by a fever of 37.8°C to 39°C that can last 4 to 16 hours. The breasts are firm or tense and warm on palpation bilaterally.

Management

For women who have breast engorgement and are breast-feeding, more regular feedings, and a warm compress or warm shower to enhance milk removal are recommended to empty the breast. Massage or pumping can be used to help empty the breast if the engorgement is causing the infant to have difficulty in latching on and nursing. Alternating the breast that the infant starts nursing with and breast-feeding from both breasts at each feeding can help equally empty the breasts. For women who are not breast-feeding, one sixth to one half of patients will experience moderate-to-severe milk leakage, and pain can be expected to occur in two thirds of these women.

Currently, lactation suppressants are not recommended in the United States. Analgesics such as acetaminophen and ibuprofen are recommended for pain. Wearing a sports bra, cool cabbage leaves, and using ice packs between feedings are commonly recommended. As mentioned before, some patients will experience symptoms for up to 2 weeks. Reassuring the patient that the engorgement will resolve is important.

TIPS TO REMEMBER

- Breast-feeding is the preferred nutrition for the first 6 months of a child's life.
- Vitamin K is absent, and vitamin D is deficient in colostrum and milk. These will need to be supplemented in exclusively breastfed infants.
- Breast engorgement occurs 1 to 4 days postpartum with a peak in symptoms at days 3 to 5 postpartum. Mastitis is more common 3 to 4 weeks postpartum.
- Management for breast engorgement is supportive with analgesics and ice packs. In breast-feeding women, continued emptying of the breasts is recommended.

COMPREHENSION QUESTIONS

1. Ms R presented to labor and delivery in active labor at 34 weeks pregnant and delivered a healthy baby boy. She has a known diagnosis of hepatitis C, and is being treated for active tuberculosis. Her urine drug screen returns positive, as well as the confirmatory test for HIV. Which of the following medical problems of Ms R is *not* a contraindication to breast-feeding in the United States?

   A. HIV infection
   B. Hepatitis C
   C. Active tuberculosis treatment
   D. Maternal cocaine use

2. Ms C undergoes a cesarean delivery after a long, drawn-out labor during which she stopped dilating at 8 cm. She developed an intra-amniotic infection during

labor and finished antibiotic treatment. She tried to breast-feed, but it hurt too much and she would rather bottle-feed. It is postoperative day #3 and she is ready to go home but complains of bilateral breast swelling. You diagnose breast engorgement. Which of the following is the least effective management for her breast engorgement?

A. Lactation suppressants.
B. Warm compress to the area to enhance let down and empty the breast.
C. Cold compress between feedings.
D. Analgesics to decrease discomfort.

Answers

1. **B**. Hepatitis C is not a contraindication for breast-feeding as the transmission rate has been shown to be the same between breast- and bottle-fed infants. HIV can be transmitted through the breast milk to the infant. Therefore, it is contraindicated in industrialized nations where replacement feeding is readily available and safe. However, recommendations may differ in countries that have a high neonatal and infant death rate due to infections and malnutrition. In addition, maternal street or illicit drug use and uncontrolled alcohol use are reasons to not breast-feed the infant.

2. **D**. The goal is effective removal of the milk. Lactation suppressants are not recommended for engorgement. Analgesics, cabbage leaves, a warm shower to enhance let down, or cold compress between feedings are all options for breast engorgement.

SUGGESTED READINGS

American Academy of Pediatrics. Breastfeeding and the use of human milk: section on breastfeeding. *Pediatrics*. 2012;129(3):e827–e841.

American College of Obstetricians and Gynecologists. Committee Opinion Number 361: breastfeeding: maternal and infant aspects. *Obstet Gynecol.* 2007;109:479–480.

Roser DM. Breast engorgement and postpartum fever. *Obstet Gynecol.* 1966;27(1):73–77.

Spitz AM, Lee NC, Peterson HB. Treatment for lactation suppression: little progress in one hundred years. *Am J Obstet Gynecol.* 1998;179(6 pt 1):1485–1490.

The puerperium. In: Cunningham GF, Leveno KJ, Bloom SL, Hauth JC, Rouse DJ, Spong CY, eds. *Williams Obstetrics*. 23rd ed. New York, NY: The McGraw-Hill Companies Inc; 2010.

World Health Organization. *Protecting, Promoting and Supporting Breastfeeding: The Role of Maternity Services*. Geneva: WHO; 1989.

Perinatal Depression

Sarah Mallard Wakefield, MD

A 28-year-old G2P1 presents to clinic for her initial prenatal visit. Her last menstrual period was 9 weeks prior to presentation. Her first pregnancy resulted in an uncomplicated term vaginal delivery. She denies any history of medical problems until asked specifically about a history of depression, anxiety, or other psychiatric illness. She begins to tear up and reports that after her first baby was born, she felt alone and frustrated, and had thoughts that she was inadequate as a mother. She states that "it got pretty bad." She and her husband have been married for 6 years. He is in the military, and she stays at home to provide the primary care for their daughter. Prior to trying to conceive this time, she reports social use of alcohol once every 1 or 2 weeks. She denies any history of substance abuse.

1. What is in your differential diagnosis for emotional dysregulation after delivery?

2. What are the next steps you need to take in the management of this patient?

Answers

1. Your differential diagnosis should include normal adjustment, postpartum blues, major depressive disorder with postpartum onset (postpartum depression), and major depressive disorder (with onset during pregnancy or prior to pregnancy).
2. Your next step, in addition to typical initial prenatal screening and education, is to get a more detailed history of depressive symptoms including onset, severity, treatment, and resolution. You should also assess the patient's current psychosocial support system, risk for depression during and following this delivery, and need for referral to psychiatric services.

CASE REVIEW

You tell her you would like to get more information about her symptoms after the delivery of her daughter. She reports that she felt very alone after the birth of her child. You ask what kind of support she had during labor and delivery and after going home. Her husband was deployed for overseas duty during her second trimester. Her mother flew in for the birth of her baby, but she was only able to stay for a week. The patient often found herself crying when her baby cried, and she began to wonder if it had been a good decision for her to become pregnant. You ask her about specific neurovegetative symptoms. She felt very tired and without energy to perform daily tasks of caring for herself and her home. When you ask specifically if she ever had thoughts of harming herself or her baby during this time, she tears up again. She reports that she did have fleeting thoughts that she might drop her baby or cause her some harm. She denies any thoughts about intentional harm to herself or her baby. You ask her when these symptoms first began, how long they lasted, and when they resolved. She reports excitement at the beginning of her pregnancy, but as she entered her third trimester, she began to feel sad most days of the week and began to perseverate about her husband's absence from the birth of their child. She began to have significant trouble sleeping and low energy during the day. She reported these symptoms to her doctor who assured her that these were normal symptoms of the third trimester of pregnancy. She began to stay home more often and to not participate in the events planned among members of her military wives' support club. She became increasingly anxious about her delivery and wondered if she would be a good mother. These symptoms worsened significantly after her mother returned to her own home about a week postpartum. Her husband returned home when their daughter was 3 months old. He became very concerned about the patient and finally convinced her to talk to their assigned family practice physician on base. She was diagnosed with postpartum depression and prescribed sertraline. However, she did not start this medication due to concerns about its excretion in her breast milk. At 9 months postpartum, her milk supply decreased and she began to supplement with formula. At that time she began the sertraline that was very helpful for her mood symptoms. She took sertraline for approximately 1 year with good effect, and then was tapered off this medication. She has not been on any antidepressant for the last 3 years and denies any relapse of mood symptoms during that time. Her husband has been very helpful in caring for their daughter, and they were recently transferred to a base closer to her family. You explain how common depression is in women during childbearing years and inquire whether she was ever diagnosed with depression or had significant neurovegetative symptoms prior to this described episode. She reports having some mood dysregulation and mild neurovegetative symptoms during the time of her parents' divorce when she was in her late teenage years. You ask her if she has been having any of the aforementioned symptoms before or during this pregnancy. After a pause, she states that she is somewhat worried that her husband might have to leave again during this pregnancy, although he has taken a job where that is very unlikely. She then states, "No! You know, I am very happy and excited about this baby. It's the right thing for our family, and my little girl is going to be the best big sister. I don't even want to think about that sad time in my life right now." You express your congratulations but add that you want her to monitor her mood symptoms throughout this pregnancy and you will be checking in with her about this during her care. You advise her that the prenatal packet provided by the clinic includes a handout about depression in pregnancy and during the postpartum period. You emphasize that early treatment is the best treatment.

PERINATAL DEPRESSION

Diagnosis and Treatment

Pregnancy is thought to be a time of emotional well-being for women. However, around 10% of women experience symptoms that meet criteria for a depressive disorder during pregnancy and 50% to 80% of women experience postpartum blues. The first year postpartum represents the lifetime peak of psychiatric admissions for women. Postpartum blues are characterized by anxiety, mood lability, and crying spells and typically resolve within 2 weeks postpartum. Depression, on the other hand, changes thoughts, feelings, and behaviors and is defined as having either: (a) sad or depressed mood, or (b) loss of interest or pleasure in previously enjoyable activities for most of the day, every day for a period of at least 2 weeks. These symptoms must also be accompanied by at least 5 of the following: decreased energy or fatigue, worthlessness or guilty feelings, trouble with concentration or making decisions, recurrent thoughts about death or suicide, or changes in appetite, weight, sleep, or movement.

Postpartum depression has a usual onset of 1 to 3 weeks after delivery and is further characterized by increasing sadness, doubt, guilt, and helplessness that interfere with caring for oneself or baby or interferes in completing routine tasks at home or work. Many women experience intense concerns about their babies, and some fear that they will harm their babies or themselves.

Lifetime risk factors for developing a depressive illness include; family history, hormonal changes, and stressful life events. Risk factors more specific to the perinatal period include a history of depression, marital discord, poor support, loss of freedom, an adverse life event, or an unwanted or complicated pregnancy. Women are at further risk of postpartum depression in instances of premature child birth, having a child born with a birth defect, prolonged hospital stay, or having difficulties breast-feeding.

During pregnancy and the postpartum period many depressive symptoms are often overlooked due to their similarity with common symptoms of that time. For instance, fatigue, appetite disturbance, decreased libido, and decreased energy may all be symptoms common to pregnancy not complicated by depression, but they could very well be symptoms of an impending or current depressive illness. Therefore, diagnosis and treatment of perinatal depression begins with a thorough history that should include at least a brief psychiatric history. In addition to any current depressive symptoms, you should inquire about any family history of depressive illness, previous depressive episodes, and their onset, severity, duration, and treatment. The most appropriate time to have this conversation is during prepregnancy planning.

Screening with a validated tool such as the Edinburgh Postnatal Depression Scale takes less than 3 minutes to complete and has been validated on pregnant and postpartum populations with good sensitivity and specificity. If a patient screens positive, greater investigation is required. It is important to have a referral process in place for appropriate mental health care follow-up. Your goal is not to dictate the direction of treatment but to appropriately inform your patient about both the risks of maternal depression and the benefits of treatment so that you can work as a team to maximize maternal–fetal or maternal–neonate well-being.

Maternal mental illness is associated with problematic mother–infant attachment, decreased cognitive competence of the infant, developmental delays, and behavioral problems in the infant even in cases where the mother exhibits only mild-to-moderate depressive symptoms. A major depressive illness in the mother is further associated with poor prenatal care compliance, poor nutrition, decreased fetal growth and low birth weight, increased crying, and a rise in neonatal intensive care unit admissions.

While mild depression may be treated with nonpharmacological interventions such as interpersonal therapy and increasing support around the patient, antidepressant medication is indicated for symptoms that interfere with maternal well-being and functioning. Severe depressive symptoms during either pregnancy or the postpartum period may necessitate treatment with hospitalization and/or electroconvulsive therapy (ECT). All psychotropic medications cross the placenta, are found in amniotic fluid, and are excreted in breast milk. Despite conflicting studies over the years, it is more appropriate to protect the fetus and neonate from moderate to severe depression than to avoid the use of medication. A single medication at a higher dose is preferred over multiple medications at lower doses in order to limit the fetus and neonate's medication exposure. Medication selection should be based on a history of efficacy in your particular patient or at least in the population at large if the patient has no prior history of treatment. Prior exposure during pregnancy should be taken into consideration, and medication switches should be avoided if possible. Medications with fewer metabolites, high protein binding to decrease placental crossing, and fewer interactions are preferred. Paroxetine has been linked to fetal cardiac defects and is currently the only antidepressant contraindicated during pregnancy. Any fetus exposed to paroxetine should be referred for fetal echocardiogram. However, even studies involving paroxetine have been inconsistent, and the overall risk of cardiac defects is increased only to 2/1000 births.

TIPS TO REMEMBER

- You should specifically ask about mood symptoms when taking a prenatal history.
- Perinatal depression, unlike postpartum blues, has multiple negative sequelae for both mother and fetus/neonate and warrants appropriate screening and intervention.
- A team effort is the best approach for treatment of perinatal depression.

- Nonpharmacological interventions including aerobic exercise and support groups can be beneficial for mild depressive symptoms.
  - Antenatal classes and labor/delivery support decrease the onset of postpartum depression.
  - Interpersonal therapy is an evidence-based therapy for perinatal depression.
- Antidepressant medication can be the safest choice in pregnancy and the postpartum period, especially when weighed against the effects of maternal depression.
- To minimize medication exposure of fetus/neonate, the use of 1 medication at a higher dose with proven efficacy and safety for the patient or overall population is preferred over several medications at lower doses.
- Paroxetine is an antidepressant medication that is not recommended for use during pregnancy due to an increased risk of cardiac defects.

COMPREHENSION QUESTIONS

1. Ms Smith is a 27-year-old female who presents to clinic for follow-up 2 weeks after her cesarean section. Her baby is home doing well, but she reports great anxiety over the last 2 weeks about her baby ending up in the NICU for a few hours after birth and wonders if there is something she did wrong during her pregnancy. She reports frequent crying episodes over the last 2 weeks especially during breast-feeding but often without any provocation. She does report that these symptoms seem to be improving, and she is beginning to get a handle on what it is to "be a mom." She has never known anyone with postpartum depression, but she wants to make sure that is not what is going on with her. Of the following statements to convey to Ms Smith which is most accurate?

   A. Her symptoms are consistent with postpartum or baby blues, and she has nothing to worry about as these symptoms will continue to resolve.

   B. Her symptoms are consistent with major depressive disorder with postpartum onset, and you recommend starting an SSRI medication immediately.

   C. Her symptoms are consistent with postpartum or baby blues, and will most likely continue to resolve. However, you do encourage her to monitor these symptoms and call the clinic if they worsen.

   D. Her symptoms are consistent with major depressive disorder and you carefully question her about symptoms of mood symptoms during pregnancy that she did not previously report.

2. Ms Reynolds is a 34-year-old female who presents for her initial prenatal visit. She is currently 9 weeks gestational age by dates and ultrasound. She is excited about this pregnancy but states concerns about her history of depression. She

has been on fluoxetine for many years for recurrent depressive symptoms. Each time she has tapered or stopped this medication, her depressive symptoms have relapsed. She wants to do what is best for her baby and has thought about stopping her medication. She is fearful of the relapse of her severe depressive symptoms. You advise her to do which of the following?

A. Stop her medication immediately and warn her about the potential for teratogenic effects of being on this type of medication during embryogenesis.
B. Slowly taper her medication to avoid the side effects of stopping this medication immediately.
C. Continue her current medication since this medication is completely safe.
D. Consider continuing her medication at the current dose, and discuss the risks/benefits with her.

3. Ms Thompson presents for a typical second trimester prenatal care visit during her first pregnancy. She reports concerns about postpartum depression due to recently finding out that her cousin suffered with severe depressive symptoms after delivering her baby. She denies any personal history of depression, but she is curious about any medications to prevent postpartum depression. You advise her to do which of the following?

A. Start an antidepressant medication due to her concerns and her family history of postpartum depression.
B. Not worry about postpartum depression, because her cousin's history is unlikely to have anything to do with her.
C. Not worry about postpartum depression because it is so uncommon.
D. Participate in antenatal classes in preparation for the birth of her child and to have a support structure in place for labor and delivery and during her postpartum period.

Answers

1. **C**. Her symptoms of mood lability with crying episodes and anxiety are consistent with postpartum or baby blues. You recommend that she continue to monitor her mood for improvement and to not hesitate to call the clinic with worsening symptoms.

2. **D**. Due to her recurrent episodes of severe depression, it is highly likely that her depression would relapse with discontinuation of her medication at this time. You discuss with her that overall this type of medication is thought to be safe during pregnancy, but there are always risks to taking medications during pregnancy. You also discuss the known sequelae of maternal depression and invite her to openly discuss her worries with both you and her mental health care provider. You assure her that you will work together for the best outcome for both her and her baby. If

she does decide to continue medication to prevent depression relapse, you would advise her to stay on this medication as it is known to be efficacious for her symptoms, and her baby has already been exposed to this agent.

3. **D.** This patient does not have a personal or family history of depression and denies any current symptoms. Therefore, initiating medication at this time would be inappropriate. Antenatal classes and labor/delivery support have been shown to prevent the onset of postpartum depression.

SUGGESTED READINGS

ACOG Committee on Practice Bulletins—Obstetrics. ACOG Practice Bulletin: clinical management guidelines for obstetrician-gynecologists number 92, April 2008 (replaces practice bulletin number 87, November 2007). Use of psychiatric medications during pregnancy and lactation. *Obstet Gynecol.* 2008;111:1001–1020.

American College of Obstetricians and Gynecologists. Committee on Obstetric Practice. Committee Opinion no. 453: Screening for Depression During and After Pregnancy. *Obstet Gynecol.* 2010;115:394–395 [reaffirmed 2012].

Kornstein S, Clayton A. *Women's Mental Health, a Comprehensive Textbook.* New York, NY: The Guilford Press; 2002.

Wisner K. Perinatal depression: the most common complication of childbirth. <http://www.acog.org/~/media/Sections/PA/Perinatal%20Depression.pdf?dmc=1HYPERLINK>, <http://www.acog.org/~/media/Sections/PA/Perinatal%20Depression.pdf?dmc=1&ts=20130730T0022330448"&HYPERLINK>, <http://www.acog.org/~/media/Sections/PA/Perinatal%20Depression.pdf?dmc=1&ts=20130730T0022330448"ts=20130730T0022330448>; Accessed July 8, 2013.

Section III.
Ambulatory Care

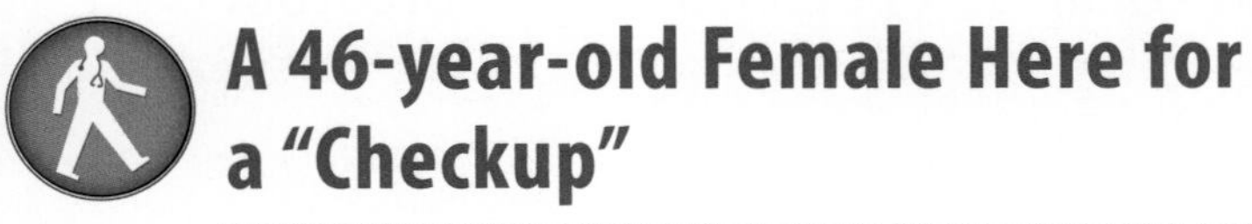

A 46-year-old Female Here for a "Checkup"

Jennifer R. Hamm, MD

The patient is a 46-year-old G2P2 who has not seen a physician since the delivery of her last child 6 years ago. She has no complaints at today's visit. She has no significant past medical, surgical, or family history. She does not smoke, drinks socially 1 to 2 times per month, and denies use of recreational drugs. She has been sexually active with 1 partner, her husband, for the last 15 years. On examination, her blood pressure is 117/76. Her weight is 205 lb and her height is 5 ft 5 in, resulting in a BMI of 34.

1. What preventive testing is appropriate for this patient?

2. What additional screening and counseling should be performed?

Answers

1. Given the patient is 46 years old and hasn't seen a doctor in the last 6 years, she is due for cervical cancer screening. The preferred method for this is cotesting with cervical cytology (Pap smear) and HPV testing. Breast cancer screening is also recommended. ACOG recommends a clinical breast examination be performed and a screening mammogram be ordered. Given her age, and her obesity, screening for diabetes and dyslipidemia should be performed as well.
2. You should review the patient's immunization history and encourage any immunizations that may be due (influenza, Tdap). Additional screening and counseling regarding sexuality, nutrition and fitness, psychosocial issues, cardiovascular health, and overall health/risk assessments (genetic risks, breast health, UV protection and skin health, safety in the workplace and home, safe driving) should be performed.

WELL WOMAN EXAMINATION

The well woman examination (WWE) is one of the most frequent, and important, patient encounters you will have as an Ob-Gyn. It is an excellent opportunity to screen patients for known risk factors of disease, ensure immunization status is up to date, and provide recommended preventive counseling and testing. Recommendations vary based on age and risk factors.

The foundation of the WWE is a comprehensive history and physical examination combined with age- and risk-based screening, immunization, and evaluation and counseling recommendations.

Diagnosis

While the WWE is not a diagnostic problem, per say, you may still "diagnose" numerous areas where your patient has significant risk factors for disease or harm.

Important areas of historical screening:

1. Gynecologic and obstetric:
    - Menstrual history and characteristics
    - Reproductive and contraceptive history or plans
    - Sexual practices
    - Sexual function
    - History of infections, HPV immunization, and cervical cancer screening
    - Fecal or urinary incontinence or issues of pelvic prolapse
2. Medical and surgical:
    - Current or past diagnoses and procedures
    - Medications, vitamins, and supplements
    - Immunization history
    - Use of complementary or alternative medicine
    - Allergies
3. Family:
    - Hx of malignancies
    - Cardiovascular disease
    - Diabetes or thyroid disease
    - Obesity
4. Psychosocial:
    - Alcohol, tobacco, and drug use
    - Past or present hx of abuse or neglect, intimate partner violence
    - Physical activity
    - Diet and nutrition
    - Occupational risks or exposures
    - Stress and sleep disorders
    - Depression history or symptoms
    - Safe driving

The extent and contents of the physical examination will vary based on the setting and the patient's age and risk factors. Key areas include:

1. Vitals:
   - Height
   - Weight
   - BMI
   - Blood pressure
2. Oral cavity (dentition)
3. Neck:
   - Thyroid enlargement or nodularity
   - Adenopathy
4. Breasts:
   - Clinical breast examination every 1 to 3 years in patients aged 20 to 39
   - Clinical breast examination annually in women aged 40 and above
5. Abdomen:
   - Masses
   - Hernias
   - Organ enlargement
6. Pelvic examination:
   - To begin at age 19 to 20 if indicated by medical history
   - Annual pelvic examination in women aged 21 and above
7. Additional physical examination as clinically appropriate

Treatment

For our purposes, "treatments" can be thought of as the screening tests, immunizations, or counseling conversations that should occur as a result of the "diagnostic" process above.

- Preventive testing: A comprehensive summary of preventive screen recommendations by age group is given in Table 36-1. Below are those that you will order most frequently:
  1. Cervical cancer screening:
     - Before age 21—none
     - Age 21 to 29—cervical cytology every 3 years

Table 36-1. Preventive Care Assessment Time Schedule

Screening Tests	AGE			
	13-18	**19-39**	**40-64**	**≥65**
Complete H&P	X	X	X	X
Cervical Cancer	Start at age 21, no matter when first sexual activity	X 21-29: Q 3 y cytology alone ≥30: Q 5 y cytology and HPV (preferred) **or** Q 3 y cytology alone (acceptable)	X Q 5 y cytology and HPV (preferred) **or** Q 3 y cytology alone (acceptable)	X No screening necessary after adequate negative prior screening results
Breast Cancer		X >20: Q 1-3 y Clinical breast examination Consider mammo: if hx, first degree relative with, or many relatives with, premenopausal breast/ovarian CA	X Q 1 y Clinical breast examination Q 1-2 y[a] Screening mammogram	X Q 1 y Clinical breast examination Q 1-2 y[a] Screening mammogram
Colon Cancer	Colon Ca/Aden Polyps in first-degree relative <60, or >2 first degree rel any age, or fam hx nonpolyp colon CA, CRCA, or IBD	Colon Ca/Aden Polyps in first degree rel <60, or >2 first degree rel any age, or fam hx nonpolyp colon CA, CRCA, or IBD	X Start age 50[b]: Q 10 y **Colonoscopy** (preferred) or Q 5 y Flex Sig, double contrast BE, or CT colonograph or Q 1 y FOB (2-3 samples) or stool DNA	X Q 10 y **Colonoscopy** (preferred) or Q 5 y Flex Sig, double contrast BE, **or** CT colonograph or Q 1 y FOB (2-3 samples) or stool DNA
Osteoporosis (DEXA)		**If menopausal and:** hx of fragility fx, weight <127 lb, medical causes of bone loss, parental hx of hip fx, current tobacco use, alcoholism, rheumatoid arthritis, or FRAX fracture risk >9.3%	**If menopausal and:** hx of fragility fx, weight <127 lb, medical causes of bone loss, parental hx of hip fx, current tobacco use, alcoholism, rheumatoid arthritis, or FRAX fracture risk >9.3%	X Start age 65: Repeat Q 15 y if T-score ≥–1.5 and low FRAX. Repeat Q 5 y if T-score –1.5 to –1.99. Repeat Q 1 y if T-score –2.0 to –2.49

Diabetes	Inc BMI; first degree rel with DM; sedentary; HR race; PCOS; Hx GDM; HTN; HDL <35; TG >250	Inc BMI; first degree rel with DM; sedentary; HR race; PCOS; Hx GDM; HTN; HDL <35; TG >250	**X** Start age 45: Q 3 y fasting blood sugar (ADA preferred)	**X** Q 3 y fasting blood sugar (ADA preferred)
Hyperlipidemia	Fam hx early CVD or PVD, hyperlipidemia, personal hx- DM, obesity, CVD risk factors (HTN/tobacco)	Fam hx early CVD or PVD, hyper-lipidemia, personal hx- DM, obesity, CVD risk factors (HTN/tobacco)	**X** Start age 45: Q 5 y fasting lipid profile	**X** Q 5 y fasting lipid profile
Thyroid Dysfunction		Hx autoimmune disease; strong fam hx thyroid disease	**X** Start age 50: Q 5 y TSH	**X** Q 5 y TSH
Chlamydia	**X** Q 1 y If sexually active	**X** ≤25: Q 1 y >25: if at risk	If sexually active; multiple partners; hx std; IV drug use; entering a detention facility	If sexually active; multiple partners; hx std; IV drug use; entering a detention facility
HIV Testing	If sexually active or entering a detention facility	If sexually active; >1 partner since last-test; IV drug use; prostitution; hx cervical ca; preconceptual	If sexually active; >1 partner since last-test; IV drug use; prostitution; hx cervical ca; preconceptual	If sexually active; >1 partner since last-test; IV drug use; prostitution; hx cervical ca
STD Testing	If sexually active; multiple partners; hx std; IV drug use; entering a detention facility	If sexually active; multiple partners; hx std; IV drug use; entering a detention facility	If sexually active; multiple partners; hx std; IV drug use; entering a detention facility	If sexually active; multiple partners; hx std; IV drug use; entering a detention facility
Bacturia	Diabetic patients			**X**
Anemia (Hgb)	Hx menorrhagia; ancestry—Caribbean; Latin American; Asain; Mediterranean; African			
Rubella Titer	Childbearing age and no evidence of immunity (preconceptual)			
Hepatitis C Testing	Hx IV drug use; receive clotting factors before 1987; hemodialysis; persistent elevation of AST/ALT; hx transfusion or transplant before 1992; occupational percutaneous or mucosal exposure to HCV + pt			
TB Testing	HIV+; close contact with TB; endemic area; IV drug use; alcoholism; long-term care; health care workers			

[a]American Congress of Obstetrics and Gynecology, the American Cancer Society, and the National Comprehensive Cancer Network recommend yearly screening mammograms starting at age 40. The National Cancer Institute recommends screening mammograms starting at age 40, every 1 to 2 years. USPSTF 2009 recommendations call for biennial mammograms in women aged 50 to 74.

[b]The American College of Gastroenterology recommends routine colon cancer screening for African Americans to start at 45 due to the increased incidence and earlier age of onset of colon cancer in this population.

- Age 30 to 64—cotesting with cervical cytology and HPV every 5 years (preferred) or cytology alone every 3 years (acceptable)
- Age ≥65—no further screening if adequate negative prior screening and no history of cervical intraepithelial neoplasia (CIN) 2 or higher:
  - Adequate prior screening: 3 consecutive negative cytology results or 2 consecutive negative cotest results within the previous 10 years, with the most recent test performed within the past 5 years
- Prior total hysterectomy (no cervix) with no history of CIN 2, CIN 3, or adenocarcinoma—none
- High-risk populations that require additional screening:
  - HIV-positive or immunocompromised women—annual cytology (for newly diagnosed HIV+ patients cytology every 6 months in first year of diagnosis)
  - History of CIN 2, CIN 3, or adenocarcinoma in situ—age-based screening for at least 20 years following the initial posttreatment surveillance period, even if it requires screening to continue past age 65

2. Breast cancer screening (ACOG, ACS, NCI recommendations):
   - Age 20 to 39—clinical breast examination every 1 to 3 years
   - Age ≥40—annual clinical breast examination and screening mammography
   - High-risk populations that require earlier screening:
     - A personal history of breast cancer
     - A first-degree relative, or many second-degree relatives, with premenopausal breast/ovarian CA
3. Colon cancer screening:
   - Age ≥50 (or age ≥45 if African American, as recommended by the American Gastroenterology Association)
   - Preferred screening—colonoscopy every 10 years
   - Other acceptable screening tests:
     - Flexible sigmoidoscopy every 5 years
     - Double-contrast barium enema every 5 years
     - CT colonography every 5 years
     - Fecal occult blood (FOB) testing annually:
       - Must perform on several different samples
     - Stool DNA testing annually

- High-risk populations that require earlier screening:
  - History of colon cancer or adenomatous polyps in:
    - A single first-degree relative <60
    - >2 first-degree relatives of any age
  - Family history of nonpolypoid colon CA, CRCA, or IBD

4. Sexually transmitted infection and HIV screening:
   - All women should be offered STI and HIV screening, especially if they engage in high-risk behaviors or have multiple sexual partners.
   - Routine screening for chlamydia should be performed in all women under 26 years of age who are sexually active.
5. Osteoporosis screening:
   - Routine screening with DEXA scan to begin at age 65
   - High-risk populations that may need earlier screening:
     - If the patient is menopausal and has:
       - A history of fragility fracture
       - Weighs <127 lb
       - Medical causes of bone loss (eg, chronic steroid use, rheumatoid arthritis)
       - A parental history of hip fracture
       - Current tobacco use or alcoholism
       - FRAX fracture risk >9.3%
6. Diabetes screening:
   - Routine screening every 3 years to begin at age 45
   - High-risk populations that may need earlier screening:
     - Obesity
     - History of gestational DM
     - History of PCOS
     - Sedentary lifestyle
     - Hypertension
     - Dyslipidemia (HDL <35; TG >250)
     - First-degree relative with adult-onset DM
   - Acceptable screening tests:
     - Fasting BS (recommended by ADA)
     - Hemoglobin A1C
     - Two-hour GTT

7. Hypercholesterolemia screening:
   - Routine screening every 5 years to begin at age 45.
   - High-risk populations that may need earlier screening:
     - Those patients with a personal history of diabetes, obesity, or CVD risk factors (including hypertension or tobacco)
     - A family history of early CVD or PVD, or hyperlipidemia
   - Fasting lipid panel is the recommended screening method.
8. Thyroid dysfunction screening:
   - Routine screening every 5 years to begin at age 50.
   - High-risk populations that may need earlier screening:
     - History of autoimmune disease
     - Strong family history of thyroid disease
   - TSH is the recommended screening method.

- Immunizations: The full list of immunization recommendations is given in Table 36-2. Below are those that you will provide most frequently:
  1. HPV:
     - There are currently 2 vaccines available for use in the United States. Cervarix is a bivalent HPV vaccine that protects against HPV 16 and 18 (seen in 70% of cervical cancers). Gardasil is a quadrivalent vaccine that prevents infection from 4 HPV types—16, 18, 6, and 11 (seen in 90% of genital warts). It has also been shown to protect against cancers of the anus, vagina, and vulva.
     - Vaccination with a single series (3 doses) is recommended for girls and women between the ages of 9 and 26.
       - CDC recommends the vaccine routinely be given to 11- to 12-year-old girls.
  2. Tdap:
     - Pertussis, "whooping cough," remains a major health concern, with 41,000 cases reported to the CDC in 2012 and 18 deaths (most occurring in infants less than 3 months of age).
     - Vaccination recommendations:
       - One dose between age 11 and 18.
       - Adults above the age of 18 should receive a single dose of Tdap to replace a single dose of Td.
       - Pregnant women should be vaccinated with every pregnancy, with optimal dosing between 27 and 36 weeks gestation.

Table 36-2. Preventive Care Assessment Time Schedule

	AGE			
Vaccinations	**13-18**	**19-39**	**40-64**	**≥65**
Hep B	**X** One series if not already immunized	If HR—dialysis; clot factor recipient; immunosupp; worker/students; IV drug user; hx STD; household contact; prison/long-term care; travelers	If HR—dialysis; clot factor recipient; immunosupp; worker/students; IV drug user; hx STD; household contact; prison/long-term care; travelers	If HR—dialysis; clot factor recipient; immunosupp; worker/students; IV drug user; hx STD; household contact; prison/long-term care; travelers
Menningococcal	**X** Once between 11 and 18, if not previously immunized	If HR—military recruit; first-year college students in dorms; asplenia; terminal complement def; travel to endemic area	If HR—military recruit; first-year college students in dorms; asplenia; terminal complement def; travel to endemic area	If HR—military recruit; first-year college students in dorms; asplenia; terminal complement def; travel to endemic area
HPV	**X** One series if not already immunized (age 9-26)	**X** One series if not already immunized (up to age 26)		
Tetanus	**X** Once between age 11 and 18—TDaP	**X** One dose Tdap for Td booster, and then q 10 y from last booster One dose Tdap in each pregnancy between 27 and 36 weeks gestation	**X** One dose Tdap for Td booster, and then q 10 y from last booster One dose Tdap in each pregnancy between 27 and 36 weeks gestation	**X** One dose Tdap for Td booster, and then q 10 y from last booster
Flu	**X** Yearly	**X** Yearly for anyone who wants to decrease risk, but especially HR	**X** Yearly age 50 or as above	**X** Yearly

(continued)

Table 36-2. Preventive Care Assessment Time Schedule (*Continued*)

Vaccinations	AGE			
	13-18	**19-39**	**40-64**	**≥65**
Pneumococcal	If HR—chronic disease; asplenia; CVD; Resp Dx; Immunosupp; chronic liver Dx; CSF leak second dose in 5 years in certain groups	If HR—chronic disease; asplenia; CVD; Resp Dx; Immunosupp; chronic liver Dx; CSF leak second dose in 5 years in certain groups	If HR—chronic disease; asplenia; CVD; Resp Dx; Immunosupp; chronic liver Dx; CSF leak second dose in 5 years in certain groups	**X** Once
Hep A	If HR—chronic liver dx; clotting dx; drug use; travelers; HAV researchers	If HR—chronic liver dx; clotting dx; drug use; travelers; HAV researchers	If HR—chronic liver dx; clotting dx; drug use; travelers; HAV researchers	If HR—chronic liver dx; clotting dx; drug use; travelers; HAV researchers
Varicella	All susceptible adolescents and adults	All susceptible adolescents and adults	All susceptible adolescents and adults	All susceptible adolescents and adults
Zoster (Shingles)			**X** Age ≥60: Single dose	**X** If not already immunized, single dose
MMR	Second dose if—entering college; health care worker; travelers; RNI and postpartum	Second dose if—entering college; health care worker; travelers; RNI and postpartum	Second dose if—entering college; health care worker; travelers; RNI and post-partum; or born between 1963 and 1967	

3. Influenza:
   - Recommended annually for everyone over 6 months of age
4. Pneumococcal:
   - Vaccination with a single dose is routinely recommended in women 65 years of age and older.
   - High-risk populations that may require earlier immunization include patients with:
     - Asplenia
     - Cardiovascular or respiratory disease
     - Immunosuppression
     - Chronic liver disease
     - CSF leak

- Evaluation and counseling:
  1. Reproductive health:
     - Contraceptive options
     - Procreative and preconception counseling/screening
     - Safer sex practices and STI prevention
     - Sexuality and intimacy counseling
     - Menopausal symptom management and treatment options
  2. Medical and surgical:
     - Counseling on risk factor modifications and lifestyle changes related to disease
     - Encouraging compliance with recommended immunizations
     - Medication safety
  3. Family history:
     - Counseling or referral for genetic assessment of familial cancers
     - Counseling and methods of risk factor modification for familial-associated conditions such as cardiovascular disease, diabetes, and obesity
  4. Psychosocial:
     - Counseling on tobacco cessation
     - Counseling on drug or alcohol abuse with discussion of treatment options and local resources
     - Identification of depression or depressive symptoms and discussion of treatment options and local resources

- Safety:
  - Domestic violence resources or referrals within your community
  - Proper gun safety
  - Safe driving (seat belts, no texting)
  - Use of proper protective gear at home or at work
- Exercise and nutrition:
  - Importance of maintaining a healthy weight
  - Regular weight-bearing exercise
  - Calcium supplementation
  - Stress management

TIPS TO REMEMBER

- The WWE provides us with an opportunity to conduct a comprehensive assessment of a woman's health. It should serve as a time to encourage our patients to adopt or maintain a healthy lifestyle.
- No 2 women are exactly alike, therefore no 2 WWEs will be. Each patient has her own risks based on age and history (medical, social, family) that will require you to assess what testing, immunization, or counseling is appropriate for her.

COMPREHENSION QUESTIONS

1. What is the purpose of the WWE?

A. Identify risk factors for disease
B. Provide preventive counseling
C. Identify medical problems
D. Build upon the physician–patient relationship
E. All of the above

2. What is the **preferred** method of cervical cancer screening in patients aged 30 to 64?

A. Cervical cytology every 3 years
B. Cervical cytology every 5 years
C. Cervical HPV testing every 2 years
D. Cervical cytology and HPV cotesting every 5 years
E. Cervical cytology and HPV cotesting every 3 years

3. Which of the following screening tests is not routinely recommended for a 50-year-old woman?

A. Screening for thyroid dysfunction with TSH
B. Osteoporosis screening with DEXA scan

C. Breast cancer screening with mammography
D. Colon cancer screening with colonoscopy
E. Screening for diabetes with fasting blood sugar

4. Which of the following immunizations would routinely be recommended for a 65-year-old woman, who hadn't received any immunizations in the last 10 years?
A. Varicella zoster (shingles vaccine)
B. Td booster
C. Influenza
D. Pneumococcal
E. All of the above are recommended immunizations for this patient

Answers

1. **E.** The WWE is a key time for the identification of medical conditions and risk factors for conditions. It gives the clinician an opportunity to perform preventive counseling, while further establishing the relationship between the physician and patient.

2. **D.** While it is acceptable to perform cytology alone every 3 years, the preferred screening for cervical cancer in this age group is cotesting with cytology and HPV every 5 years.

3. **B.** In a 50-year-old patient, screening mammography, colonoscopy, TSH, and fasting blood sugar would be recommended. Routine screening for osteoporosis with a DEXA scan, however, is not recommended until age 65.

4. **E.** All of these immunizations would be recommended. See Table 36-2.

SUGGESTED READINGS

ACOG. Well-woman care assessments and recommendations. <http://www.acog.org>; July 2013.

Centers for Disease Control & Prevention. MMWR Morbidity and Mortality Weekly Report. Recommended adult immunization schedule for persons aged 0 through 18 years and adults aged 19 and over—United States 2013. Vol 62(1). January 28, 2013.

Committee on Gynecologic Practice and the American Society for Reproductive Medicine Practice Committee. Committee Opinion No. 532: compounded bioidentical menopausal hormone therapy. *Obstet Gynecol.* 2012;120:411–415.

Committee on Practice Bulletins—Gynecology, The American College of Obstetricians and Gynecologists. ACOG Practice Bulletin No. 129. Osteoporosis. *Obstet Gynecol.* 2012;120:718–734.

USPSTF Recommendations. <http://www.uspreventiveservicestaskforce.org>.

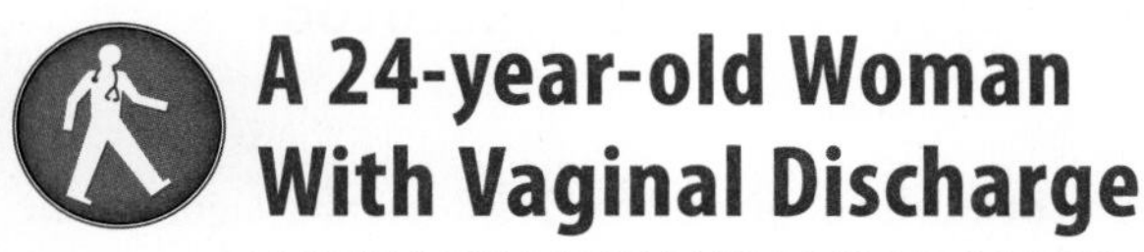

A 24-year-old Woman With Vaginal Discharge

Dana S. Phillips, MD

A 24-year-old G0 presents to your office with a complaint of a vaginal discharge.

1. How do you assess her complaint by history and physical examination?

2. How do you manage this patient's complaint?

Answers

1. Information you should obtain on history includes characteristics of discharge (color, odor), and vaginal or vulvar symptoms such as itching, burning, dysuria, swelling, or dyspareunia.

   On physical examination, examine the external genitalia for discharge or lesions, and then perform a speculum examination and assess the vaginal vault and cervix. Obtain a specimen for a wet prep from the vaginal mucosa. Consider obtaining a cervical specimen for gonorrhea and chlamydia testing. Remove the speculum and perform a bimanual examination (it is important to complete this examination, especially if the patient's complaint includes pain).

2. Treatment should be based on the history and physical examination findings. The most common causes of vaginal symptoms include bacterial vaginosis (BV), vulvovaginal candidiasis, and trichomoniasis, and treatment should be geared to treat these specific causes.

CASE REVIEW

Vaginal discharge is one of the most common reasons for patient visits to the general gynecology clinic. An intern should be able to obtain an appropriate history, perform a physical examination, and manage this gynecologic condition.

VAGINITIS

Diagnosis

History: Using open-ended questions the intern should clarify the patient's symptoms. She may complain of itching, burning, irritation, discharge, swelling, dysuria, and/or dyspareunia. Information about the location of symptoms, duration, prior treatment used (including home remedies), menstrual history, and sexual history also provides diagnostic clues. Typical symptoms of vulvovaginal candidiasis include itching and burning, or irritation and burning with urination; for

BV the patient often complains of a fishy odor, and for *Trichomonas vaginalis* she may report discharge, itching and burning, or postcoital bleeding. However, a reliable diagnosis cannot be made on the basis of history alone.

Physical examination: The pelvic examination begins with visual inspection of the vulva. The physician should assess for skin changes such as erythema and edema, or any lesions. The vaginal examination also begins with inspection, noting the presence or absence of a vaginal discharge. A specimen should be obtained for vaginal pH, the amine "whiff" test, a saline "wet" mount, and 10% potassium hydroxide (KOH) microscopy. Visual inspection of the cervix for erythema, color of discharge from the cervix, if present, or other lesions should be noted. A cervical culture or polymerase chain reaction test could be obtained for gonorrhea/chlamydia screening if indicated, or infection is suspected by history. Ancillary tests for diagnosing specific types of infection (*T. vaginalis*, *Gardnerella vaginalis*, and candidal vulvovaginitis) may be available as a lab study at your facility.

Bimanual examination should be performed as part of the assessment of a patient with this complaint to assess for cervical and uterine tenderness, as well as adnexal size and tenderness.

Vaginal specimen: Evaluation of the specimen should be done immediately after it is obtained, and is performed in a stepwise fashion:

1. Check the pH of the specimen using appropriate pH paper.
2. Obtain a glass slide, and place a small amount of the vaginal discharge with saline on the right side of the slide and cover with a coverslip.
3. On the left side of the slide place a small amount of discharge and add a small amount of 10% KOH.
4. Inspect for the following findings on the saline side:
   a. Clue cells are vaginal epithelial cells studded with adherent coccobacilli.
   b. Trichomonads are tear-shaped organisms that are smaller than an epithelial cell, and exhibit spinning or jerky motion.
   c. Budding yeast, hyphae, or pseudohyphae.
5. Inspect for the following findings on the KOH side:
   a. Blastospores or pseudohyphae (note that the KOH will lyse the squamous cells, allowing the pseudohyphae to be seen more easily)
6. Perform a "whiff" test by adding a small amount of KOH to the test tube with the vaginal discharge, and assess for a fishy odor caused by release of amines when KOH is applied; the test is positive if fishy odor is encountered.

Table 37-1 notes the components of a wet preparation and expected results based on infecting agent. FDA-cleared tests for trichomoniasis in women include the OSOM Trichomonas Rapid Test (Genzyme Diagnostics, Cambridge, Massachusetts), an immunochromatographic capillary flow dipstick technology, and the Affirm VPIII (Becton Dickenson, San Jose, California). A nucleic acid probe test

Table 37-1. Components of Wet Preparation

	Discharge	pH	Feature	"Whiff"
Normal	Mucousy, white to clear	3.0-4.5	Lactobacilli	–
Candidal vulvovaginitis	Curdy, thick, yellow to white	3.0-4.5	Hyphae, spores	–
Bacterial vaginosis	Gray, yellow	>5.0	Clue cells	+
Trichomonas vaginalis	Green, yellow, bubbly	>5.0	Motile trichomonads	–

evaluates for *T. vaginalis*, *G. vaginalis*, and *C. albicans*. These tests have a higher sensitivity than the wet prep for diagnosis of vaginitis, and may be used in your institution.

Treatment

Vulvovaginal candidiasis

The choice of medication and route of administration often depends on patient preference. Systemic side effects (gastrointestinal intolerance, liver function test elevations, allergic reactions) of oral therapy are rare, and usually mild and self-limited. A repeat dose of oral fluconazole, 3 days after the first dose, may increase the cure rate of complicated candidiasis. Maintenance therapy (after initial therapy to achieve mycologic remission) for those patients with recurrent vulvovaginal candidiasis with fluconazole 150 mg for 6 months has been effective.

In pregnancy low-dose, short-term use of fluconazole is not associated with known birth defects (Category C for the 150 mg ×1 regimen); however, higher doses 400 to 800 mg per day have been linked to birth defects (Category D for all other indications/doses).

Bacterial vaginosis

Clinical diagnosis requires the presence of 3 of 4 of Amsel criteria: abnormal gray discharge, vaginal pH >4.5, +amine ("whiff") test, or >20% of epithelial cells are clue cells.

BV is associated with PID, posthysterectomy infection, and acquisition of HIV/HSV. In pregnancy it has been associated with prematurity, premature rupture of membranes, and low birth weight. Both metronidazole and clindamycin can be used safely in pregnancy (both Category B).

Trichomoniasis

Diagnosis requires visualization of motile trichomonads on saline microscopy, or positive results on laboratory study. Metronidazole is the mainstay of treatment and is safe in pregnancy. When using either metronidazole or tinidazole, the patient should be advised to avoid alcohol (disulfiram-like effect).

Cervicitis due to *Neisseria gonorrhoeae* or *Chlamydia trachomatis* may present as a yellow vaginal discharge. Appropriate studies for these organisms should be obtained in patients as clinically indicated (friable cervix, purulent discharge, pelvic pain/fever) or in patients in high-risk groups. See Table 37-2 for the treatment of vaginitis.

Table 37-2. Treatment of Vaginitis

Indication	Medication	Dosage	Route	Duration
Candidiasis	Fluconazole	150 mg	Oral	1 day
	Terconazole	0.4% cream (5 g/day)	Vaginal[a]	7 days
		0.8% cream (5 g/day)	Vaginal	3 days
	Miconazole	2% cream (5 g/day)	Vaginal	7 days
		100 mg suppository	Vaginal	7 days
		200 mg suppository	Vaginal	3 days
	Nystatin	100,000 U tablet	Vaginal	14 days
	Clotrimazole	1% cream (5 g/day)	Vaginal	7 days
		2% cream (5 g/day)	Vaginal	3 days
		100 mg suppository	Vaginal	7 days
		200 mg suppository	Vaginal	3 days
		500 mg suppository	Vaginal	1 day
	Butoconazole	2% sustained release		
		Cream (5 g/day)	Vaginal	1 day
Bacterial vaginosis	Metronidazole[b]	0.75% gel	Vaginal	5 days
		500 mg 2×/day	Oral	7 days
Trichomoniasis	Metronidazole	500 mg (4 tablets at once)	Oral	1 day
		500 mg 2×/day	Oral	7 days
	Tinidazole[b]	500 mg (4 tablets at once)	Oral	1 day

[a]Vaginal dosing usually at bedtime.

[b]Provide alcohol precautions as prescription has disulfiram-like effects (nausea and vomiting).

TIPS TO REMEMBER

- A good history is important in formulating a differential diagnosis for vaginal discharge, but history alone cannot make the diagnosis.
- Important steps in evaluating a vaginal discharge are determining the pH of the sample, examining the sample under the microscope, and performing a "whiff" test.
- Treatment options depend on patient preference, and can be administered orally or vaginally (with the exception of trichomoniasis).

COMPREHENSION QUESTIONS

1. Amsel criteria for the diagnosis of BV are which of the following?
   A. Abnormal gray discharge
   B. Vaginal pH >4.5
   C. Positive amine "whiff" test
   D. >20% clue cells
   E. All of the above

2. Which of the following statements is *true*?
   A. One should avoid the use of metronidazole in pregnancy.
   B. Trichomoniasis is a sexually transmitted disease.
   C. BV is a sexually transmitted disease.
   D. Diagnosis of vulvovaginal candidiasis is best made on symptoms alone.

3. Disulfiram-like effects can be seen with which of the following medications?
   A. Metronidazole
   B. Tinidazole
   C. Both
   D. Neither

Answers

1. **E**. These are the 4 Amsel criteria, 3 of which should be positive to make the diagnosis of BV.

2. **B**. Metronidazole is safe to use in pregnancy; BV is a polymicrobial infection of overgrowth of facultative anaerobic organisms, and these are part of the normal vaginal flora; diagnosis of vulvovaginal candidiasis should be based on history, physical examination, and wet prep.

3. C. Both of these medications can be associated with nausea/vomiting as a side effect, similar to disulfiram when alcohol is also consumed.

SUGGESTED READINGS

American College of Obstetricians and Gynecologists. ACOG Practice Bulletin No. 72. Vaginitis. *Obstet Gynecol.* 2006;107:1195–1206.

Centers for Disease Control and Prevention. Sexually transmitted disease treatment guidelines. <cdc.gov>; 2010.

A 22-year-old With a 2-day History of Urinary Frequency, Urgency, and Dysuria

Charlie C. Kilpatrick, MD

Ms S, a 22-year-old woman, presents for a new patient visit complaining of frequency, urgency, and dysuria that began 2 days ago. She had a urinary tract infection (UTI) 6 months ago and believes that she has another one. She is sexually active, with the same male partner for a year, and uses condoms. She feels that her symptoms began 1 or 2 days after the last time they had vaginal intercourse. She has no other complaints, and denies vaginal discharge. She is a nulligravid, with no medical or surgical history. She has no drug allergies, and does not smoke. Her gynecologic history reveals an LMP of a week ago, no abnormal cervical cytology results, and no history of sexually transmitted infections. Her vital signs are stable, and she is afebrile. On physical examination she has some suprapubic tenderness, no costovertebral angle tenderness, and her urinalysis reveals moderate leukocytes, positive leukocyte esterase, positive nitrites, negative blood, and negative protein.

1. What is your differential diagnosis? What is most likely?

2. What is your next step?

Answers

1. The patient has a UTI based on her symptoms (frequency, urgency, and dysuria), recent history (prior UTI within the last 6 months, and timing in relation to recent vaginal intercourse), and urine dipstick results (positive leukocyte esterase and nitrites). Other causes of urinary frequency and urgency are overactive bladder syndrome and urgency incontinence. Dysuria can be caused by urolithiasis, bladder pain syndrome, vaginitis, urethritis from a sexually transmitted infection, or a urethral diverticulum.

2. Your next step is to treat in order to reduce symptoms, which can be done with oral antibiotics. No further diagnostic steps are required. You also suggest lifestyle and behavioral interventions that may reduce the risk of infection in the future.

CASE REVIEW

You treat her with nitrofurantoin 100 mg twice a day for 5 days that clears up her symptoms. She calls 2 months later with similar symptoms (3 UTIs within a year, each beginning 1 to 2 days after sexual intercourse). You treat her again, this time with trimethoprim–sulfamethoxazole 160 mg/800 mg twice a day for 3 days, and talk with her about recurrent UTIs, and prevention. The 2 of you decide to continue the behavioral modifications that you suggested the last time she developed a UTI. These strategies include the following: try not to delay urination, urinate soon after intercourse, adequate hydration with the addition of cranberry juice, and do not douche or wear tight-fitting undergarments. You also decide to begin single-dose prophylactic trimethoprim–sulfamethoxazole 40 mg/200 mg after coitus. If she develops any other UTIs with this regimen in place, it will be necessary to culture the urine and consider a different antibiotic for treatment. She seems happy with the treatment plan, and lets you know that she will call if symptoms develop.

URINARY TRACT INFECTION

Etiology

A UTI is the most common infection that presents to the ambulatory clinic, so you will see, diagnose, and treat many of these during your career and must become familiar with how to do so. Uncomplicated cystitis and pyelonephritis are considered UTIs. The former, on which we will focus our discussion, describes the lower urinary tract (bladder), while the latter involves the upper urinary tract (ureter and kidney). As long as the infections don't involve women who are pregnant, or involve urinary obstruction, diabetes, immunosuppression, neurogenic bladder, renal insufficiency, or a renal stone, the infections remain uncomplicated. These infections most often occur after organisms from the bowel colonize the urethra, and then subsequently the bladder, and, rarely, the upper urinary tract. Risk factors include vaginal intercourse, prior UTI, new sex partner, use of spermicides, and a first-degree relative with a history of UTI. Wiping patterns after urination, postcoital voiding patterns, douching, type of underwear, and frequency of urination have all been suggested as risk factors for UTI, but there are no solid data to support these theories. The most common organism responsible for UTI is *Escherichia coli* (75%-95% of the time), with other enteric gram-negative bacteria (*Pseudomonas aeruginosa*, *Proteus mirabilis*, *Klebsiella pneumoniae*) and gram-positive organisms (*Staphylococcus saprophyticus*, *Enterococcus faecalis*, and *Streptococcus agalactiae*) accounting for the majority of the rest.

Diagnosis

As in our case, diagnosis can usually be made with the symptoms with which your patient presents: dysuria, urgency, frequency, suprapubic pain, or hematuria. Fever, chills, flank pain, nausea, or vomiting are more associated with upper UTI. Urine dipstick revealing positive nitrites or leukocyte esterase has above-average sensitivity and specificity for diagnosing a UTI, and the presence of either of these lends more confidence to the diagnosis. Their absence though, especially in a patient with clear symptoms, does not rule out UTI. Gram-negative organisms convert urinary nitrates to nitrites, so this may be present with gram-negative infection but not gram-positive infection. Leukocyte esterase is an enzyme produced by white blood cells, so its presence indicates pyuria. This history can be obtained even without a visit to the physician's office, and in many cases patients can be given a refill on an antibiotic, to fill when they develop symptoms. This strategy can decrease health care costs, and improve patient satisfaction without compromising care. Microscopic urinalysis (sending the urine specimen to the lab for formal interpretation) is not usually necessary to aid in the diagnosis, although if performed and pyuria is not present, the diagnosis of UTI is doubtful. Urine culture should not be performed routinely either, but is helpful in the following situations: relapsing or recurrent infections, infection not responding to antibiotics, suspected pyelonephritis, uncertain diagnosis (eg, sexually transmitted infection or vaginitis), or in the presence of a complicated infection. The CDC still considers a UTI diagnosis a positive urine culture of $\geq 10^5$ colony-forming units/mL with no more than 2 species of microorganisms. Recurrent UTI is defined as 2 infections diagnosed within 6 months, or 3 infections within a year. A relapsing UTI is one that recurs within 2 weeks of the completion of treatment, and with the same organism.

Prevention

Most prevention strategies are aimed at reducing risk factors: abstaining from, or urinating soon after, sexual activity (to decrease inoculation of the organism), discontinuing the use of spermicides, consuming cranberry juice or D-mannose products, applying topical estrogen to the vagina in postmenopausal women, wiping front to back after urination, and avoiding tight-fitting underwear and douching. Spermicides can alter the vaginal flora, increasing uropathogen colonization. Besides the use of vaginal topical estrogen in postmenopausal women, none of these strategies has proven efficacy in prospective trials. Due to their low risk and cost-effectiveness, however, these strategies make for good first-line attempts at prevention of UTI.

Treatment

Table 38-1 highlights recommended antibiotic regimens for treatment of uncomplicated and recurrent cystitis proposed by the Infectious Diseases Society of America. The progression of uncomplicated cystitis to pyelonephritis is rare, even without antibiotic treatment, so the goal of treatment is to alleviate symptoms, while being mindful not to encourage antibiotic resistance, or increase "ecologic adverse effects." Fluoroquinolones are strongly discouraged as first-line treatment for uncomplicated UTI as organisms are beginning to develop resistance to their

Table 38-1. Antibiotic Treatment for Acute Uncomplicated Cystitis

Antibiotic	Dosage and Frequency
First-line agents	
Nitrofurantoin monohydrate	100 mg po BID for 5 days
TMP-SMX	160 mg/800 mg po BID for 3 days[a]
Fosfomycin trometamol	3 g po in a single dose
Second-line agents	
Ciprofloxacin, levofloxacin	250 mg po BID for 3 days, 250 or 500 mg po QD for 3 days
Beta-lactams (amoxicillin–clavulanate, cefdinir, cefaclor, cefpodoxime)	3-7 days

[a]If local resistance is >20%, consider another agent.

use, and local antibiotic resistance patterns will guide the use of trimethoprim–sulfamethoxazole (do not employ if resistance prevalence is known to exceed 20%). Second-line agents are used due to the following: local antibiotic resistance patterns, patient allergies, price, and availability. Recurrent uncomplicated cystitis can be treated with the same antibiotic regimen as a primary infection. If the infection recurs within 6 months, you should consider a different first-line agent. If primary preventive strategies fail, you should consider postcoital or continuous antibiotic prophylaxis, which can be started after self-diagnosis. In this case, you should make it clear that if symptoms do not resolve within 48 hours of treatment, further evaluation is necessary.

TIPS TO REMEMBER

- The diagnosis of uncomplicated UTI can be made on patient symptoms alone, with urine dipstick, urinalysis, and culture needed in certain circumstances.
- Treatment of UTI should balance the development of antimicrobial resistance within the community with cost-effective treatment for the patient.
- The goal of UTI treatment is amelioration of symptoms, as progression to pyelonephritis in the uncomplicated patient is rare.
- If conservative measures fail to decrease recurrent UTI, postcoital or continuous prophylactic antibiotics dramatically lower the incidence of recurrent UTI.
- Self-diagnosis and treatment of UTI should be considered, as this can lower health-care costs.

COMPREHENSION QUESTIONS

1. A 23-year-old healthy female, with no medical history, presents with sudden onset of dysuria, urgency, and frequency of urination. She has no other symptoms. On urine dipstick there is no evidence of nitrites or leukocyte esterase. The next best step would be which of the following?

   A. Ciprofloxacin 250 mg 1 po BID for 3 days.
   B. Send urine for culture.
   C. Send urine for microscopic urinalysis.
   D. Nitrofurantoin monohydrate 100 mg po BID for 5 days.

2. A 24-year-old healthy female calls the office complaining of frequency, urgency, and dysuria, and believes she has a UTI. She saw you 8 months ago and you treated her for a UTI that resolved her symptoms. The next best step is which of the following?

   A. Come to the office for a full history and physical examination.
   B. Drop off a urine sample for urine culture in order to tailor antibiotic treatment.
   C. Drop off a urine sample in order to perform urine dipstick.
   D. Call out a prescription for uncomplicated cystitis.

3. Which of the following is not considered a *primary* strategy to prevent recurrent UTI?

   A. Topical estrogen therapy in a postmenopausal woman
   B. Cranberry juice or D-mannose consumption
   C. Postcoital antibiotic prophylaxis
   D. Sexual abstinence

Answers

1. **D.** Given the patient's symptoms, urinalysis and urine culture are not needed to confirm the diagnosis of uncomplicated cystitis. The rapidity of onset, absence of other symptoms, and incidence of UTI all favor this diagnosis. The fact that the urine dipstick is negative should not lead you to believe that she does not have infection of the bladder, and first-line treatment is nitrofurantoin, not ciprofloxacin. Ciprofloxacin is reserved for recurrent or complicated cases given the rising prevalence of antibiotic resistance.

2. **D.** The patient has another episode of uncomplicated cystitis that should respond to antibiotics. There is no need to come into the office for a full H and P, and a urine dipstick, given her symptoms, is not likely to aid you in diagnosis. A urine culture would be helpful if the infection was recurrent (2 UTIs in 6 months, or 3 within a year), not responding to treatment, you were unsure of diagnosis,

the infection was complicated, or you suspected pyelonephritis. None of these scenarios exist in this case.

3. **C**. Primary preventive strategies include the following: abstaining from, or urinating soon after, sexual activity (to decrease inoculation of the organism), discontinuing the use of spermicides, consuming cranberry juice or D-mannose products, applying topical estrogen to the vagina in postmenopausal women, wiping front to back after urination, and avoiding tight-fitting underwear and douching. Antibiotic prophylaxis should be reserved for instances where these strategies fail.

SUGGESTED READINGS

Gupta K, Hooton TM, Naber KG, et al. International clinical practice guidelines for the treatment of acute uncomplicated cystitis and pyelonephritis in women: a 2010 update by the Infectious Diseases Society of America and the European Society for Microbiology and Infectious Diseases. *Clin Infect Dis*. 2011;52(5):e103–e120.

Hooton TM. Clinical practice. Uncomplicated urinary tract infection. *N Engl J Med*. 2012;366(11): 1028–1037.

Raz R, Stamm WE. A controlled trial of intravaginal estriol in postmenopausal women with recurrent urinary tract infections. *N Engl J Med*. 1993;329(11):753.

Roberts JR. Urine dipstick testing: everything you need to know. *EMN*. 2007;29(6):24–27.

A 23-year-old Sexually Active Female in Clinic for an Annual Examination

Charlie C. Kilpatrick, MD

A 23-year-old G0 presents to the clinic for an annual examination. She reports that she is doing well since her last annual examination, but has noticed that she does experience spotting in between her cycles and after vaginal intercourse. In review of her history she has no medical, obstetrical, or surgical history, and denies any drug allergies. She takes combination oral contraceptive pills, and occasionally ibuprofen for menstrual cramps. She has regular menses that last 4 to 5 days, and are crampy in nature. She has noticed vaginal spotting in between cycles and after intercourse for the past 4 months. She denies any history of abnormal cervical cytology or sexually transmitted infections (STIs) and has a male sexual partner whom she has been with for 4 months. She works 2 jobs, during the day doing accounting work, and nights and weekends waiting tables. She smokes occasionally, drinks socially once or twice a week, and denies illicit drug use.

1. **What is in your differential diagnosis for spotting in between cycles and after intercourse, and what are the next steps you need to take in the management of this patient?**

Answer

1. Your differential diagnosis should include unscheduled bleeding while on oral contraception, cervicitis (infectious and noninfectious), cervical dysplasia/cancer, cervical polyp, cervical ectropion, and endometritis/pelvic inflammatory disease. Your next steps are to get a comprehensive sexual history, perform a pelvic examination, which includes speculum and bimanual examination to assess for anatomic pathology, and screen for STIs that could lead to cervicitis, endometritis, or upper genital tract infection.

CASE REVIEW

You perform a comprehensive sexual history that includes information concerning her partners, prevention of pregnancy, protection from STIs, sexual practices, and past history of STIs. The sexual history reveals that she currently has a male partner, participates in oral and vaginal sex with men (no sex with women, and no anal sex), has had 3 partners since her last annual examination, uses condoms but not consistently, relies on oral contraceptive pills for birth control, and is not sure about her partners' STI history or how many partners they have had. You perform a pelvic examination and document the following: normal external female genitalia, shaved mons and labia majora, nulliparous introitus, vaginal sidewalls without lesion, and some scant discharge. The cervix is friable and bleeds when the speculum makes contact with it, but no excessive cervical ectropion is present. You perform a swab of the endocervical canal to test for gonorrhea and chlamydia, and a saline wet mount of the discharge to look for evidence of trichomoniasis. You examine the wet mount under the microscope and do not see trichomonads. You give her the results of the wet mount, counsel her on the consistent use of condoms, and decide to await the results of the swab before embarking on a treatment plan to address her intermenstrual and postcoital spotting. She inquires about being tested for other STIs, and you also offer her testing for syphilis, and counseling and testing for HIV.

The results of her HIV test and syphilis test come back negative in a day, and the swab results return in 3 days positive for chlamydia, and negative for gonorrhea. You call her to discuss the results and then call her and her partner out a prescription for azithromycin 1 g orally. You recommend that her partner is tested for the same STIs, explain that it is difficult to tell how long she has had chlamydia due to the fact that it is often asymptomatic in men and women, and encourage her to be retested for chlamydia in 3 months. Your ancillary staff also reports the results to the local health department as required by law.

SEXUALLY TRANSMITTED INFECTIONS

Diagnosis and Treatment

Diagnosing and treating STIs begin with a comprehensive sexual history in a nonjudgmental fashion using open-ended questions. Your goal is to uncover any possible risk factors for STIs that would require screening. The sexual history is very similar to what is outlined above, inquiring about the number and gender of partners, prior history of STIs in the patient and her partner(s), sexual practices (oral, vaginal, or anal sex), and the use of condoms and method of birth control. Risk factors for acquiring STIs include the answers to the sexual history as well as contact with sexual workers or engagement in high-risk sexual behavior, Internet dating, younger age (adolescence to mid-20s), any illicit drug use, or prior time in a correctional facility. The geographical location that you work in will also guide your screening efforts, and communication with your local public health department is important to determine STI prevalence.

Screening for STIs is an important step in diagnosing infection given that many of them are completely asymptomatic, especially in the female patient. Screening may limit the sequelae that can occur from untreated infection. STI screening intervals change based on whether you uncover risk factors in your history. Table 39-1 outlines risk factors, proposed screening intervals, screening tools, and treatment recommendations for 4 common STIs.

TABLE 39-1. STI Risk Factors, Screening, and Treatment Recommendations

STI	Risk Factors	Screening Tool	First-line Treatment
Chlamydia[a]	• Age <25 and sexually active • Prior STI or partner with STI • New sex partner or more than 1 partner in prior 60 days • Unmarried • Inconsistent condom use • Pregnant • Sex work or drug use	• NAAT of the vagina, endocervix, or first voided urine specimen • Culture	• Azithromycin 1 g po single dose • Doxycycline 100 mg po BID × 7 days
Gonorrhea[b]	• Risk factors and screening recommendations are the same as chlamydia	• NAAT • Culture	• Ceftriaxone 250 mg IM × 1
Syphilis	• At the time of diagnosis with another STI • Admitted to correctional facility • Commercial sex workers • Pregnant women	• Nontreponemal tests (RPR and VDRL) • Treponemal tests (MHATP, FTA-ABS, TP-EIA)	• Benzathine penicillin G 2.4 million U IM
Trichomoniasis[c]	• New or multiple partners • Prior STI or partner with STI • Injection drug use • Women who trade sex for drugs or money	• Wet mount • OSOM Trichomonas Rapid Test	• Metronidazole 2 g po single dose • Metronidazole 500 mg po BID × 7 days

NAAT, nucleic acid amplification test.

[a]Annual screening in asymptomatic women <25, and in older women with risk factors.
[b]Cotreatment for chlamydia is recommended.
[c]Based on risk factors, annual screening is not recommended for asymptomatic patients.

Chlamydia is the most common STI diagnosed in the United States. The infection is often asymptomatic, but symptoms include a change in vaginal discharge, postcoital spotting, intermenstrual spotting, dysuria, and mucopurulent discharge. In those with dysuria, a urinalysis that reveals pyuria without bacteriuria should raise suspicion for chlamydial urethritis. Testing with a nucleic acid amplification test (NAAT) has replaced culture as the gold standard, and can be performed on an endocervical or vaginal swab, or from a first voided urine specimen (the first 10 cm^3). The latter 2 allow diagnosis without a pelvic examination that may improve screening access. Given the serious sequelae (infertility, ectopic pregnancy, pelvic inflammatory disease) that can come from upper genital tract infection with chlamydia, screening sexually active asymptomatic women <25 years of age is recommended. Directly observed therapy with a single dose of azithromycin improves compliance and partner treatment is recommended. The patient and her partner should wait 7 days after completion of treatment prior to resuming sexual activity. Additional STIs should be screened for, and rescreening in 3 months is recommended given the high rate of reinfection. The presentation, sequelae, screening recommendations, testing, and rescreening guidelines for gonorrhea are very similar to chlamydia. Recently, antibiotic resistance to gonorrhea treatment has emerged, so a culture may better delineate antibiotic treatment in recalcitrant cases. Cotreatment for chlamydia is recommended in those who test positive for gonorrhea.

Syphilis is also often asymptomatic after infection, besides the chancre at the site of inoculation. The chancre is painless and usually resolves within a few weeks, so many often go untreated. Screening is based on risk factors, outlined in Table 39-1, and the initial diagnostic tool is a nontreponemal test, followed by a confirmatory treponemal test. There has been little antibiotic resistance developed by syphilis over the years to penicillin and thus it is the first-line treatment.

Trichomoniasis is the most common nonviral STI worldwide. Screening for this depends on risk factors, outlined in Table 39-1, and it is diagnosed most commonly by wet mount. There are more sensitive tests to diagnose *Trichomonas*, but the wet mount is cheap, and quick. You will learn very quickly in the intern year how to perform a wet mount and screen for trichomoniasis. Treatment is with a single dose of metronidazole, and infection in the female is not often associated with the serious sequelae of the aforementioned STIs.

Once a STI is diagnosed, the patient should be counseled on treatment for her and her partner, and prevention of STI acquisition in the future. The patient should be rescreened for STIs at 3 months following treatment. The use of condoms should be reinforced, and an adequate birth control method confirmed. Also, the following STIs require notification to your local health department: acute hepatitis B and C, chancroid, chlamydia, gonorrhea, HIV, and syphilis.

TIPS TO REMEMBER

- Open-ended questions and a nonjudgmental attitude are important in conducting a comprehensive sexual history.
- Many STIs in women are asymptomatic, so screen for them based on risk factors.
- Serious sequelae of genital gonorrhea and chlamydia include infertility, ectopic pregnancy, and pelvic inflammatory disease.
- After testing positive for an STI, rescreening after treatment should be done at 3 months given the high rate of reinfection.
- STIs that require health department notification include chancroid, chlamydia, gonorrhea, acute hepatitis B and C, syphilis, and HIV.

COMPREHENSION QUESTIONS

1. Ms Jones presents to the clinic complaining of a diffuse, malodorous, yellow-green vaginal discharge. It began a week or so ago, and is irritating to the outside of her vagina. On examination of the pelvis, the vagina is erythematous, and there is some frothy discharge. You perform a wet mount slide that reveals numerous white blood cells, and oval-shaped cells that are moving in a spinning and jerky fashion. What is it?

A. Clue cells: bacterial vaginosis
B. Hyphae: candidal vaginitis
C. Lice: pediculosis pubis
D. Trichomonads: trichomoniasis vaginalis
E. Chlamydia infected endocervical cells: chlamydia trachomatis cervicitis

2. Ms Johnson is a 24-year-old female who presents to clinic with complaints of a foul-smelling vaginal discharge. She has a new partner and a history of prior chlamydial infection 2 years ago, and uses condoms (but not consistently). You perform a saline wet mount that reveals trichomoniasis. You think she should be tested for syphilis given this result. Which test would you order?

A. Fluorescent treponemal antibody absorption (FTA-ABS)
B. *Treponema pallidum* enzyme immunoassay (TP-EIA)
C. Dark field microscopy
D. Rapid plasma reagin (RPR)
E. Culture with Mansfield's medium

3. Ms Barnes is a 22-year-old sexually active female who presents to clinic for an annual examination, cervical cytology, and questions in regard to STIs. You

answer many of her questions and perform a pelvic examination that reveals a nulliparous introitus, vaginal side wall and cervix without lesion, bimanual examination consistent with small mobile uterus, no adnexal masses or fullness, and no tenderness on examination. You get an endocervical sample for cytology and for gonorrhea and chlamydia. Which of the following statements in regard to chlamydial infections is *least accurate*?

A. Annual screening for chlamydia is not necessary in sexually active women ≤25 years of age.
B. Asymptomatic chlamydial infection is common among women.
C. Chlamydial genital infection is the most frequently reported infectious disease in the United States.
D. Sequelae of chlamydial infection in women include PID, ectopic pregnancy, and infertility.
E. Screening for chlamydia in women can be performed with a urine sample or a swab of the endocervix.

Answers

1. **D.** The description of oval-shaped cells that are spinning and have a jerky motion is one of trichomonads on a wet mount. A wet mount is performed by taking the vaginal discharge onto the slide, placing a drop of saline on it, and adding a coverslip. This can be viewed under the microscope. Trichomonads will be motile as long as they are viewed shortly after creating the slide, about 10 to 20 minutes.

2. **D.** Screening for syphilis begins with a nontreponemal test (RPR or VDRL) and then is confirmed with a treponemal test (MHA-TP, FTA-ABS, TP-PA, or TP-EIA). Once a patient has tested positive for syphilis, the treponemal test will remain positive for a lifetime. A 4-fold increase in the nontreponemal test indicates active infection.

3. **A.** Annual screening for chlamydia *is recommended* for sexually active women ≤25 years of age. This is due to the fact that the infection is commonly asymptomatic, the sequelae from infection can be devastating, and screening can be facilitated by the use of vaginal swab or urine collection.

SUGGESTED READING

<http://www.cdc.gov/std/treatment/2010/default.htm>; accessed April 9, 2013.

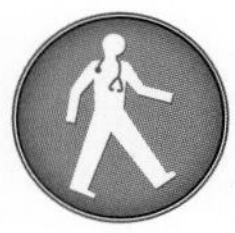

A 34-year-old Female Who Desires Oral Contraception

Susan M. Leong-Kee, MD

Ms R, a 34-year-old G1P1001, presents 3 months postpartum to restart oral contraceptive pills (OCPs). She is ready to go back to work, would like to wean from breast-feeding, and has been using condoms for contraception since delivery. She has a history of migraine headaches but no other major medical or surgical history. Her pregnancy was notable for induction of labor for gestational hypertension, and her blood pressures postpartum have remained normal. She has not yet resumed her menses, but has a long history of irregular and painful periods. Menarche started at age 13, every 21 to 45 days with moderate-to-severe cramping. She denies any abnormal pap smears or sexually transmitted diseases. She had been on combined oral contraceptives (COCs) in the past. Her only side effect was breakthrough bleeding. She denies any allergies but takes Imitrex as needed for migraines. She has been married for 3 years and works as an executive assistant. She does report a history of smoking 0.5 pack per day since age 20 but quit after she found out she was pregnant. She would like to conceive again in the next 1 to 2 years and would like to restart COCs. Her vitals and general examination are within normal limits. Weight noted to be 180 lb and height 5 ft 2 in (BMI = 32.9).

1. How would you counsel this patient on her options for contraception based on her history?

Answer

1. You counsel the patient on all options for reliable and reversible hormonal contraception, including combination contraceptives (eg, pills, patches, rings), progesterone-only methods (pills, injections, implants), and intrauterine devices (IUDs). Medical conditions that should be considered in this patient include her age, smoking history, postpartum state, gestational hypertension, and migraines. You further question whether her migraines are associated with any aura or focal neurological deficits, encourage her to not resume smoking on COCs, and ask her to monitor her blood pressures once she restarts COCs to avoid potential cardiovascular risks. You discuss some potential side effects of COCs including breast tenderness, nausea/vomiting, menstrual irregularities, mood changes, and changes in libido. Since she reports issues with breakthrough bleeding on a particular COC in the past, you suggest a COC that may have a better bleeding profile. Finally, you discuss possible noncontraceptive benefits to restarting COCs for this patient, including regulation of her menses, decreased dysmenorrhea, and the fact that the risk of COCs is less than the alternative, pregnancy.

CASE REVIEW

OCPs, which include both COCs and progestin-only pills (POPs), are considered a very effective and safe method of contraception and would be an appropriate choice for this patient. A patient's medical conditions or particular characteristics are important elements that need to be considered when choosing an appropriate and safe contraceptive method. Examples of medical conditions that should be considered in this patient's case that could represent an unacceptable health risk for use of COCs include obesity, smoking >35 years of age (with >15 cigarettes per day), migraine with aura or focal neurological deficits, and uncontrolled or severe hypertension. Of note, the American Congress of Obstetricians and Gynecologists (ACOG) recommends caution with the use of COCs in obese women over the age of 35 due to independent risk factors for venous thromboembolism (VTE). This patient does not meet any of these criteria to preclude her from restarting COCs so you begin her on them, and schedule a follow-up phone call in a few months to assure that this choice of contraception continues to be an appropriate method and that she is satisfied.

ORAL CONTRACEPTIVE PILLS

Contraceptive counseling and selection of an appropriate method of contraception are imperative for both initiation and continuation of any chosen contraceptive method and avoiding unintended pregnancies. Each year, more than 50% of all pregnancies are unintended, and almost half of unintended pregnancies occur among women who are using contraception. OCPs are considered an effective, safe, and easily reversible option of contraception for patients throughout the reproductive years. They are considered a "very effective" method of contraception, preventing pregnancy ~91% to 99% of the time. OCPs are user dependent and misuses are common, such as forgetting to take pills or failure to return on time for refills. Considerations in choice of contraception include effectiveness, safety, side effects, convenience, duration of action, childbearing plans, patient preference, reversibility, noncontraceptive benefits, availability (accessibility and cost), and privacy.

There are many misconceptions regarding the safety of OCPs, especially in terms of their potential cardiovascular and cancer risks. OCPs actually pose very little risk for women's health; they are generally safer than pregnancy. Mortality risk with OCP use is very low and major health risks are uncommon, but more likely to occur in those with underlying medical conditions. The *U.S. Medical Eligibility Criteria for Contraceptive Use, 2010* (adapted from the World Health Organization *Medical Eligibility Criteria for Contraceptive Use*, 4th ed.), provide evidence-based guidelines regarding which women are medically eligible for contraceptive methods to assure they are not exposed to inappropriate risks. The risk of cancers with use of OCPs has also been extensively studied and has shown an actual reduction in the risk of endometrial, ovarian, and colorectal cancers, a possible small increase in the risk of breast and cervical cancer, and an increased risk of liver cancer. The other important discussion with patients regarding OCPs is the potential side effects, the main reason for discontinuance. Potential side effects of OCPs include breast tenderness, nausea/vomiting, headaches, elevated blood pressures, bloating, mood lability (anxiety, irritability, and depression), menstrual irregularities, weight gain, skin changes, hyperlipidemia, and decreased libido. Patients should also be aware of possible drug interactions with certain medications that could reduce the effectiveness of OCPs. Some of these drugs include hepatic enzyme inducers (rifampin), anticonvulsants, antiretrovirals, and over-the-counter drugs such as St. John's wort and orlistat.

Treatment

Combined oral contraceptives

The choice of COC is based on several factors: medical conditions, patient preference, past experience with particular COCs, patient's desire for noncontraceptive benefits, and cost. COCs are usually distributed in a pack of 28 pills; 21 contain active hormone while 7 are placebo pills. COCs contain both ethinyl estradiol (EE) and 1 of 8 available progestins. The progesterone provides the contraception, while the estrogen component acts synergistically to increase the effectiveness of the pill and lessen irregular bleeding. The typical dose of EE in most COCs ranges between 20 and 35 mcg, but there are also 10 and 50 mcg EE pills. Studies have shown that COCs containing 20 mcg EE or less tend to have more breakthrough bleeding. Regarding the different types of progestins, there are some that are more androgenic or "testosterone-like" than others. The general mechanism of action of COCs includes the following: inhibiting ovulation, thickening and decreasing cervical mucus to prevent sperm penetration, reducing activity in the cilia of the fallopian tubes to prevent fertilization, and altering the endometrium making it less likely for implantation to occur.

In addition to the different doses of EE and type of progestin in each COC, providers should also consider different formulations of COCs that include monthly or extended cycling. Extended-cycling COCs are pill packs lasting longer than 28 days, typically including placebo every 3 months, theoretically allowing patients to "skip their period." Providers often extend cycling by using any brand COC and skipping the placebo. There are data to support the safety and efficacy of using other formulations with extended cycles, but the FDA has not approved this indication. Counseling must be done to reassure the patient that there is no known medical benefit to monthly bleeding and there is no buildup of the endometrial lining that would be considered unsafe or harmful with use of extended-cycle COC. The most common side effect of extended-cycle COCs, ironically, is breakthrough bleeding, but this usually lessens over time.

There are also many notable noncontraceptive benefits to COCs and they should be taken into consideration when selecting a COC for a patient. Menstrual-related health benefits of COCs include decreased dysmenorrhea, decreased menstrual blood loss and iron-deficiency anemia, and regulation of menses. Patients should be counseled that it could take several months (sometimes 4-6 months) before the benefits of COCs are noticed. COCs may also reduce the risk and symptoms of the following: endometriosis, premenstrual symptoms or cyclic mood symptoms, acne or symptoms of polycystic ovarian syndrome, menstrual migraines, ectopic pregnancies, functional ovarian cysts, benign breast conditions, vasomotor symptoms in perimenopausal patients, and pelvic inflammatory disease. For those patients who are concerned about increased cancer risk of OCPs, studies have shown a decreased risk of endometrial, ovarian, and colorectal cancer as well.

After selecting a COC for a patient, it is important to discuss the timing of pill initiation. Many protocols exist including a "First-day start" (a patient starts the pills on the first day of her next menses, which lessens the need for backup contraception when starting), "Sunday start" (a patient starts the first Sunday after her next menses begins, which may avoid withdrawal bleeding during the weekend in her next menses), or a "Quick start" (begins the pills the day prescribed, which may improve compliance). Backup contraception is needed for 7 days in the Sunday and Quick start, especially if her menses was more than 5 days before starting her pills. Several clinical studies now prefer the "Quick start" to avoid time delay in starting contraception and possibly an unintentional pregnancy. This preferred protocol does not consider time during the menstrual cycle as a factor in starting the OCPs, and the patient is counseled to start the first pill on the day of her visit, as long as she is certain she is not pregnant and does not need emergency contraception. Even if she does start the pill pack and has an unknown undetectable early pregnancy, patients can be reassured that the hormones will not adversely affect an early pregnancy. Counseling should also be done for patients on what to do with missed or late hormonal contraception. Generally, the patient should take the missed pill as soon as she remembers and the next pill at the regular time. Patients should be advised that missed pills in the first week of a pill pack pose the greatest risk of unintentional pregnancy and backup contraception should be used for 1 week if 1 to 2 pills are missed at the start of the pack or 3 or more pills in the first week of the pack. It is important to emphasize that correct initiation, continuation, and consistent use of COCs result in the lowest risk of unintentional pregnancies.

Progestin-only pills

POPs, otherwise known as the "minipill," are another option for patients who are candidates for OCPs. POPs also come in 28-pill packs; all of the pills contain active hormone, but do not contain any estrogen. Therefore, they may not hold the same risks as COCs and have fewer contraindications than COCs. POPs are useful for women who want immediately reversible hormonal contraception but for whom estrogen is contraindicated. Many providers also choose POPs during the postpartum period as lactation is not disturbed. (Studies have not shown, however, that COCs affect milk supply once good milk flow is well established.) POPs contain a lower dose of progestins with 2 available formulations of either norethindrone or norgestrel. Although many believe that POPs are less effective than COCs, data comparing the efficacy of both types of contraception are scant. POPs are highly effective if taken as directed. Patients should be counseled that they are to be taken continuously and that they should be taken within a few hours of the same time every day. If a patient misses a pill, she should take the missed pill as soon as she remembers and the next pill at the regular time. She should also use a backup method for 2 days if the pill is taken more than 3 hours past her regular time. The most common side effects of POPs include irregular bleeding/spotting, as well as other progestin-related side effects, such as bloating, and mood lability.

TIPS TO REMEMBER

- OCPs are a very effective method of contraception and pose very little health risks to most patients.
- Each patient should be screened for contraindications and potential health conditions or characteristics that preclude the safe use of OCPs.
- Patients should thoroughly be counseled on potential risks, benefits, and alternatives of using OCPs as well as potential side effects and drug interactions before initiation.
- Selection of a particular formulation/brand of the OCP as well as recommendations for monthly versus extended cycling should depend on the patient's overall clinical picture, patient preference, past experiences, desire for noncontraceptive benefits, and cost.
- Counseling on timing of pill initiation and protocol for missed or late hormonal contraception should be discussed as correct and consistent use of any contraceptive method results in the lowest risk of unintended pregnancies.
- Follow-up after initiation of OCPs should be done to assure that the patient is satisfied with the contraceptive method, does not desire any change, and has no troublesome side effects.

COMPREHENSIVE QUESTIONS

1. A 24-year-old G0 presents to your clinic desiring contraception but also complaining of heavy menses and severe dysmenorrhea. After doing a thorough H&P and discussing her options, you and the patient decide to start her on a low-dose COC. The patient calls after 2 months of using the prescribed COC and requests a change in hormonal contraception as she did not notice any change in her

symptoms. She denies any other side effects. Your next step should be which of the following?

A. Ask the patient to come in to discuss changing her method of hormonal contraception as she should have already seen a difference in her symptoms.
B. Advise the patient that it can several months before results of the OCPs may be seen and to follow-up in 4 to 6 months if there is still no change in symptoms.
C. Call in a new prescription for another brand of COC with a slightly higher dose of EE and have her follow-up in 1 month.
D. Advise the patient to discontinue her prescribed COC and use condoms only.

2. Ms R, the lady in the case question above, leaves the clinic with a prescription for COCs. She has been reliably breast-feeding every 3 hours since delivery. She calls back after she picks up the pills, because she doesn't know when to start them. Which of the following statements concerning when to start her COCs is most accurate?

A. She may follow a "First-day start" and begin them the first day of her next menses, but she will need backup contraception for the first 5 days.
B. She may follow a "Sunday start" and begin them on Sunday of the next week, in order that she can follow the descriptions on the pill pack.
C. She may follow a "Quick start" and start them today, as long as a urine pregnancy test is negative, and she needs backup contraception for 2 weeks.
D. She may follow a "Quick start" and start them today, with backup contraception for 7 days, and her reliable breast-feeding and condom use preclude a urine pregnancy test.

3. A 28-year-old G1P1001 presents 2 weeks postpartum for problem visit s/p a NSVD with a second-degree laceration. She is also requesting to restart contraception. She has used COCs in the past with good tolerance and minimal side effects and would like to restart right away. She has no major medical problems, is a nonsmoker, and is bottle-feeding. She does not want to try to conceive again for 2 to 3 years. Your next step would be which of the following?

A. Refill her COC as requested today and discuss with her the "Quick start" initiation protocol.
B. Refill COC as requested today, but caution the patient to not start for at least 3 full weeks after delivery.
C. Write a new Rx for POPs today, but caution the patient to not start for at least 3 full weeks after delivery.
D. Advise the patient to use condoms for at least 6 months before restarting COCs.

Answers

1. **B.** COCs can offer many noncontraceptive benefits, including menstrual-related health benefits such as decreasing menstrual blood loss and dysmenorrhea. Patients, however, should be counseled that it could take several months (typically up to 4-6 months) before the benefits of COCs are noticed. This patient could also benefit from extended-cycling COCs to decrease menstrual-related symptoms and should be offered this option as well.

2. **D.** The "First-day start" method doesn't require backup contraception, while the "Sunday start" is the *first Sunday after the onset of her next menses.* The "Quick start" allows for the most compliance, while decreasing unintended pregnancy rates, but does require backup contraception for a week. Reliable breast-feeding and condom use would preclude a urine pregnancy test in this situation, but one can check a urine pregnancy test if there is any doubt or concern about a potential pregnancy.

3. **B.** COCs should not be started for at least 4 to 6 weeks (minimum 3 full weeks) after delivery for non–breast-feeding women to avoid VTE risk due to the hypercoagulable state postpartum. If the patient was breast-feeding, there are theoretical concerns about the effects of COCs on breast milk production in the early postpartum period (<1 month) when milk flow is being established. POPs could also be prescribed today and safely initiated immediately postpartum, but the patient's preference is to start the COC that she used previously with minimal side effects.

SUGGESTED READINGS

ACOG Committee on Practice Bulletins—Gynecology No. 73. Use of hormonal contraception in women with coexisting medical conditions. *Obstet Gynecol.* 2006;107:1453–1472.

ACOG Committee on Practice Bulletins—Gynecology No. 110. Noncontraceptive uses of hormonal contraceptives. *Obstet Gynecol.* 2010;115:206–218.

Anderson FD, Hait H, Seasonale-301 Study Group. A multicenter, randomized study of an extended cycle oral contraceptive. *Contraception.* 2003;68:89–96.

Burkman R, Schlesselman JJ, Zieman M. Safety concerns and health benefits associated with oral contraception. *Am J Obstet Gynecol.* 2004:190(suppl):S5–S22.

Centers for Disease Control and Prevention. U.S. Medical Eligibility Criteria for Contraceptive Use, 2010. *MMWR Recomm Rep.* 2010;59(RR-4):1–86. <www.cdc/gov/mmwr>.

Finer LB, Henshaw SK. Disparities in rates of unintended pregnancy in the United States, 1994 and 2001. *Perspect Sex Reprod Health.* 2006;38(2):90–96.

Hatcher RA, Trussell J, Nelson A, Cates W, Kowal D, Policar MS. *Contraceptive Technology.* 20th revised ed. New York: Ardent Media; 2011:45–71, 75–81, 237–247, 249–341.

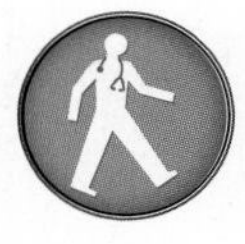

A 19-year-old G2P1011 Presents to the Office for Contraception Counseling

Naghma Farooqi, MD

A 19-year-old G2P1011 presents to the office for contraception counseling. She would like information concerning effective contraception options. She had a term vaginal delivery at age 17 and then a spontaneous miscarriage at the age of 18. Both pregnancies were unplanned and resulted from inconsistent use of oral contraceptives. She now desires long-term contraception that does not involve an ongoing effort to prevent pregnancy.

1. What options can you offer this young woman?

2. What are the risks and benefits associated with those options?

Answers

1. The first option is long-term use of IM depot medroxyprogesterone acetate (Depo-Provera). It requires less daily adherence than oral contraceptive pills (OCPs), but being late for an injection could still result in an unintended pregnancy. Two more suitable options are placement of an intrauterine contraceptive device (IUD), of which 3 different types will be reviewed in this chapter, and placement of an etonogestrel-secreting implant (Nexplanon®) in the upper arm of the patient. The term "long-acting reversible contraception" (LARC) applies to these 2 methods.
2. The benefits and risks of these options vary with the method being considered. No method is 100% effective and variable rates of patient requests for discontinuation have been reported. Benefits common to all LARCs include minimal need for patient compliance and the fact that, as the name LARC implies, they are long acting *and* reversible. Risks include irregular uterine bleeding and a low, but finite failure rate. Method-specific risks will be presented as each option is discussed.

CASE REVIEW

Contraceptive options are widely used and available in the United States. Oral contraceptives are by far the most popular among all age groups. OCPs require daily intake at approximately the same time. Irregular intake causes irregular bleeding and ovulation. Our patient has demonstrated inability to consistently use this method of birth control and would benefit from long-acting contraception that is reversible and doesn't require daily adherence.

LONG-ACTING REVERSIBLE CONTRACEPTION

Options available in the United States are:

A. IUDs:

1. ParaGard copper T 380A
2. Mirena—LNg20 levonorgestrel intrauterine system
3. Skyla—LNg13 levonorgestrel intrauterine system

B. Intradermal implantable device:

1. Nexplanon—etonogestrel single implant

IUD

The first device dates back to the early 1900s. Since then many modifications and different shapes and types of IUDs have emerged. Only 3 types are available in the United States.

ParaGard is a T-shaped device with polyethylene-wrapped copper wire around the stem and the arms (see Figure 41-1). The device is FDA approved for

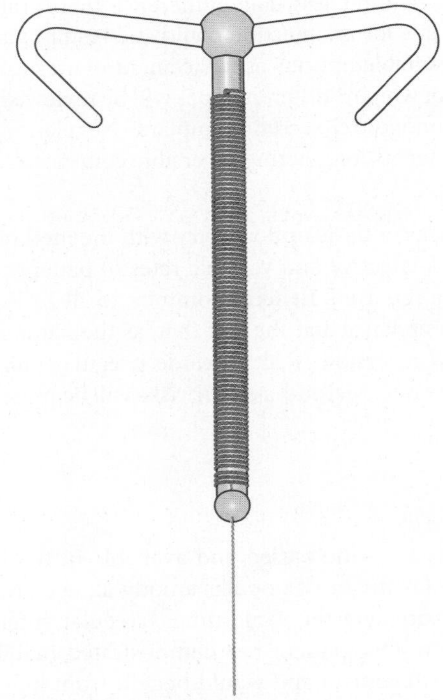

Figure 41-1. Copper T 380A—ParaGard IUD

10 continuous years. The reported failure rate at 1 year is 0.8/100 women and a 10-year failure rate of 1.9/100 women.

Proposed mechanism of action of the copper T 380A—ParaGard:

1. Prefertilization action:
   - Inhibition of sperm migration and motility
   - Reduced transport and speed of ovum
   - Damage and destruction of ovum
2. Postfertilization action:
   - Destruction of fertilized ovum

These effects are due to a sterile inflammatory reaction causing an increase in cytotoxic peptides and activation of enzymes that are detrimental to both the sperm and ovum. There is no interruption of ovulation with ParaGard use.

Common side effects of the ParaGard:

- Dysmenorrhea: An increase in cramping has been reported and this may or may not resolve with continuous use. Pain is usually during a menstrual cycle.
- Heavy menstrual cycles: Increase in duration and amount of bleeding occurs that may subside within 1 year of use, but some women continue to report abnormal bleeding for several years.
- Intermenstrual spotting: This is common to all the intrauterine devices and is thought to be due to local irritation of the endometrium.

Levonorgestrel intrauterine system LNg20—Mirena

This is a T-shaped, silicone sleeve loaded with 52 mg of levonorgestrel on the stem (see Figure 41-2). It releases 20 μg of levonorgestrel daily and is FDA approved for up to 5 years of continuous use. The 1-year failure rate is 0.2/100 women. Women with this device in place continue to ovulate normally. At 24 months 50% of users have amenorrhea, 25% have very light infrequent cycles, 11% have spotting, and the remainder report normal or heavy bleeding. In addition to contraception, it is used to treat dysmenorrhea and heavy menses.

Mechanism of action:

- Causes a sterile inflammatory mechanism similar to the copper T 380A.
- Thickens the cervical mucus, thereby creating a barrier to sperm penetration.
- Promotes endometrial decidualization and glandular atrophy, thereby making the intrauterine environment hostile to implantation.
- Increases expression of glycodelin A in the endometrial glands, thus inhibiting binding of sperm to ova.

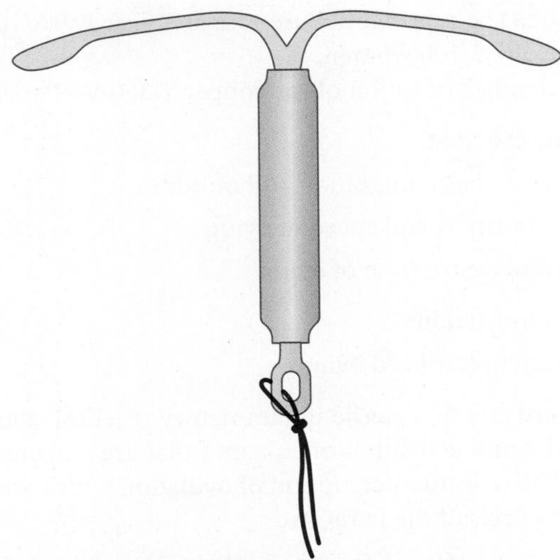

Figure 41-2. Levonorgestrel intrauterine system LNg20—Mirena

Common side effects of the Mirena:

- Irregular menses due to irregular shedding of endometrium.
- Six percent to 14% women report weight gain that may be due to the effect on carbohydrate metabolism.
- Ten percent to 14% report increasing acne, possibly due to systemic absorption of some progesterone.
- Mild insulin resistance with no significant change in serum glucose levels in normal women.

Levonorgestrel-releasing intrauterine system LNg14—Skyla

This is also a T-shaped device (see Figure 41-3). It was initially approved in 2000 and became available in 2013. It has a polyethylene frame with a steroid reservoir containing 13.5 mg of the progestin levonorgestrel. It releases 14 mcg per day and is FDA approved for contraception for 3 years. The pregnancy rate in the first year of use is 0.41 per 100 women per year and the cumulative 3-year rate is 0.9%.

The Skyla is smaller in size compared with the Mirena, 28 × 30 mm versus 32 × 32 mm, has a smaller inserter, and hence is an easier insertion in nulliparous women and in women with a stenotic cervix. Skyla contains a silver ring, which makes it easy to identify on both ultrasound and x-ray.

Mechanism of action:

- Similar to the LNg20 IUD system.
- Not much information is available about the noncontraceptive benefit of the Skyla LNg14 system.

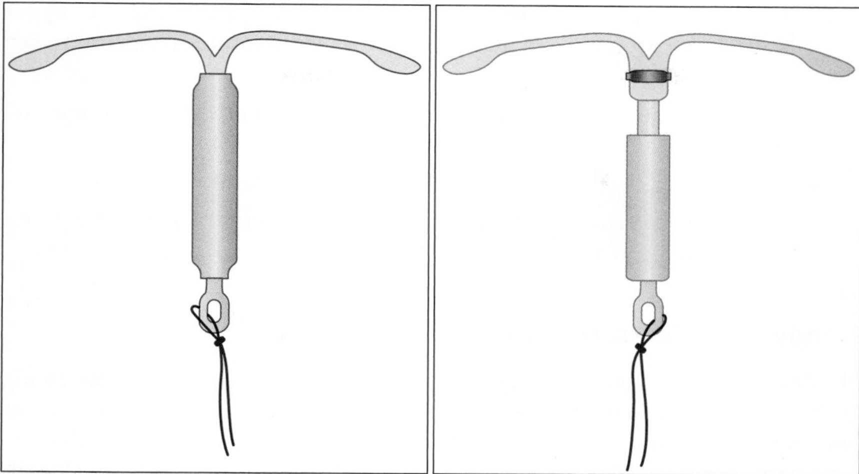

Figure 41-3. Mirena device (on left) compared with Skyla device (on right)

Side effects:

- Irregular bleeding in the first 3 to 6 months of use is the most frequent complaint among users. The same mechanism applies here as in the Mirena IUD.
- The hormonal side effects are similar to the LNg20 system.

Common side effects of all the IUDs:

- Irregular bleeding patterns.
- Expulsion of the device spontaneously in 4.4% to 9.2%.
- Retraction of the IUD string inside the cavity making removal a technical challenge.
- Perforation of the uterus at the time of insertion is a rare complication.
- If pregnancy occurs with the device in place, it is more likely to be ectopic.

Common misconceptions about the IUDs:

1. Contraception is due to repetitive expulsion of a conception.
2. Increases the rate of pelvic inflammatory disease.
3. Increases the absolute risk of an ectopic pregnancy.
4. Increases the infertility risk in nulliparous women.

Counseling prior to insertion:

- Failure and complication rates, though minimal, must be discussed in detail.
- Irregular bleeding for the first 4 to 6 weeks after insertion is to be expected.

- Increase in menstrual flow and dysmenorrhea, especially with the copper T 380A, are common and may take up to a year to subside (sometimes they do not resolve).
- Dysmenorrhea and menstrual flow decrease with the levonorgestrel system.
- A self–string check every 4 to 6 months is recommended.
- Consult a physician immediately if there is a suspicion of a pregnancy with an IUD in the uterus.

Etonogestrel Contraceptive Device: Nexplanon

The device is a 40 × 2 mm semirigid ethylene vinyl acetate rod containing 68 mg of the progestin etonogestrel (see Figure 41-4). It was initially introduced as Implanon, but later, with some modification, was remarketed as Nexplanon. The chemical composition and pharmaceutical indications for both are similar. Nexplanon is detectable by plain x-ray and does not require MRI to locate it. The failure rate reported is 0.38 pregnancies per 100 women users, making it one of the most effective LARC devices. It is FDA approved for 3 years.

The rod is placed subdermally in the inner upper arm. It has 68 mg of etonogestrel with a daily release of 60 to 70 μg initially, and then decreasing to 35 to 40 μg per day at the end of 1 year, 30 to 40 μg per day by the end of the second year, and 25 to 30 μg per day by the end of the third year.

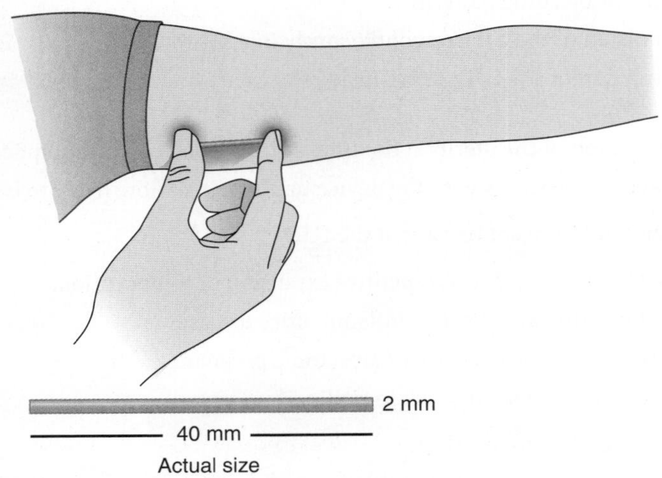

Figure 41-4. Etonogestrel contraceptive device: Nexplanon

Mechanism of action:

- Thickens the cervical mucus.
- Decreases tubal motility and inhibits fertilization.
- The progestin also inhibits gonadotropin secretion, thereby inhibiting ovulation.
- The endometrial lining is affected to a lesser extent and is not a major contributor to the contraceptive mechanism of Nexplanon.

Common side effects:

- Irregular bleeding, which may not resolve with time. Numbers of bleeding days are highest in the first 3 months of use.
- Headache, weight gain, breast tenderness, and emotional lability have been reported.
- Insertion site infection, hematoma, and pain in the first few days after insertion. Resolve with local measures and occasionally antibiotics.
- Decrease in the efficacy of contraception may occur with certain hepatic enzyme inducers such as antiretroviral medications.
- Possible decrease in contraception in overweight and obese women.
- Deep placement may make palpation and removal of the device difficult.

FOLLOW-UP OF OUR CASE

The patient in this case was presented with LARC options. She was counseled extensively on the benefits and the side effects of each. The patient opted for the etonogestrel subdermal implantable device—Nexplanon. She was brought back on day 4 of her menses and the device was inserted by a Nexplanon-certified physician. A negative urine pregnancy test on day 4 of the cycle confirmed absence of a pregnancy.

Note: Nexplanon may be inserted at any time if the physician is certain that the patient is not pregnant. Backup contraception for 7 days is advised if the patient is greater than 5 days from her last menstrual period.

TIPS TO REMEMBER

- Insertion of all of these devices requires special training.
- Detailed counseling of women regarding risks, benefits, side effects, and alternatives to LARCs may help to eliminate early discontinuation.
- Arguably one of the main benefits of LARCs is that patient adherence is *not* required.

COMPREHENSION QUESTIONS

1. Which of the following statements is *true*?
   - A. The ParaGard IUD is contraindicated in nulliparous women.
   - B. Mirena IUD use increases the rate of PID in nulliparous women.
   - C. The Skyla IUD is FDA approved for contraception for a period of 3 years.
   - D. Nexplanon is placed subdermally in a patient's arm only during her menses.

2. Which of the following is *not* a mechanism of action of the levonorgestrel intrauterine system?
   - A. Thickening of the cervical mucus
   - B. Suppression of the endometrium
   - C. Suppression of gonadotropins, and thereby suppression of ovulation
   - D. Increased expression of glycodelin A in the endometrial glands, thereby inhibiting the binding of the sperm to the ova

3. Which of the following is not a common side effect of the levonorgestrel-containing intrauterine system (Mirena)?
   - A. Irregular menses
   - B. Increased menstrual flow
   - C. Weight gain
   - D. Acne

Answers

1. **C.** Skyla is FDA approved for 3 years. At the end of year 3 the release of levonorgestrel is only 5 μg per day. This low level of progestin is not significant enough to provide effective contraception. Removal of the device after 3 years is recommended.

2. **C.** Levonorgestrel has no suppression effect on gonadotropins when placed in the uterus. It does not suppress ovulation either. Its main mechanism is a sterile chemical reaction, change in the endometrium, thickening of the cervical mucus, and glycodelin A expression.

3. **B.** The Mirena IUD is associated with weight gain, acne, and irregular menses. It is also often used in patients who complain of heavy or painful menses, as it tends to decrease and not increase the menstrual flow.

SUGGESTED READINGS

American College of Obstetricians and Gynecologists. ACOG Practice Bulletin No. 121: long-acting reversible contraception: implants and intrauterine devices. *Obstet Gynecol.* 2011;118:184–196.

Blumenthal PD, Gemzell-Danielsson K, Marintcheva-Petrova M. Tolerability and clinical safety of Implanon. *Eur J Contracept Reprod Health Care.* 2008;13:29–36.

Darney P, Patel A, Rosen K, Shapiro LS, Kaunitz AM. Safety and efficacy of single-rod etonogestrel implant (Implanon): results from 11 international clinical trials. *Fertil Steril.* 2009;91:1646–1653.

Gemzell-Danielsson K, Schellschmidt I, Apter D. A randomized, phase II study describing the efficacy, bleeding profile, and safety of two low dose levonorgestrel-releasing intrauterine contraceptive systems and Mirena. *Fertil Steril.* 2012;97:616–622.

Hubacher D, Chen PL, Park S. Side effects from copper IUD: do they decrease over time? *Contraception.* 2009;79:356–362.

Sivin I, Stem J, Diaz J, et al. Two years of intrauterine contraception with levonorgestrel and with copper: a randomized comparison of the TCu 380Ag and levonorgestrel 20mcg/day devices. *Contraception.* 1987;35:245–255.

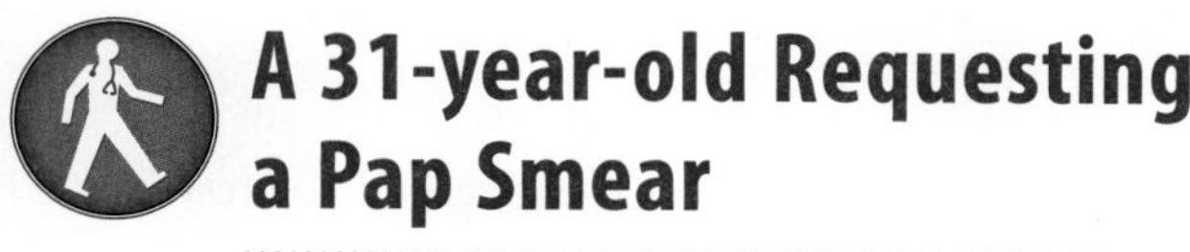

A 31-year-old Requesting a Pap Smear

Katie M. Smith, MD

A 31-year-old G3P2012 presents for a routine well woman examination. She is using a combined oral contraceptive (COC) pill for contraception, and is requesting a refill and her yearly Pap smear. She is heterosexual, recently married, and reports coitarche at age 19 with 5 lifetime sexual partners. She was treated for chlamydia in college, but denies other sexually transmitted infections (STIs). She has no history of abnormal Pap smears, and the last was normal over 2 years ago. Her menses are regular and nonpainful, and she denies heavy or intermenstrual bleeding. Her pelvic examination is normal, and you obtain a sample for cervical cytology.

You let her know that you will refill her COCs and contact her with the test results. Cytology results return atypical squamous cells of undetermined significance (ASCUS), high-risk (HR) human papillomavirus (HPV) positive.

1. **According to the ASCCP guidelines, what is the appropriate cervical cancer screening for this woman?**
2. **What is the most appropriate next step in the management of her cervical cytology?**

Answers

1. Women 30 years of age and older should be screened with cervical cytology and an HR HPV cotest. Cotesting means that an assay will be performed looking for 1 of the 13 HR types of HPV *regardless* of the result of the cytology. Patients with negative results for both tests and no history of high-grade dysplasia can be screened with both tests every 5 years until the age of 65. Alternatively, a woman 30 and over can be screened with cervical cytology alone every 3 years (no cotesting).
2. This next step is colposcopy that may lead to biopsy of the cervix and endocervical curettage (ECC).

CASE REVIEW

The patient is notified of the results, and returns for colposcopy. You obtain informed consent, perform a "time-out," and then complete a colposcopy. There are no gross lesions seen on the cervix, and you apply acetic acid. The colposcopy is adequate (which means that the transformation zone [TMZ] is visualized), and you biopsy the cervix at 5 and 9 o'clock, and perform ECC. Monsel solution is applied for hemostasis and the patient is discharged from the clinic in good condition.

Her biopsy results return as CIN1, the ECC is negative, and you recommend follow-up in a year, for a Pap and HR HPV cotest.

CERVICAL DYSPLASIA

Etiology

HPV infection is prevalent in the United States, with almost 80% of sexually active adults acquiring the infection prior to the age of 50. Infection with HR HPV is necessary for the development of cervical cancer. Thirteen HR types have been identified, and are associated with cervical dysplasia and cervical cancer. HPV types 16 and 18 account for about 70% of all cervical cancers. HPV 6 and 11 are low-risk types; they are not associated with dysplasia or cancer, but are the cause of most genital warts. Since infection with HR HPV is asymptomatic, it is important that women be screened with cervical cytology to identify abnormal cells in the cervix.

Prevention

Infection with HPV 16 and 18 can be prevented with HPV vaccination prior to the initiation of sexual activity. Quadrivalent vaccination protects against HPV 6, 11, 16, and 18. Vaccination is targeted for young women aged 11 to 12 but can be given anytime between ages 9 and 26. Prior abnormal cervical cytology is not a reason to withhold vaccination in a young woman. HPV vaccination is now also approved for young men between the ages of 9 and 26, with emphasis on vaccinating them routinely at ages 11 to 12. Recent studies have shown over a 50% decrease in HPV since introduction of the vaccine, even though routine vaccination of girls and boys has not been widespread.

Screening for Cervical Dysplasia and Cervical Cancer

Screening for cervical cancer is performed with cervical cytology; this approach is responsible for most of the reduction in the incidence and mortality from cervical cancer in the last 30 years. The majority of women who develop cervical cancer have either not been screened adequately or not been screened at all. Screening should begin at age 21. Women <21 are not recommended for screening for a number of reasons: cervical cancer is very rare in this age group, screening does not impact disease, and there is the potential for harm with treatment. For women aged 21 to 29, cytology alone is recommended every 3 years. The Pap smear should be interpreted as satisfactory or unsatisfactory and then will either be negative for intraepithelial lesion or malignancy (NILM) or return with one of many variations of abnormal epithelial cells. An unsatisfactory Pap can result if there is too much inflammation obscuring visualization of the epithelial cells, or if there are not enough cells to be evaluated. Table 42-1 lists the spectrum of abnormal Pap smear results.

Table 42-1. Abnormal Cervical Cytology

ASCUS	Atypical squamous cells of undetermined significance	HPV "reflex" testing used to determine if colposcopy is needed
LSIL	Low-grade squamous intraepithelial lesion	Colposcopy indicated except in young women where repeat cytology may be acceptable
ASC-H	Atypical squamous cells, cannot rule out high grade	Colposcopy indicated
HSIL	High-grade squamous intraepithelial lesion	Colposcopy indicated
AGC	Atypical glandular cells present (may be labeled NOS, favor endocervical, favor endometrial, or favor neoplasia)	Colposcopy, plus ECC and possible endometrial biopsy, plus HPV testing in some patients

HPV testing can be ordered as a "reflex," where it is only performed when certain cytology results are found, or as a cotest, where HPV testing is performed regardless of the result of the cytology. Reflex testing with HR HPV should be ordered for ASCUS Pap smears only in the age group 21 to 29. For women aged 30 and older, it is recommended that screening occur every 5 years with both cytology and an HR HPV cotest. Women over the age of 65 do not need further screening with cervical cytology provided they have had adequate negative screening in the past. If a woman has her cervix removed during a hysterectomy and has no history of high-grade cervical dysplasia in the previous 20 years, she no longer needs cervical cytology.

Evaluation and Management

The evaluation of abnormal cervical cytology is determined by the abnormality uncovered, HR HPV results, and the patient's age. Patients who meet a certain threshold of risk for cervical cancer based on cytology (plus HR HPV testing when indicated) are evaluated with colposcopy. Colposcopy is the application of 3% to 5% acetic acid to the surface of the cervix and using magnified light to visualize the cervix. Areas that are abnormal are likely to become "acetowhite." The use of magnification, as well as dilute acetic acid, can also be used to look for vascular changes associated with cervical dysplasia. The cervical epithelium is composed of both squamous and columnar cells and metaplasia occurs at the squamocolumnar junction (SCJ), or TMZ. During colposcopy the clinician looks for evidence of dysplasia, and ensures that the entire TMZ can be seen; a colposcopy is adequate if the entire TMZ is seen and any acetowhite lesion on the cervix can be seen in its entirety. Endocervical sampling (ECC) is recommended in any colposcopy where no lesions are seen, in any colposcopy performed after high-grade squamous intraepithelial lesion (HGSIL), and in any woman with cytology noting atypical glandular cells. ECC should not be performed in pregnant women as there is the possibility of rupture of the membranes, although biopsies of the ectocervix can safely be performed during pregnancy.

Treatment of cervical dysplasia is usually reserved for high-grade lesions (CIN2/3), although persistent low-grade dysplasia can be treated after 2 years without evidence of clearance. Treatment is usually performed with either ablation or excision of the TMZ. Ablation is usually done with cryotherapy. Its advantages are its low cost as well as low risk of bleeding or infection and minimal discomfort for the patient. Excision of the TMZ is done with either a loop electrosurgical excision procedure (LEEP) or a cold knife conization of the cervix (CKC). LEEP can be performed either in the office with local intracervical or paracervical block or in the operating room with regional or general anesthesia. It involves a wire loop and use of an electric current to remove a portion of the TMZ. CKC is performed in the operating room; a scalpel is used to remove a larger, cone-shaped portion of the cervical TMZ. Both procedures have some risk of excessive bleeding, infection, and damage to surrounding organs, although the risks are minimal. A CKC can sample more of the glandular endocervix and is preferred for glandular abnormalities including adenocarcinoma in situ.

Recommendations for follow-up after treatment vary depending on the final pathologic diagnosis and the patient's age as well as her interest in future fertility. Excisional procedures may be associated with preterm labor, preterm birth, or cervical insufficiency. Patients who have abnormal cervical cytology are no longer in a screening group; they now are in surveillance. It is important to remember that as our knowledge about HPV and cervical dysplasia and cancer increases, screening, treatment, and follow-up recommendations will change. Make sure you are following the most current screening and treatment algorithms.

TIPS TO REMEMBER

- Remember to ask your patients about her Pap screening history, such as when she was last screened and any history of cervical dysplasia.
- Utilize published guidelines to stay up-to-date on the most current screening and management guidelines.
- An adequate colposcopic examination requires that you visualize the entire TMZ or any lesion in its entirety.

COMPREHENSION QUESTIONS

1. Mrs Smith presents with her 17-year-old daughter for her first well woman examination. She has just learned that her daughter is sexually active and has had multiple sexual partners and has not consistently used condoms. The appropriate cervical cancer screening for this patient is which of the following?

   A. Screening with cervical cytology alone
   B. Screening with visual inspection of the cervix
   C. No screening
   D. Cervical cytology and HR HPV testing

2. Ms Gibson is a 40-year-old female who presents for her well woman examination. She reports she is having heavy regular menses every month. Her cervical cytology returns as HSIL. What is the next best step in the management for this patient?

   A. Repeat cervical cytology in 6 months
   B. Colposcopy, indicated cervical biopsies, and ECC
   C. Repeat cervical cytology with HR HPV cotesting in 6 months
   D. HR HPV testing alone at next visit

3. Mrs Jones is a 28-year-old G1P0 with an intrauterine pregnancy at 17 weeks; she presented 4 weeks ago for her initial prenatal visit. A Pap smear done at that time returned as ASC-H. What is the next best step in her management?

   A. Colposcopy postpartum
   B. Colposcopy with indicated cervical biopsies
   C. Colposcopy with indicated cervical biopsies, and ECC
   D. Repeat cervical cytology postpartum

Answers

1. **C**. No cervical cancer screening is recommended in patients <21 years of age. A 17-year-old does not meet guidelines for cervical cancer screening. STI testing should be performed, and counseling in regard to safe sexual practices and condom usage should be carried out.

2. **B**. Due to the patient's age and cytology result, colposcopy with indicated cervical biopsy and ECC is the right choice. Repeating cytology or cytology with/without HR HPV is not recommended in 6 months.

3. **B**. During pregnancy colposcopy can be safely done and is recommended for cervical dysplasia. Biopsies can also be taken as indicated, but an ECC should not be performed due to the potential to rupture the fetal membranes.

SUGGESTED READINGS

American Society for Colposcopy and Cervical Pathology (ASCCP) consensus guidelines on the management of women with abnormal cervical cancer screening tests and American Cancer Society. <http://www.asccp.org/ConsensusGuidelines/tabid/7436/Default.aspx>; Accessed July 29, 2013.

Saslow D, Solomon D, Lawson HW, et al; American Cancer Society; American Society for Colposcopy and Cervical Pathology; American Society for Clinical Pathology. American Cancer Society, American Society for Colposcopy and Cervical Pathology, and American Society for Clinical Pathology screening guidelines for the prevention and early detection of cervical cancer. *Am J Clin Pathol.* 2012;137(4):516–542.

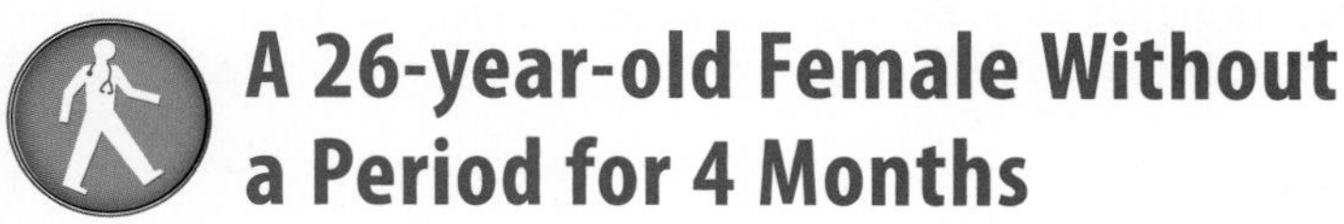

A 26-year-old Female Without a Period for 4 Months

Jaou-Chen Huang, MD

Ms M, a 26-year-old female, presents with a complaint of missing periods. Her menarche was at age 11. Her periods were irregular initially, but became regular (every 28 days, lasting 3-5 days) shortly after she turned 12. Over the past 2 years, she began to miss periods: initially the periods were delayed for 1 to 2 weeks, and lately they are "chaotic"—she may bleed twice in a month or skip up to 16 weeks before her next period. During this time, she has developed acne on her face and increased hair over her lips and around her nipples. She has also gained 60 lb over the course of 12 months—she is 5′5 and now weighs 180 lb. She is sexually active but does not want to become pregnant; she and her partner use condoms and withdrawal for protection. On physical examination you uncover the following:

Raised brown velvety pigmentation at the back of neck and moderate facial acne.

Hirsutism noted on chin, chest, and upper thighs and in a male pattern on the abdomen.

Normal breast examination; no galactorrhea.

Normal skin thickness and no abnormal bruising.

Pelvic examination revealed normal external female genitalia and clear watery mucus from cervical os. Normal size uterus, mobile.

No adnexal masses felt although difficult due to habitus.

1. What is the likely diagnosis?

2. What constitutes the initial treatment for this patient?

Answers

1. Secondary amenorrhea due to polycystic ovarian syndrome (PCOS).
2. (A) Confirm she is not pregnant (urinary human chorionic gonadotropin [hCG]).

   (B) Rule out other underlying conditions, such as thyroid dysfunction (serum TSH), prolactinoma (serum prolactin), nonclassic congenital adrenal hyperplasia (serum 17-hydroxyprogesterone level), ovarian insufficiency (serum FSH), and androgen-secreting tumors (serum testosterone level).

   (C) Endometrial protection.

CASE REVIEW

PCOS is a common cause of irregular periods and secondary amenorrhea in women of reproductive age. It is a condition where gonadotropins are "out of balance." Instead of cyclic changes leading to follicular growth and ovulation, a "steady state" is reached in affected individuals. Clinically, this manifests with irregular or no ovulation resulting in irregular bleeding or amenorrhea, and hyperandrogenism.

In our patient, you uncover on the physical examination signs of hyperandrogenism (male pattern hair growth, acne, hirsutism) and anovulation (on pelvic examination the clear mucus coming from the cervical os). The laboratory testing revealed that she was not pregnant, and had normal TSH, prolactin, FSH, 17-hydroxyprogesterone, and testosterone levels. We began her on oral contraceptive pills to normalize her cycles and improve her acne, and encouraged her to begin a weight loss regimen. She followed up in 3 months and had lost 11 lb. She also reported her cycles and acne were improved.

POLYCYSTIC OVARIAN SYNDROME

Diagnosis

A diagnosis of PCOS is made in women with clinical signs of hyperandrogenism, oligo-ovulation, and the elimination of other conditions that may cause irregular periods and hyperandrogenism. These conditions include pregnancy, thyroid dysfunction, hyperprolactinemia, ovarian insufficiency, and adrenal dysfunction (late-onset congenital adrenal hyperplasia and Cushing syndrome). Usually, urine hCG, TSH, prolactin, 17-hydroxyprogesterone, and FSH are requested. In those with features of Cushing syndrome, a dexamethasone suppression test is performed.

The overnight dexamethasone suppression test consists of taking 1 mg dexamethasone at 23:00 and determining serum cortisol level at 8:00 in the following morning. A value of <50 nmol/L essentially rules out Cushing syndrome. A value of >50 nmol/L requires a 24-hour urine collection to determine the total free cortisol. Those who secrete >200 μg free cortisol over 24-hour period need further workup—they have Cushing syndrome.

Although it is not required for the diagnosis of PCOS, an endometrial biopsy, to look for endometrial hyperplasia or cancer, is recommended for women with irregular menses >45 years of age or in younger women with risk factors for these conditions (obesity, chronic anovulation). A determination of diabetes or impaired glucose tolerance is also reasonable for the patient. A fasting blood sugar and/or HbA1C are usually requested too.

A positive progesterone withdrawal bleed is part of the initial management, and ensures that amenorrhea is a "functional" disorder, that is, hormonal imbalance, rather than an "organic" disorder (such as pituitary adenoma, adrenal tumor, or tumor of the central nervous system). A negative withdrawal bleed may also be caused by disorders of the hypothalamus, pituitary, or the uterus (such as Asherman syndrome).

Pathophysiology

PCOS is a complex and heterogeneous endocrine disorder. The complexity of this condition can be appreciated from the number of diagnostic criteria currently in use: NIH (1990), Rotterdam (2003), and AE-PCOS (2006). Nonetheless, it is fair to say that the end result is a "steady state" of gonadotropins, which leads to oligo-ovulation or anovulation. Elevated LH increases the androgen production by the ovarian stroma leading to androgen excess. Thus, some patients report excess facial hair, or hair around nipples or over the lower abdomen.

A steady state of gonadotropins does not propel follicles through the maturation process. This leads to anovulation or unpredictable ovulation and irregular periods or amenorrhea. Multiple follicles produced by unchanging gonadotropins create the characteristic ultrasound image of the "necklace sign"—numerous small follicles beneath the ovarian cortex resembling a necklace.

Treatment

If the patient has not had a menstrual cycle for greater than 6 weeks, a progesterone withdrawal bleed to confirm an intact hypothalamic–pituitary–ovarian axis is achieved by prescribing medroxyprogesterone acetate (Provera) 10 mg daily for 5 days. This paves the way for ovulation induction with clomiphene citrate in those who desire pregnancy (details below). The length of the initial progesterone administration may be extended to 10 or 12 days to ensure a complete shedding of the uterine lining, that is, a "medical curettage." This extended regimen is appropriate in patients with a long history of irregular bleeding/amenorrhea, and, thus, unopposed estrogen. It may take 14 days before bleeding starts; any amount/duration of bleeding is considered positive. Disorders of the hypothalamus, pituitary, and uterus are in the differential diagnoses for those who do not bleed after Provera challenge.

The first-line treatment for overweight PCOS patients is lifestyle modification, including exercise, diet alteration, and weight reduction. It is an effective nonmedical intervention, but few are successful, because it takes great determination and persistence. If nonmedical intervention does not reach the goal, medical management is applied.

After a withdrawal bleed, medical management depends on a patient's symptom(s) and her desire for fertility. For those desiring pregnancy, ovulation induction is accomplished by clomiphene citrate. For those not desiring pregnancy, protection of the endometrium is achieved via cyclic progesterone or combination oral contraceptive (COC) pills.

The starting dose of clomiphene citrate is 50 mg daily on cycle days 5 to 9—cycle day 1 being the first day of progesterone withdrawal bleeding. Evidence of ovulation includes pregnancy, or spontaneous onset of menstruation with a serum progesterone >3 ng/mL 1 week after ovulation (which can be determined by urinary LH test or documentation of dominant follicles by a transvaginal ultrasound). In the case of a confirmed ovulation but no pregnancy, the same dose is given in subsequent months. In the case of anovulation, the dose is increased by 50 mg, to 100 mg daily. The maximum dose is 200 mg daily. There is no consensus on how many months a patient may receive clomiphene citrate, but most would agree an investigation for other causes of infertility should be initiated after 12 months, if not sooner.

In addition to protecting the endometrium and the other benefits that COCs provide (see Chapter 40), they help to reduce excess hair growth and/or acne. COCs achieve this through reducing testosterone production by the ovarian stroma and increasing sex hormone–binding globulin production by the liver; both contribute to a lower level of circulating free testosterone.

TIPS TO REMEMBER

- PCOS patients normally present with irregular periods, but some may present with amenorrhea.
- In many patients weight is an important factor. In overweight teenagers the symptomatology may follow menarche immediately. In others, the symptoms occur after weight gain.
- PCOS is a heterogeneous condition of various etiologies. It is a diagnosis of exclusion, and the end result of hormonal imbalance (or steady state of gonadotropins)—a functional derangement.
- Pregnancy must be considered in women of childbearing age complaining of irregular periods/amenorrhea.
- Endometrial hyperplasia or cancer should be ruled out in patients >45 years of age with irregular menses, or in younger women with risk factors (chronic anovulation, obesity).
- Cushing syndrome is rare (5 cases per million per year), but the consequence of missing the diagnosis is serious. The symptomatology of PCOS and Cushing syndrome overlaps: weight gain, irregular periods, and amenorrhea.
- The dose of clomiphene citrate is maintained in subsequent months if ovulation is confirmed, but the patient does not become pregnant.

COMPREHENSION QUESTIONS

1. You diagnosed Ms M with PCOS and begin lifestyle modification as treatment. She returns in a few months and notes an improvement in her cycles and acne. Which of the following statements in regard to PCOS is/are true?

   A. PCOS is a functional derangement caused by a steady state of gonadotropins.

   B. A positive progesterone withdrawal bleed confirms an intact hypothalamic–pituitary–ovarian axis.

C. The first-line treatment for overweight PCOS patients is lifestyle modification, including exercise, diet alteration, and weight reduction.
D. All are correct.

2. Ms M would also like to improve her acne and hirsutism. You explain to her that the COCs will help with both of these complaints. Which of the following statements concerning COCs is correct in regard to improving Ms M's acne and hirsutism?
A. COCs bind up excess free testosterone, thereby decreasing the availability of active testosterone that leads to hirsutism/acne.
B. COCs increase androgen production by the ovaries.
C. COCs increase sex hormone–binding globulin by the liver.
D. COCs decrease the peripheral conversion of testosterone to its more active form dihydrotestosterone.

3. Ms M tells you that she is interviewing for medical schools, and she has been doing some reading on PCOS. She is curious how you made the diagnosis of PCOS so quickly. Of all the following statements, which is *false* in regard to diagnosing PCOS?
A. PCOS is a clinical diagnosis manifest by hyperandrogenism and oligo-ovulation.
B. PCOS is a diagnosis of exclusion after a number of other disorders are ruled out.
C. Other disorders that should be tested for when diagnosing PCOS include the following: thyroid disease, prolactinoma, and nonclassic congenital adrenal hyperplasia.
D. PCOS does not require laboratory analysis in most cases as the physical examination findings are pathognomonic.

Answers

1. **D.** All are correct.

2. **C.** COCs increase sex hormone–binding globulin production by the liver, which in turn reduces free testosterone in the circulation. They do not bind testosterone, nor decrease the ovarian production of it, and do not decrease its conversion to a more active form.

3. **D.** PCOS is manifested by signs of hyperandrogenism and oligo-ovulation, and is made clinically after other disorders are ruled out by laboratory analysis.

SUGGESTED READINGS

Casper RF, Mitwally MF. A historical perspective of aromatase inhibitors for ovulation induction. *Fertil Steril.* 2012;98:1352–1355.

Legro RS, Barnhart HX, Schlaff WD, et al. Clomiphene, metformin, or both for infertility in the polycystic ovary syndrome. *N Engl J Med*. 2007;356:551–566.

Nieman LK, Biller BM, Findling JW, et al. The diagnosis of Cushing's syndrome: an Endocrine Society clinical practice guideline. *J Clin Endocrinol Metab*. 2008;93:1526–1540.

NIH Evidence-based Methodology Workshop on Polycystic Ovary Syndrome. <http://prevention.nih.gov/workshops/2012/pcos/default.aspx>; December 3–5, 2012.

Speroff L, Glass RH, Kase NG. Anovulation and the polycystic ovary. In: *Clinical Gynecologic Endocrinology and Infertility*. 6th ed. Philadelphia, PA: Lippincott Williams & Wilkins; 1999: 487–522.

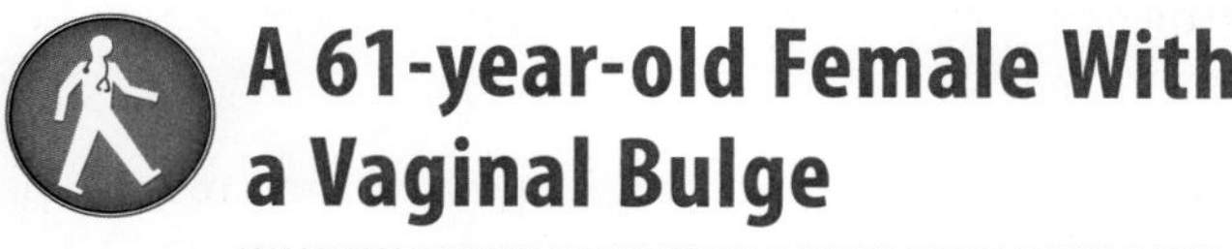

A 61-year-old Female With a Vaginal Bulge

Charlie C. Kilpatrick, MD

A 61-year-old P4014 presents to the clinic complaining of a vaginal bulge that she has noticed for a number of years but has recently worsened after performing some chores around the house. She can now see the bulge, it is bothering her, and she is concerned that it may be cancer. In review of her history she has no relevant past medical or surgical history, and delivered all of her children vaginally. She denies any allergies, is not taking any medication, does not smoke, and has occasional alcohol intake. She has not had menses for 10 years, denies abnormal cervical cytology or sexually transmitted infections, and has a healthy sexual relationship with her spouse of 40 years. She relates a history of leaking urine with coughing, sneezing, and heavy lifting that has recently decreased in frequency, but at the same time she has developed some difficulty with emptying her bladder. She urinates 4 times a day, and once at night. She denies any difficulty with incontinence of flatus or feces. Her vital signs are within normal limits and examination of the pelvis reveals the following: atrophic external female genitalia, parous introitus, vagina also with signs of atrophy, parous cervical os without lesion, no active bleeding or discharge, a uterus that is freely mobile, and no adnexal fullness. Pelvic Organ Prolapse Quantification (POP-Q) examination of the patient supine while straining, and then while standing and straining reveals the following: Aa +2 Ba +3 C −3 TVL 9 GH 3 PB 3 Ap −2 Bp −2 D −6. The transverse diameter of the introitus is 2.5 cm, the urethra is mobile, and with reduction of the prolapsed tissue she leaks urine with coughing. Rectovaginal examination is within normal limits, without evidence of enterocele or rectocele.

1. **What is in your differential diagnosis, and what are the next steps you need to take in the management of this patient?**

Answer

1. Your differential diagnosis should include pelvic organ prolapse (POP), and stress urinary incontinence. Few ancillary tests are needed in the assessment of POP, and in this case a urinalysis and postvoid residual given her voiding symptoms would help. You should also administer a self-assessment questionnaire to determine the severity and impact of her pelvic floor symptoms.

CASE REVIEW

The number 1 reason for hysterectomy in the postmenopausal patient in the United States is POP, and the anterior vaginal wall is typically the most common area affected. When reviewing a cohort of women who presented for a routine gynecologic examination, 35% of women had Stage 2 prolapse, and most clinicians would agree that prolapse beyond the hymenal ring is clinically significant. Childbirth, age, and obesity are the 3 leading risk factors, and the most common symptom specific to prolapse is the feeling, or visual confirmation, of a bulge in the vagina. The rest of this chapter will review diagnostic steps and treatment recommendations for POP.

PELVIC ORGAN PROLAPSE

Diagnosis

POP is descent of the pelvic organs resulting in protrusion of the uterus, vagina, or both. A vaginal bulge is the most specific symptom in women who present with POP. Evaluation begins with a detailed history taking into account symptoms that could accompany POP related to the vagina, bladder or lower urinary tract, bowels, and sexual function. Table 44-1 lists common symptoms grouped by anatomic location that are useful to document in the history of present illness.

Table 44-1. Common Symptoms in Women With POP

Bowel
Incontinence of gas or stool
Splinting to start or complete defecation
Urgency to defecate
Incomplete emptying or straining to defecate
Lower urinary tract
Urinary incontinence
Urinary urgency
Hesitancy with urination, difficulty emptying her bladder, prolonged urinary stream
Urinary frequency
Incomplete bladder emptying
Manual compression to void or change in position to void
Vaginal
Feeling or seeing a bulge in the vagina
Heaviness or pressure in the vagina

anterior wall Aa	anterior wall Ba	cervix or cuff C
genital hiatus GH	perineal body PB	total vaginal length TVL
posterior wall Ap	posterior wall Bp	posterior fornix D

Figure 44-1. Pelvic organ prolapse grid.

In the case above, this patient's stress incontinence has recently improved, but she has now developed obstructive urinary symptoms, which is common as the POP stage worsens. A self-assessment of pelvic floor symptoms and/or quality of life (Pelvic Floor Distress Inventory, Pelvic Floor Impact Questionnaire) is important in setting expectations for, and establishing a baseline prior to, treatment.

Physical examination should include assessment of the patient in a supine and standing position in order to visualize the prolapse in its most severe stage, and quantify it using the POP-Q classification system (Figure 44-1). There are 3 points along the anterior and posterior vaginal wall that are recorded with a +/– to denote their relationship to the hymen *at the moment of greatest prolapse.* Aa is a fixed point 3 cm proximal to the urethral meatus (meant to represent the urethrovesical junction), Ba the most distal point of the anterior vaginal wall, and C represents the cervix or vaginal cuff. Posteriorly, Ap is a fixed point 3 cm proximal to the posterior vaginal hymen, Bp is the most distal portion of the posterior vaginal wall, and D is the posterior fornix (meant to represent the insertion of the uterosacral ligaments to the cervix, but only estimated in women with a uterus). The letter system can be quite confusing when you begin, but a helpful hint is to *think of the "big A" as a "big F" or fixed, and think of the "big B" as a "big D" or distal.* The "little a" represents the anterior vaginal wall, and the "little p" represents the posterior vaginal wall. The last 3 measurements are not expressed with +/– and are the perineal body (PB, from the midanal opening to the posterior vaginal hymen), genital hiatus (GH, from the midurethral opening to the posterior vaginal hymen), and total vaginal length (TVL, from the cuff or posterior fornix to the hymen). This examination can be done at the time of every gynecologic examination and with practice won't take much time at all. The stage of prolapse refers to the most distal prolapse of the anterior or posterior vaginal wall and is expressed from Stage 0 (little or no prolapse) to Stage 4 (total eversion of the vagina, or ≥TVL –2). Stage 2 is at the level of the hymen (within 1 cm of the hymen in either direction), while Stage 1 is minimal prolapse (between Stages 0 and 2), and Stage 3 is past the hymen, but not complete eversion of the vagina, and is considered clinically significant prolapse. The easiest way to remember the stages is to remember that Stage 2 is at the level of the hymen, keeping in mind that Stages 0 and 4 represent the extremes. With practice this will become second nature. Noting stress incontinence, condition of the vaginal tissue, urethral hypermobility, and a rectovaginal examination to determine the presence of enterocele/rectocele and tone of the anal sphincter completes a thorough examination for POP.

Treatment

Treatment goals depend on symptom severity, and patient expectations. Observation, pelvic floor exercises, pessary use, and surgical management are the current treatment options. Observation can be used for the patient who does not desire any intervention, with closer surveillance for those with severe prolapse to avoid renal dysfunction caused by kinking of the urethra. There are little data on pelvic floor exercises, but in general these are more successful with a highly motivated patient with less severe POP stage. Pessary use is an option that should be offered to all patients, but is generally preferred for patients who would like to avoid surgical management. The most commonly used pessary is the ring with support, but there are numerous pessary types. Ideally, the patient should be able to insert and remove the pessary herself, but in some cases this is not possible. Complications with pessary use include vaginal erosions and vaginal discharge. Erosions arise from direct pressure of the pessary on the vaginal wall and are more common in patients with vaginal atrophy. Vaginal estrogen application can prevent atrophy and limit erosions. Vaginal discharge is more common with certain pessary types and with a longer duration of use. Pessary removal and cleaning should ideally be done nightly, but at least once or twice a week. In patients who physically cannot remove their pessaries, more frequent clinic visits are necessary. Pessaries are rarely associated with severe complications except in cases of neglect, noncompliance, or patients lost to follow-up. After pessary placement in the office it is important to ensure the pessary fits snugly but allows a finger to pass comfortably between the pessary and vaginal side wall. With the pessary in place, the patient should be comfortable, and able to empty her bladder. The pessary should remain in place during Valsalva, walking, and standing prior to leaving the clinic.

Surgical management of POP, for those patients who decline or fail pessary usage, can either reconstruct vaginal support or obliterate the vagina. Obliterative procedures completely close off the vaginal canal moving prolapsed organs back into the pelvis. These procedures (LeFort colpocleisis) are reserved for patients who have no desire for future vaginal intercourse. They have low recurrent prolapse rates, and are associated with fewer complications than reconstructive procedures. Reconstructive procedures can be performed abdominally (abdominal sacrocolpopexy, culdoplasty, paravaginal repair) or vaginally (high uterosacral ligament suspension, McCall culdoplasty, iliococcygeus ligament fixation, anterior or posterior colporrhaphy), or a combination of both.

TIPS TO REMEMBER

- POP is common and will be more common in the future as the population ages.
- A vaginal bulge is the most specific symptom associated with POP, but associated symptoms should be established at the initial visit.
- It is important for physicians to evaluate patient expectations and baseline symptoms prior to treatment.
- The POP-Q provides objective measurement of POP, and allows for staging of the prolapse. "Big A" references a fixed point, while "big B" references the most distal point along the anterior or posterior vaginal wall.
- Stage 2 prolapse is at the level of the hymen.
- Treatment options consist of observation, pelvic floor exercises, pessary use, and surgery.

COMPREHENSION QUESTIONS

1. All of the following are proven risk factors for POP, *except* which one?
   A. Childbirth
   B. Age
   C. Obesity
   D. African American race

2. The patient in the clinical scenario above has what stage of POP (Aa +2 Ba +3 C −3 TVL 9 GH 3 PB 3 Ap −2 Bp −2 D −6)?
   A. Stage 1
   B. Stage 2
   C. Stage 3
   D. Stage 4

3. The following POP Q measurement represents what pelvic organ support stage?

   Aa +1 Ba +1 C −5 GH 3 PB 3 TVL 9 Ap −1 Bp −1 D −7
   A. Stage 1
   B. Stage 2
   C. Stage 3
   D. Stage 4

4. All of the following statements in regard to pessary management are true, *except* which one?

A. You should be able to insert a finger between the pessary and the walls of the vagina.

B. After pessary placement in the office, the patient should be able to void, Valsalva, walk, and perform various other activities without the pessary dislodging.

C. Follow-up after pessary placement depends on a women's ability to place and remove the pessary.

D. Daily vaginal estrogen is mandatory for all patients with a pessary in place.

Answers

1. **D.** African American race is not a risk factor for POP. Hispanic and Asian races have higher rates of POP. Childbirth (with each vaginal birth the incidence of prolapse increases), increasing age, and obesity are the risk factors most often associated with POP.

2. **C.** Stage 3 prolapse. The patient's most severe prolapse is along the anterior vaginal wall, Ba of +3. This is greater than >+1 but less than [TVL −2], which corresponds to Stage 3.

3. **B.** Stage 2 prolapse. The most distal measurement in this scenario is Aa and Ba, both of which are +1. Remember that Stage 2 is ≥−1 and ≤+1 or, in other words, *Stage 2 = hymen.* Keep this in mind and then work either back to less severe prolapse or forward for more severe prolapse.

4. **D.** Vaginal estrogen cream helps to avoid vaginal erosion and can be applied up to 3 times a week, but daily use is not mandatory. The rest of the statements are true.

SUGGESTED READINGS

Barber MD. Symptoms and outcome measures of pelvic organ prolapse. *Clin Obstet Gynecol.* 2005;48(3): 648–661.

Bump RC, Mattiasson A, Bø K, et al. The standardization of terminology of female pelvic organ prolapse and pelvic floor dysfunction. *Am J Obstet Gynecol.* 1996;175(1):10–17.

Jelovsek JE, Maher C, Barber MD. Pelvic organ prolapse. *Lancet.* 2007;369(9566):1027–1038 [review].

Swift SE, Tate SB, Nicholas J. Correlation of symptoms with degree of pelvic organ support in a general population of women: what is pelvic organ prolapse? *Am J Obstet Gynecol.* 2003;189:372–377.

A 52-year-old Postmenopausal Patient Presents for a Well Woman Examination

Charlie C. Kilpatrick, MD

You are seeing a patient who presents for a well woman examination. She is postmenopausal, and her last menstrual cycle was 2 years ago. She has occasional hot flushes, and night sweats, and also complains of vaginal dryness. Otherwise she is doing well, with no medical problems, has 3 children that she delivered vaginally, a laparoscopic appendectomy, and has no known drug allergies. She takes a vitamin daily and occasionally something for acid reflux. She has never had an abnormal Pap smear (most recent one was last year), and denies sexually transmitted infections. She is happily married and with the same partner for over 30 years. She urinates 3 to 4 times per day, and once at night, and denies urinary urgency or leaking urine with coughing and sneezing. She had a mammogram 3 months ago and it was normal. You get prepared to complete a breast and pelvic examination and ask if she has any other concerns. She hesitates and then admits that her desire to have intercourse lately has declined, and it has begun to bother her. She states that initially she began to have pain with intercourse that just got worse, and because of the pain she is hesitant to have vaginal intercourse. She states the pain is with penetration, and she has tried lubricants that helped some but not completely. She would like to know if there is anything that she could do to restore her sexual life with her husband of 30 years.

1. **What is your differential diagnosis for your patient's painful vaginal intercourse?**
2. **What is your next step in the workup and treatment of this patient?**

Answers

1. Painful intercourse, or dyspareunia, can be due to a number of factors. The patient described above likely has vaginal atrophy. This can make intercourse uncomfortable, and in our case has led to a decrease in desire for sexual relations that bothers her, or hypoactive sexual desire disorder (HSDD). She may also have bladder pain syndrome, depression, vulvodynia, history of sexual abuse, uterine pathology, uterine retroversion, pelvic inflammatory disease, or pelvic adhesive disease.
2. Your next step is to elicit a more complete sexual history or administer a female sexual dysfunction (FSD) questionnaire in order to document her baseline

sexual function, and determine what is bothering her. This can be filled out at home and returned or completed before she leaves the office. You also need to perform an examination of the vagina and pelvis looking for signs of vaginal atrophy, palpate her levator muscles, and perform a bimanual examination to pinpoint where her pain is located (superficial, deep, along the bladder, or posteriorly near the rectum).

CASE REVIEW

You give her a questionnaire that she completes in the office. It reveals that for the past 6 months she has not been satisfied with her sexual function, due to problems with pain during intercourse and now low desire to have intercourse. You then perform a visual/physical inspection of the vagina that reveals thin, friable vaginal tissue that is a faded dull pink, unlike what you have seen during other examinations in pregnant patients. The vagina is tender with insertion of the speculum, and you notice a small tear after the examination along the posterior vaginal wall with some spotting. The bimanual examination is normal, the uterus is small and mobile, and there is no pain with manipulation of the uterus. The levator muscles are not tense or tender to touch, and the anterior vagina near the bladder does not cause her pain with touch, nor does the posterior vagina overlying the rectum.

You diagnose her with vaginal atrophy and begin her on topical estrogen to apply a pea-sized amount to the vagina nightly for 2 weeks, and then every other night for another 2 weeks, and she is given a follow-up examination for a repeat examination in 1 month.

You follow up with the resident on the service and find out that her vaginal tissue regained a more pinkish hue after topical estrogen, and her complaints of vaginal dryness improved. She began to have intercourse again with her husband and at first there was some pain, but over time and with continued topical estrogen this improved. The vaginal atrophy improved which lessened her pain with intercourse and her desire for sexual activity returned.

FEMALE SEXUAL DYSFUNCTION

Sex is complicated. This discussion will very briefly review some salient points. It is appropriate, when you are seeing a patient who presents with sexual complaints, to get the best history and create the best differential you can, and then refer the patient to someone who is skilled and knowledgeable in this clinical arena. Although it may make you feel uncomfortable at first, approaching the topic of sexual function with your patients will be well received. FSD is prevalent, peaking in a woman's fifth to sixth decades of life. As women age their need and desire for sexual activity declines.

There are 4 types of FSD: sexual pain disorder, HSDD, arousal disorder, and orgasmic disorder. These conditions are considered a dysfunction when they create marked distress or interpersonal difficulty in the patient's life. It is therefore important to determine how this condition affects your patient's life. Also, keep in mind that one dysfunction may be linked to another, and often are. For example, in our clinical scenario the patient had pain with intercourse, which then led to a decrease in desire creating distress within the patient. The interrelated nature of the sexual dysfunctions highlights the need for a thorough and complete sexual history.

HSDD is a deficiency or absence in desire for sexual activity that creates distress. HSDD in older patients is often an isolated event, while in younger patients is more often linked to situational circumstances (relationship issues, depression, medication use, chronic disease). Treatment is directed at the inciting condition; there are numerous medications linked with decreased sexual desire. Those with the most data include SSRIs, COCs, and steroids. A thorough medication history is essential. In postmenopausal women there are prospective data that demonstrate transdermal testosterone improves sexual desire and function. Although used in Europe, the FDA has not approved the medication for this indication because there are little long-term data supporting the safety of testosterone in women.

Sexual pain disorders include dyspareunia and vaginismus and should not be the result of inadequate lubrication. Dyspareunia is genital pain associated with intercourse, while vaginismus is involuntary spasm of the outer one third of the vagina that interferes with sexual intercourse. Treatment of dyspareunia is directed at the inciting factors, and a thorough history and pelvic examination are crucial to the diagnosis. In postmenopausal women (or after surgical menopause) vaginal atrophy (due to a lack of estrogen) can cause pain and discomfort with intercourse. Topical estrogen, rather than oral estrogen, alleviates the atrophy and decreases pain with intercourse. Because of the systemic effect that estrogen can have, the smallest dose for the shortest amount of time is recommended. Vaginismus is rare, and treatment is often cognitive and behavioral psychotherapy. Patients with vaginismus often relate that they are unable to use tampons during their menstrual cycle because it is too painful. Sexual pain disorders are often associated with arousal and desire disorders.

Arousal disorders refer to the inability to complete sexual activity that causes distress. They are often best treated by altering medication dosages or addressing an underlying gynecologic or medical condition. There are some devices that can be placed over the clitoris in order to improve vaginal blood flow and lubrication, improving arousal and orgasm.

Orgasmic disorders refer to an absence or delay in attaining orgasm that causes distress. They can be caused by a number of factors: history of abuse, religious and cultural beliefs, age, personality, and relationship status. Addressing anxiety issues, improving self-image, and behavioral techniques (masturbation techniques) can all help to improve these disorders.

TIPS TO REMEMBER

- Practitioners who care for women should inquire about sexual function and perform a sexual history. A questionnaire that a patient can complete in the waiting room can suffice.
- The prevalence of FSD peaks between 40 and 60 years of age.
- Medications may cause FSD and a thorough medication history is recommended.
- Testosterone is effective in improving HSDD, but is not currently FDA approved due to a lack of long-term safety data.
- Topical estrogen can improve the vaginal mucosa after menopause and decrease painful intercourse.

COMPREHENSION QUESTIONS

1. Ms R presents to the office for an annual examination. She is 22 and has not had vaginal intercourse nor undergone a Pap smear test. She is nervous and anxious about seeing a gynecologist. She has regular cycles and uses pads (not tampons as these hurt), and denies any history of STIs. You begin the pelvic examination and cannot place a speculum or even perform a digital examination as the patient is very tense, and she complains of pain. Which of the following would best describe this patient's condition?

   A. HSDD
   B. Vaginal atrophy
   C. Orgasmic disorder
   D. Vaginismus

2. What would be the preferred treatment option for Ms R?

   A. Transdermal testosterone
   B. Topical estrogen
   C. Behavioral techniques including directed masturbation
   D. Cognitive and behavioral psychotherapy

3. Ms K is a 28-year-old female who comes to clinic for a Pap smear. She has no history of STIs, has a male partner, and all of her Pap smears have been normal. She was using a progesterone-containing IUD for birth control but developed some irregular bleeding and switched to a COC pill about 3 months ago. Since then, she has noticed that her desire for sexual activity with her partner has

diminished and it is affecting their relationship. She is wondering if there is anything she can do about it. Which of the following is the best choice?

A. Begin transdermal testosterone that should improve her sexual desire.
B. Recommend couples counseling.
C. Reassure her that this is common in relationships and should get better with time.
D. Discuss with her switching her birth control method.

Answers

1. **D.** Vaginismus is the involuntary contraction of the outer one third of the vagina that can make vaginal intercourse almost impossible. None of the other choices are outlined in the scenario.

2. **D.** Vaginismus is treated with behavioral and cognitive psychotherapy, most often with desensitization techniques. Topical estrogen is appropriate for vaginal atrophy, transdermal testosterone is appropriate for postmenopausal patients with HSDD (but not currently in the United States), and masturbation is used in orgasmic disorders.

3. **D.** Medications are often the cause of HSDD. In this case it looks as though her COC pills may be the culprit. Switching her birth control method would be a good first start associated with relatively little harm. Testosterone is not approved in the United States for HSDD, and the data that are available are mainly for use in postmenopausal patients.

SUGGESTED READINGS

American College of Obstetricians and Gynecologists Committee on Practice Bulletins—Gynecology. ACOG Practice Bulletin No. 119: female sexual dysfunction. *Obstet Gynecol.* 2011;117(4):996–1007.

Hatzichristou D, Rosen RC, Derogatis LR, et al. Recommendations for the clinical evaluation of men and women with sexual dysfunction. *J Sex Med.* 2010;7(1 pt 2):337–348 [review].

Shifren JL, Monz BU, Russo PA, Segreti A, Johannes CB. Sexual problems and distress in United States women: prevalence and correlates. *Obstet Gynecol.* 2008;112(5):970–978.

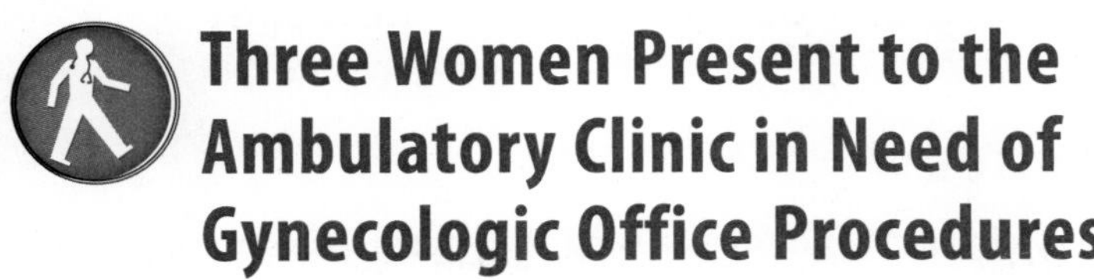

Three Women Present to the Ambulatory Clinic in Need of Gynecologic Office Procedures

Naghma Farooqi, MD and
Edward R. Yeomans, MD

One of the factors that attracts students to the field of obstetrics and gynecology is the opportunity to perform procedures in the ambulatory clinic. These procedures can be accomplished under either local or no anesthesia and may be either diagnostic or therapeutic. In this chapter, 3 common gynecologic office procedures are described.

A 55-year-old Woman Presenting With Vulvar Itching

A 55-year-old postmenopausal female presents complaining of itching near the vagina. Vulvar examination revealed atrophic-appearing tissue with some excoriated skin bilaterally near the labia minora and clitoris, as well as some edema around the clitoris.

1. What is your differential diagnosis?

2. What procedure will you perform?

Answers

1. The differential diagnosis for vulvar pruritus includes lichen planus, lichen sclerosus (LS), genital wart/condyloma accuminatum, contact dermatitis, irritants/allergens, and vulvar neoplasia/malignancy.
2. A vulvar biopsy is indicated for diagnosis and appropriate management, especially in women who are in this patient's age group.

CASE REVIEW

You suspect this is LS and perform a 3-mm punch biopsy of one of the excoriated areas. A day later this returns as hyperkeratosis, thinning, and loss of normal rete ridge pattern. You communicate with the patient that this is LS and what the course of the disease is, and recommend a topical high-potency steroid ointment to be applied in a thin layer nightly. Follow-up is in a month to review the area. She sees you in a month and the pruritus is much better, and you switch her to a lower-potency steroid with scheduled follow-up.

VULVAR PRURITUS

Lichen planus is a chronic condition causing tiny flat papules to appear on mucus membranes and on the vulva. These lesions are painful and pruritic. Topical steroids help alleviate the symptoms and biopsy is necessary only if local treatment fails. LS is a vulvar abnormality characterized by thinning of the epithelium, hyalinization of the dermis, and lymphocytic infiltration below the dermal zone. Pain, burning, and pruritus are the main complaints. Local steroids are helpful and biopsy is necessary if the condition persists. Genital warts and condyloma accuminata are viral diseases of the vulva, vagina, cervix, and rectum and are caused by the human papillomavirus (HPV). The most frequent HPV types involved are 6 and 11. Raised cauliflower-like lesions are sometimes seen that bleed upon touch or friction. Biopsy is needed to rule out cancer. Vulvar intraepithelial neoplasia (VIN) may progress to carcinoma in situ or invasive cancer. The risk of invasive cancer is higher in older women, and the immunosuppressed. More commonly, though, genital warts are the lesions found on presentation. HPV types 16, 18, 31, 33, and 35 are more frequently associated with VIN or invasive cancer.

Vulvar biopsy is one of the more common gynecologic office procedures. It is performed most commonly using a Keyes punch (Figure 46-1) and scalpel. The vulva includes the labia majora, labia minora, clitoris, hymen, vestibule, Bartholin glands, and the paraurethral glands. The epithelium covering the vulva is squamous. Indications for biopsy include:

1. Visible lesion
2. Concern for malignancy
3. Recurrence of lesion after treatment
4. Discolored dermis/epidermis

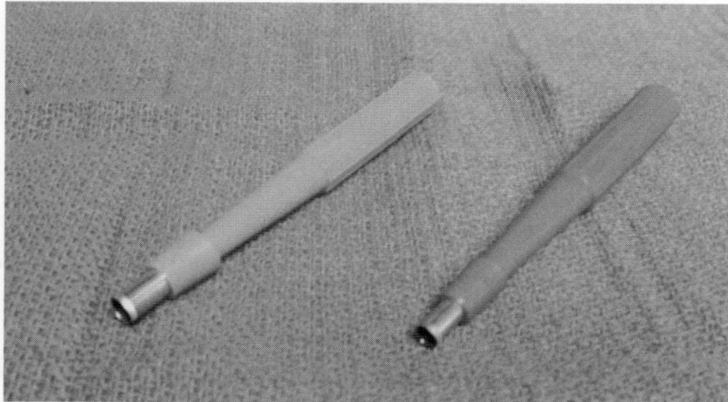

Figure 46-1. Different sizes of Keyes punches.

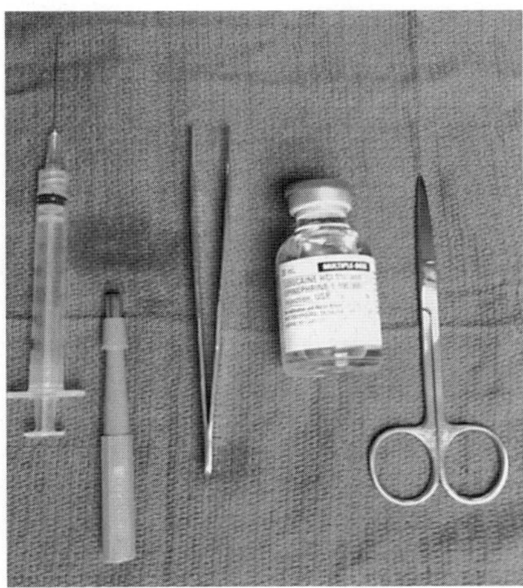

Figure 46-2. Supplies needed for vulvar biopsy.

Procedure

For supplies, see Figure 46-2.

1. Informed consent is obtained, the patient is placed in dorsal lithotomy position, and a 'time out' is performed.
2. Area to be biopsied is cleaned with antiseptic solution ×3.
3. One percent or 2% anesthetic is injected locally with a 26-gauge needle.
4. The wheal should be larger than the intended biopsy.
5. Test the area and assure that patient is adequately anesthetized.
6. Take the Keyes punch and place over the area of interest and with light pressure rotate into the vulva.
7. Hold punched out area with pickups and use scalpel to remove the round biopsy specimen.
8. Place in 10% formalin specimen bottle and send to pathology.
9. Hemostasis on the biopsy site can be achieved by pressure, application of silver nitrate, or a small suture using 4-0 Vicryl, monocryl, or chromic.

Postprocedure Precautions

1. The site should be kept clean and dry.
2. Sitz baths and the local application of antibacterial cream may be used.
3. If pain, bleeding, and/or increased swelling occurs, tell the patient to call the office for evaluation.

A 26-year-old Woman With Swelling in her Left Labium Minus

A 26-year-old G3P2012 presents to the office with the complaint of swelling in her vagina. She denies any trauma, new partner, discharge, or fever. The patient gives a history of a similar swelling and spontaneous resolution via drainage about a year ago. This new swelling appeared a month ago and has increased in size causing discomfort during intercourse and now on ambulation. A recent physical examination and Pap smear is normal as per her records.

1. What is your likely diagnosis?

2. What treatment will you offer to this patient?

Answers

1. The most likely diagnosis is a Bartholin gland cyst or abscess.
2. The 2 most frequently used treatments are placement of a Word catheter and marsupialization.

CASE REVIEW

You explain to the patient that this is a Bartholin gland cyst and provide her with information on treatment. She elects to have a Word catheter. After informed consent you place the Word catheter. She returns in 2 weeks and is doing well. You let her know that you will deflate the balloon and remove the catheter in a month. She returns in a month and you remove the catheter.

BARTHOLIN GLAND CYST AND ABSCESS

The Bartholin glands are located at the 4- or 8-o'clock position of the vulva on each side of the introitus. Each gland is the size of a pea. The Bartholin ducts open into a space between the hymen and the labia minora. Sometimes the opening of one of the ducts gets blocked. This causes a buildup of secretions leading to formation of a cyst. Two percent of women will develop this in their lifetimes. If they remain small, no treatment is needed. Treatment is indicated if the patient is symptomatic from the cyst. Infections resulting in an abscess may occur. Antibiotics are necessary if surrounding cellulitis develops with an abscess or you suspect gonorrhea/chlamydia infection. Drainage of a Bartholin cyst is achieved by creating a fistulous tract from the cyst to the epithelial surface by placing a Word catheter or by marsupialization. Placement of a Word catheter is a simple office procedure, whereas marsupialization may require anesthesia in the operating room. The recurrence rate of Bartholin cysts and abscesses is about 20%. Repeated recurrences may require marsupialization or even removal of the entire gland.

Placement of a Word Catheter Procedure

1. Informed consent is obtained.
2. The patient is placed in dorsal lithotomy position, and a 'time out' is performed.
3. The Bartholin duct cyst is exposed.
4. The entire vulva and the swollen cyst are cleaned with antiseptic solution ×3.
5. The most fluctuant point on the cyst is marked.
6. Local anesthetic is injected using a 26-gauge needle.
7. A scalpel is used to make a small stab incision in the most prominent, dependent, fluctuant area, usually on the medial side of the cyst. The incision must be large enough to place the catheter but not larger than the catheter to avoid spontaneous expulsion.
8. Fluid or pus will drain freely. Cultures are usually obtained. A small curved hemostat is introduced to break loculations inside the cyst.
9. The Word catheter (Figure 46-3) is then introduced and the bulb is inflated with saline through a syringe to 5 cm^3 capacity.
10. Patient is cleaned and the tubing of the catheter is tucked into the vagina to avoid friction with clothing or the possibility of being pulled out.

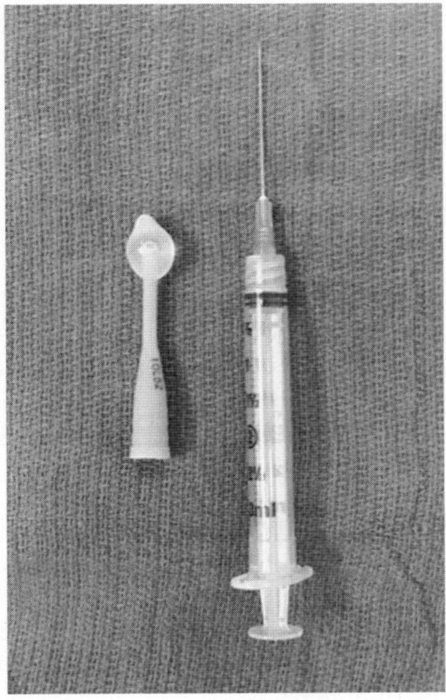

Figure 46-3. Word catheter with balloon partially inflated.

Postprocedure Precautions

1. The Word catheter, ideally, should stay in place for 4 to 6 weeks.
2. Patient is advised to perform sitz baths 2 to 3 times per day. She may use Epsom salts in her baths.
3. Increased discharge may require use of panty liners.
4. Sexual intercourse and tampons should be avoided while the catheter is in place.
5. Follow up immediately if pain increases, fever or chills occur, and/or swelling is increased.

A 30-year-old Woman Referred for an Abnormal Pap Smear

A 30-year-old G2P2002 is referred to the clinic for evaluation of a high-grade squamous intraepithelial lesion (HSIL) cervical cytology. This is the patient's first abnormal pap. She doesn't report any sexually transmitted infections (STIs) and has had 6 lifetime partners. She has been with her current partner for 6 months. The patient is on oral contraceptive pills for birth control and has no medical or health problems.

1. What is the next step for this patient?

Answer

1. HSIL cervical cytology is further investigated with a colposcopy, endocervical curettage (ECC), and directed biopsies in order to look for evidence of invasive cancer.

CASE REVIEW

Your patient undergoes colposcopy, ECC, and biopsies at the 2-, 5-, and 8-o'clock positions. The results return cervical intraepithelial neoplasia (CIN) II–III for all 3 biopsies, and the ECC is negative. You communicate this to her and schedule her for loop electrosurgical excision procedure (LEEP) in the clinic.

COLPOSCOPY/CERVICAL BIOPSY/ENDOCERVICAL CURETTAGE

Colposcopy is an office procedure and usually doesn't require anesthesia. The colposcope (Figure 46-4) magnifies the cervical image. The entire squamocolumnar junction needs to be fully visualized—this is the junction of the normal

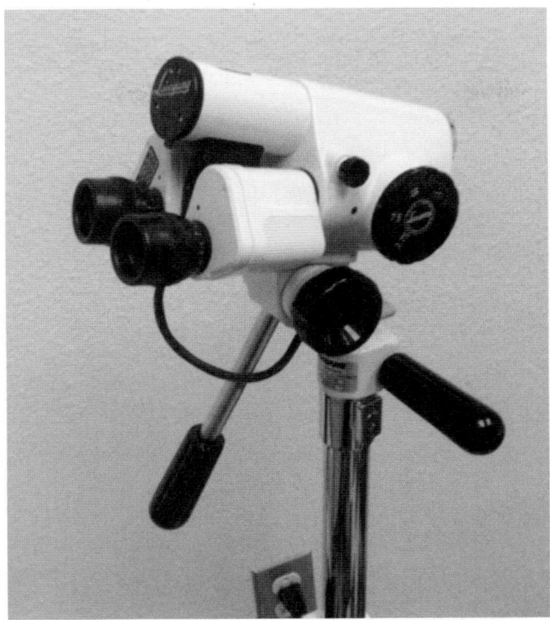

Figure 46-4. Colposcope used to magnify cervix.

endocervical columnar epithelium and ectocervical squamous epithelium. The magnification used is 10 to 16×.

Procedure

1. Informed consent is obtained, the patient is placed in dorsal lithotomy position, and a 'time out' is performed.
2. Bivalve speculum placed and cervix visualized entirely.
3. Three percent acetic acid applied to the cervix.
4. Colposcope focused and the cervix visualized again.
5. Abnormal areas may be identified as white tissue with sharp borders, atypical sharp-bordered lesions with blood vessels (mosaic pattern) or red areas with stippling (punctation).
6. Acetowhite epithelium after application of acetic acid results from cells with an increased nuclear–cytoplasmic ratio.
7. Biopsies are taken from any abnormal area (atypical vessel, punctate lesions, and mosaicism). Punch biopsy forceps (Figure 46-5) are used to obtain a specimen.

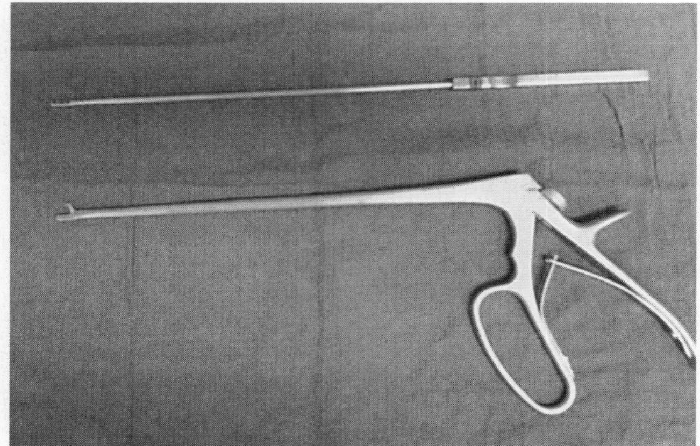

Figure 46-5. Top: endocervical curette; bottom: cervical biopsy instrument.

8. ECC is performed even if the entire transformation zone (TZ; squamocolumnar zone) is seen. This helps in the evaluation of dysplastic tissue in the endocervical canal. An endocervical curette (Figure 46-5) is used for this.
9. At the end of the procedure, Monsel solution or silver nitrate is used to achieve hemostasis.
10. The specimens are placed in formalin and usually labeled as biopsy taken from 1, 2, 3 o'clock, etc.
11. ECC is sent separately.

Postprocedure Precautions

1. No intercourse, or tampon use for 3 days.
2. If bleeding, foul-smelling discharge, or increasing pain occurs, contact the office immediately.

A 30-year-old With CIN II–III (Continuation)

The biopsy results were CIN II–III and the ECC was negative. The patient is here today to undergo a LEEP procedure.

1. How do you perform a LEEP procedure?

Answer

1. A wire loop acts as a surgical knife when connected to an electrical source. An electrosurgical unit with both cutting and coagulation currents is attached to

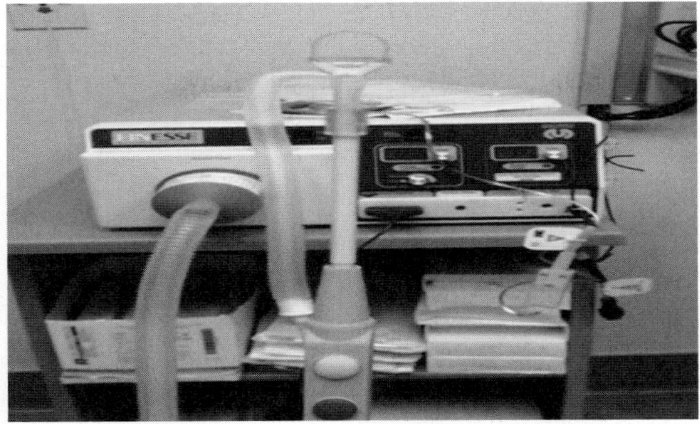

Figure 46-6. The LEEP machine.

the wire loop (Figure 46-6). Different sizes of the wire loop are available and are used according to the size of the TZ or the lesion. The width and depth of the loops can be adjusted. After the procedure a roller ball cautery, attached to the same electrosurgical unit, may be used to coagulate and cauterize the base of the incision for hemostasis. Ferric subsulfate solution (Monsel) is also used for this purpose. The goal of this procedure is to remove the entire TZ. The advantage of a LEEP that utilizes cautery over a "cold knife cone" (standard scalpel blade) is that the LEEP provides a tissue sample as well as providing treatment to the surrounding area.

CASE REVIEW

The patient tolerated the procedure without problem and went home. You called her back in 2 days to give her the results—CIN II–III without evidence of cancer, and schedule follow-up.

LEEP Procedure

1. Informed consent is obtained, the patient is placed in dorsal lithotomy position, and a 'time out' is performed.
2. A special colposcope speculum is placed in the vagina. There is a suction device attached to the speculum to remove smoke and improve visualization of the operating field.
3. The entire cervix is visualized.
4. A paracervical block using local anesthesia with epinephrine is injected circumferentially.

5. The cervix is painted with acetic acid or Lugol's iodine to delineate the TZ. White discoloration occurs with the acetic acid and no uptake of red-brown color occurs in the TZ with Lugol's.
6. The electrosurgical unit is adjusted to the physician's preferred setting of cut and coagulation (50/50, 70/30, etc).
7. The loop is moved across the TZ in a transverse or vertical fashion using fluid movements.
8. The specimen is removed from the cervix.
9. Hemostasis is achieved using roller ball cautery or Monsel solution.
10. The speculum is removed and the patient is asked to sit up.
11. The specimen is sent to pathology in formalin with correct anatomic orientation.

Postprocedure Precautions

1. Avoid excessive physical activity for 48 hours.
2. Abstain from sexual intercourse, and avoid tampons for 4 weeks.
3. Vaginal discharge or spotting is normal for 1 to 3 weeks.
4. Contact your physician if bleeding increases and requires pad changes, fever greater than 100.4°F, severe pain, or foul discharge.

TIPS TO REMEMBER

- All office procedures require a signed informed consent document, and verbal 'time out' prior to beginning. This document should be witnessed, and checked by the operator before starting the procedure.
- Assemble all necessary equipment before starting the procedure, to avoid sending your nurse or assistant out of the room to get what you need.
- Remember that the patient is awake for all of these procedures. Be careful what you say and offer verbal reassurance to the patient that things are going well.
- Carefully explain to the patient what she should watch for and call you for before she leaves your office.

COMPREHENSION QUESTIONS

1. You are performing colposcopy on a patient for HSIL cervical cytology. You visualize the cervix under magnification and are deciding where to biopsy. Which of the following is the best area to biopsy?

A. Mosaicism at 9 o'clock

B. Atypical blood vessels at 3 o'clock

C. Punctate lesions at 5 o'clock
D. All of the above

2. Which of the following steps should be completed before performing Word catheter placement in the office?
A. Obtain informed consent.
B. Perform a verbal 'time out'
C. Provide adequate pain control.
D. All of the above.

3. You perform a LEEP procedure and send your patient home. You communicate to her to alert the office if which of the following occurs?
A. The patient develops a grayish discharge.
B. The patient develops vaginal spotting.
C. The patient develops a vaginal discharge.
D. The patient develops a fever, vaginal pain, and increased bleeding.

Answers

1. **D.** Colposcopy is an inexact science, and in general the more biopsies performed the more sensitive the procedure is, regardless of skill. All of the findings listed are indications for biopsy.

2. **D.** Informed consent is a routine part of *all* office procedures. Lithotomy position will allow adequate visualization and pain control is a must before any surgical procedure.

3. **D.** Fever, pain, and an increase in vaginal bleeding all require your patient to notify the office. The other symptoms listed are common after LEEP.

SUGGESTED READINGS

Noller KL. Intraepithelial neoplasia of the lower genital tract (cervix, vulva): etiology, screening, diagnostic techniques, management. In: Katz VL, Lentz GM, Lobo RA, Gershenson DM, eds. *Comprehensive Gynecology*. 5th ed. Philadelphia, PA: Mosby Elsevier Inc; 2007:743–758.

Nichols DH, Sweeney PJ. *Ambulatory Gynecology*. 2nd ed. Philadelphia, PA: JB Lippincott Company; 1995:416–517.

Rock JA, Thompson JD. *TeLinde's Operative Gynecology*. 8th ed. Philadelphia, PA/New York, NY: Lippincott Raven Publishers; 1997:891, 1404–1405.

Schorge JO, Schaffer JI, Halvorson LM, Hoffman BL, Bradshaw KD, Cunningham FG. *Williams Obstetrics*. 23rd ed. New York, NY: The McGraw-Hill Companies Inc; 2008:87.

Urman RD, Punwani N, Bomboaugh M, et al. Safety considerations for office-based obstetric and gynecologic procedures. *Rev Obstet Gynecol*. 2013;6:e8–e14.

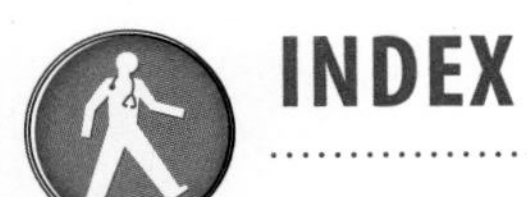

INDEX

Page numbers followed by *f* or *t* indicate figures or tables, respectively.

W